Pharmaceuticals in the Environment

Springer

Berlin
Heidelberg
New York
Barcelona
Hong Kong
London
Milan
Paris
Singapore
Tokyo

Klaus Kümmerer (Ed.)

Pharmaceuticals in the Environment

Sources, Fate, Effects and Risks

With 35 Figures and 51 Tables

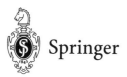 Springer

Editor

Assoc. Prof. Dr. Klaus Kümmerer
Universitätsklinikum Freiburg
Institut für Umweltmedizin und Krankenhaushygiene
Hugstetter Straße 55
D-79106 Freiburg i. Br., Germany
E-mail: kkuemmerer@iuk3.ukl.uni-freiburg.de

ISBN 3-540-41067-8 Springer-Verlag Berlin Heidelberg New York

Library of Congress Cataloging-in-Publication Data

Pharmaceuticals in the environment : Sources, fate, effects and risks / Klaus Kümmerer [editor].-- 1st ed.
  p. cm
  Includes bibliographical references and index.
  ISBN 3540410678 (alk. paper)
  1. Drugs--Environmental aspects. I. Kümmerer, Klaus, 1959-

TD196.D78 P43 2001
363.738--dc21

2001020498

Springer-Verlag Berlin Heidelberg New York
a member of the BertelsmannSpringer Science+Business Media GmbH
© Springer-Verlag Berlin Heidelberg 2001
Printed in Germany

The use of general descriptive names, registered names, trademarks, etc. in this publication does not imply, even in the absence of a specific statement, that such names are exempt from the relevant protective laws and regulations and therefore free for general use.

Cover Design: *design & production*, Heidelberg
Dataconversion: Büro Stasch (*www.stasch.com*) · Uwe Zimmermann, Bayreuth

SPIN: 10744981 – 30/3130/xz – 5 4 3 2 1 0 – Printed on acid-free paper

Foreword

When the first green wave appeared in the mid and late 1960s, it was considered a feasible task to solve pollution problems. The visible problems were mostly limited to point sources, and a comprehensive "end of the pipe technology" (= environmental technology) was available. It was even seriously discussed in the US that what was called "zero discharge" could be attained by 1985.

It became clear in the early 1970s that zero discharge would be too expensive, and that we should also rely on the self purification ability of ecosystems. That called for the development of environmental and ecological models to assess the self purification capacity of ecosystems and to set up emission standards, considering the relationship between impacts and effects in the ecosystems. This idea is illustrated in Fig. 0.1. A model is used to relate an emission to its effect on the ecosystem and its components. The relationship is applied to select a good solution to environmental problems by application of environmental technology.

Meanwhile, it has been disclosed that what we could call the environmental crisis is much more complex than we initially thought. We could, for instance, remove heavy metals from wastewater, but where should we dispose the sludge containing the heavy metals? Resource management pointed towards recycling to replace removal. Nonpoint sources of toxic substances and nutrients, chiefly originating from agriculture, emerged as new threatening environmental problems in the late 1970s. The focus on global environmental problems such as the greenhouse effect and the decomposition of the ozone layer added to the complexity. It was revealed that we use as much as about 100 000 chemicals, which may threaten the environment due to their more or less toxic effects on plants, animals, humans and entire ecosystems. In most industrialised countries comprehensive environmental legislation was introduced to regulate the wide spectrum of different pollution sources. Trillions of dollars have been invested in pollution abatement on a global scale, but it seems that two or more new problems emerge

Fig. 0.1. The strategy applied in environmental management in the early 1970s is illustrated. An ecological model is used to relate an emission to its effect on the ecosystem and its components. The relationship is applied to select a good solution to environmental problems by application of environmental technology

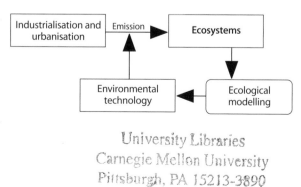

for each problem that we solve. Our society does not seem geared toward solving environmental problems, or is there perhaps another explanation?

Recently, standards for environmental management in industries and green accounting have been introduced. The most widely applied standards today for industrial environmental management are the ISO 14000-series. These initiatives attempt to analyse our production systems to find new ways and methods to make our production more environmentally friendly. More than 100 countries have backed up the international standards for effective management of environmental impacts.

Figure 0.2 illustrates how complex environmental management is today. The first figure shows that a simultaneous application of environmental technology, ecotechnology, cleaner technology and environmental legislation is needed in environmental management.

Environmental technology offers a wide spectrum of methods that are able to remove pollutants from water, air and soil. These methods are particularly applicable to coping with point sources.

Cleaner technology explores the possibilities of recycling by-products or the final waste products or attempting to change the entire production technology to obtain reduced emissions. It attempts to answer the pertinent question: couldn't we produce our product using a more environmentally friendly method? It will to a great extent be based on environmental risk assessment, LCA and environmental auditing. The ISO 14000-series and risk reduction techniques are among the most important tools in the application of cleaner technology. The environmental risk assessment of chemicals is in this context a very important tool, as it results in a quantification of the environmental risk.

Ecotechnology covers the use of ecosystems to solve pollution problems, including the erection of artificial ecosystems. It also encompasses the technology that is applicable to the restoration of more or less deteriorated ecosystems. The mentioned classes of technologies cover a wide spectrum of methods. We have, for instance, many environmental technological methods to cope with different wastewater problems, and to

Fig. 0.2. The use of environmental models in environmental management, which, today, is very complex and must apply environmental technology, cleaner technology and ecotechnology. Models are used to select the right environmental management strategy. In addition, the global environmental problems, which also require the use of models as a synthesizing tool, play an increasing role

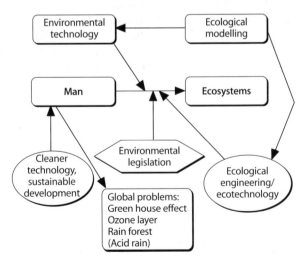

select the right method or most often the right combination of methods, a profound knowledge of the applicability of the methods and of the processes and characteristics of the ecosystem receiving the emission is necessary.

Environmental legislation and green taxes may be used in addition to these classes of technology. They may in principle be used as regulating instruments in every step of the flow from raw materials and energy to final waste disposal of the used product.

The 20th century has introduced more than 100 000 chemicals that are used in our every day life, either in households, industries or agriculture. We have "blindly" introduced these chemicals without realising the consequences for the environment and directly and indirectly for human health. EU started to list these chemicals in the late 1970s, and since the mid 1980s it has been compulsory to set up an environmental risk assessment for all new chemicals. It was the idea, meanwhile, to make environmental risk assessments for the chemicals already in use, but it is going very slowly, and at the present rate, we shall not be able finish ERAs for all the applied chemicals in this century. Probably, it is necessary to speed up the evaluation of the chemicals in use, for instance by forging a closer cooperation between the environmental agencies and the chemical industry, in order to obtain a realistic picture of the environmental risk associated with the many chemicals we apply today.

It is strange that drugs were not included when a compulsory environmental risk assessment was introduced for new chemicals, because drugs have properties that cause suspicion about environmental effects. Drugs are

- biologically active.
- often mobile as the water solubility is high relative to the molecular weight. This is particularly true for metabolites of the drugs that can be found in urine and therefore also in the wastewater.
- not readily biodegradable.

Drugs have, in other words, properties that make them environmentally interesting.

Today, an environmental risk assessment is required for all new medical compounds used in veterinary drugs, but it is expected that this will also be required for human drugs in the near future.

This volume focuses on what we know but also what we don't know about drugs, or rather what we ought to know to understand the occurrence, the fate and the effect of the about 4 000 medical compounds that we are using in the drugs applied today. What basic knowledge do we have today about drugs to be able to set up ERAs for the medical compounds?

Recently (February 2000) Chemosphere published a special issue on "drugs in the environment." This issue contained several interesting papers on these topics. This volume is, however, the first book to review "drugs in the environment." A book can, of course, give more detailed information than scientific papers, and also make links to what is known more generally about chemical compounds in our environment. The publication of this book is therefore an important step forward in our effort to

1. understand the environmental occurrence and processes of drugs,
2. quantify their effects and risks and

3. properly abate the associated pollution problem by trying to give an answer to the following two pertinent questions:
   - Which medical compounds should be phased out and substituted by other compounds?
   - Could we solve some of the problems with environmental or cleaner technology? How?

At least a decade will pass before we have a proper overview of the many environmental problems that are associated with medical compounds discharged into the environment. At that time – ten or fifteen years from now? – we may have substituted the most environmentally harmful chemicals with other compounds as a concluding result of the performed ERAs. The focal point is, however, that we have a realistic knowledge about the risk involved in the use of medical compounds and can phase out the most risky compounds. This process has already started – slowly but surely – because the medical industry is very concerned today about the fate and effect of antibiotics and recommendations on which antibiotics to use from an environmental point of view can already to a certain extent be given today.

Sven Erik Jørgensen[1]

---

[1] *Current address*: Prof. Sven Erik Jørgensen, The Royal Danish School of Pharmacy, Department of Analytical and Pharmaceutical Chemistry, Universitetsparken 2, DK-2100 Copenhagen, Denmark, E-mail: SEJ@mail.dfh.dk.

Preface

All of us use pharmaceuticals for ourselves or for our pets, in husbandry, in agriculture or in aquaculture. But who knows what will happen to the compounds after their administration or use? Are they distributed in the environment or are they eliminated beforehand? What are the possible effects and risks for humans and the environment in connection with the emission of pharmaceuticals into the environment? Pharmaceuticals, diagnostic aids as well as disinfectants used in medicine enter municipal sewage and the aquatic environment. Drugs and growth promoters used in veterinary medicine and husbandry are excreted by animals and emitted into soil via manure or can be part of the runoff from soils after heavy rain fall, which then passes into surface water. Drugs used in aquaculture are passed directly into surface water. Some, such as X-ray contrast media, are excreted completely unchanged, while others are metabolised either into metabolites, which are still active or inactive metabolites. Outdated medications or their remnants are sometimes disposed of down household drains or as (household) waste. The fate, occurrence and effects of pharmaceuticals in the aquatic and terrestrial environment is still mainly unknown.

The disposal of pharmaceuticals in the environment means that a huge number of different substances in different amounts, products and modes of action have to be considered. Therefore, it is difficult to obtain an appropriate overview on the ongoing research. It is even more difficult to identify the most important questions for a systematic approach. The information available is still scarce and not sufficient for sound assessment and decision-making. For this reason, the European Science Foundation (ESF), located in Strasbourg (France), commissioned the workshop "Pharmaceuticals in the Environment." It was held in July 1999 in Freiburg (Germany). The core of the book consists of issues discussed and explored in depth during this workshop. Some other authors, not present at the workshop, have been added.

The book does not claim to give a complete review of the state of the art related to pharmaceuticals in the environment. There is a lot of literature, symposia, international networking and research organising on EDSs. This is still lacking for pharmaceuticals other than hormones. This book gives a short review of the fate, occurence and effects of pharmaceuticals using examples of some typical compounds to highlight the most important questions and issues related to pharmaceuticals in the environment. Input, occurence, fate and effects as well as the possible risks and their assessment are addressed. The book also gives an introduction to this new field of environmental chemistry, ecotoxicology and environmental hygiene.

This book would not have been realised without the workshop "Pharmaceuticals in the Environment" commissioned by the European Science Foundation (ESF). Dr. A. Moth-

Wiklund and her team from the Life and Environment Standing Commitee (LESC) at the ESF always gave good support whenever necessary. All the participants of the workshop contributed to the lively discussions and the identification of the important questions of research in the future. The contributors to this volume were very patient with the editor. The workshop and the book would have not been realised without the support of the director of the Institute of Environmental Medicine and Hospital Epidemiology at the Freiburg University Hospital, Prof. Dr. med. Franz Daschner, and of all my co-workers in the field of pharmaceuticals in the environment. Tina Kümpel and Birgit Stadel helped with the manuscripts. Dr. Witschel from Springer Verlag (Heidelberg) created the opportunity to publish this book. Special thanks to my wife and my children for their encouragement and their support.

Thank you!

Klaus Kümmerer
Freiburg, January 2001

Contents

Contributors

Alexy, Radka, Dipl.-Ing.
Universitätsklinikum Freiburg
Institut für Umweltmedizin und Krankenhaushygiene
Hugstetter Straße 55
D-79106 Freiburg i. Br., Germany
E-mail: ralexy@iuk3.ukl.uni-freiburg.de

Bagnati, Renzo, MSc
"Mario Negri" Institute for Pharmacological Research
Department of Environmental Health Sciences
Via Eritrea 62
I-20157 Milan, Italy
E-mail: bagnati@marionegri.it

Benfenati, Emilio, Dr.
"Mario Negri" Institute for Pharmacological Research
Department of Environmental Health Sciences
Via Eritrea 62
I-20157 Milan, Italy
E-mail: benefati@marionegri.it

Calamari, Davide, Prof. Dr.
University of Insubria
Department of Structural and Functional Biology
Environmental Research Group
Via J. H. Dunant 3
I-21100 Varese VA, Italy
E-mail: davide.calamari@unimi.it

D'Haese, Isabel
University of Gent
Department of Agricultural and Applied Biological Sciences
Laboratory of Microbial Ecology and Technology (LabMET)
Coupure Links 653
B-9000 Gent, Belgium
E-mail: IDE@analis.be

Di Guardo, Antonio, Dr.
University of Insurbia
Department of Structural and Functional Biology
Via J.H. Dunant 3
I-21100 Varese VA, Italy
E-mail: antonio.diguardo@uninsurbia.it

Dietrich, Daniel, Prof. Dr.
Universität Konstanz
Jacob-Burckhardt-Straße 25
D-78457 Konstanz, Germany
E-mail: daniel.dietrich@uni-konstanz.de

Fanelli, Roberto, Dr.
"Mario Negri" Institute for Pharmacological Research
Department of Environmental Health Sciences
Via Eritrea 62
I-20157 Milan, Italy
E-mail: fanelli@marionegri.it

Fioretti, Francesca, MSc
"Mario Negri" Institute for Pharmacological Research
Department of Environmental Health Sciences
Via Eritrea 62
I-20157 Milan, Italy
E-mail: fioretti@marionegri.it

Frimmel, Fritz Hartmann, Prof. Dr.
Universität Karlsruhe
Engler-Bunte-Institut
Engler-Bunte-Ring 1
D-76131 Karlsruhe, Germany
E-mail: fritz.frimmel@uni-karlsruhe.de

Gremm, Thomas, Dr.
Universität Karlsruhe
Engler-Bunte-Institut
Engler-Bunte-Ring 1
D-76131 Karlsruhe, Germany
E-mail: thomas.gremm@ciw.uni-karlsruhe.de

Halling-Sørensen, Bent, Dr.
The Royal Danish School of Pharmacy
Institute of Analytical and Pharmaceutical Chemistry
Universitetsparken 2
DK-2100 Copenhagen, Denmark
E-mail: bhs@mail.dfh.dk

Hartemann, Philippe, Prof. Dr.
Université Henri Poincaré
Département Environnement et Santé Publique
9, Avenue de la Forêt de Haye
F-54505 Vandoeuvre-lès-Nancy, France
E-mail: p.hartemann@chu-nancy.fr

Hubner, Peter, Dr.
Universität Freiburg
Institut für Umweltmedizin und Krankenhaushygiene
Hugstetter Straße 55
D-79106 Freiburg i. Br., Germany
E-mail: phubner@iuk3.ukl.uni-freiburg.de

Jensen, John
National Environmental Research Institute
Department of Terrestrial Ecology
Vejlesøvej 25
DK-8600 Silkeborg, Denmark
E-mail: JJE@dmu.dk

Knacker, Thomas, Dr.
ECT Ökotoxikologie GmbH
Böttgerstraße 2–14
D-65439 Flörsheim, Germany
E-mail: th-knacker@ect.de

Kozak, Ruth G.
University of Gent
Department of Agricultural and Applied Biological Sciences
Laboratory of Microbial Ecology and Technology (LabMET)
Coupure Links 653
B-9000 Gent, Belgium

Kümmerer, Klaus, Dr., Assoc. Prof.
Universitätsklinikum Freiburg
Institut für Umweltmedizin und Krankenhaushygiene
Hugstetter Straße 55
D-79106 Freiburg i. Br., Germany
E-mail: kkuemmerer@iuk3.ukl.uni-freiburg.de

Kümpel, Tina, Dipl.-Ing. (FH)
Universitätsklinikum Freiburg
Institut für Umweltmedizin und Krankenhaushygiene
Hugstetter Straße 55
D-79106 Freiburg i. Br., Germany
E-mail: tkuempel@iuk3.ukl.uni-freiburg.de

Midtvedt, Tore, Prof. Dr.
Karolinska Institute
Department of Cell and Molecular Microbiology
Laboratory of Medical Microbial Ecology
Box 285
SE-17177 Stockholm, Sweden
E-mail: tore.midtvedt@cmb.ki.se

Montforts, Mark, Dr.
Centre for Substances and Risk Assessment (CSR)
National Institute for Public Health and the Environment
P.O. Box 1
NL-3720 BA Bilthoven, the Netherlands
E-mail: mark.montforts@rivm.nl

Natangelo, Marco, MSc
"Mario Negri" Institute for Pharmacological Research
Department of Environmental Health Sciences
Via Eritrea 62
I-20157 Milan, Italy
E-mail: natangelo@marionegri.it

Pfluger, Paul
Universität Konstanz
AG Umwelttoxikologie
Jacob-Burckhardt-Straße 25
D-78457 Konstanz, Germany
E-mail: paul.pfluger@uni-konstanz.de

Römbke, Jörg
ECT Ökotoxikologie GmbH
Böttgerstraße 2–14
D-65439 Flörsheim, Germany
E-mail: j-roembke@ect.de

Teichmann, Hanka
Umweltbundesamt
Bismarckplatz 1
D-14191 Berlin, Germany
e-mail: hanka.teichmann@uba.de

Tjørnelund, Jette, Dr., Ass. Prof.
The Royal Danish School of Pharmacy
Institute of Analytical and Pharmaceutical Chemistry
Universitetsparken 2
DK-2100 Copenhagen, Denmark
E-mail: jt@mail.dfh.dk

Verstraete, Willy, Prof. Dr.
University of Gent
Department of Agricultural and Applied Biological Sciences
Laboratory of Microbial Ecology and Technology (LabMET)
Coupure Links 653
B-9000 Gent, Belgium
E-mail: Willy.Verstraete@rug.ac.be

Webb, Simon, Dr.
Procter & Gamble Eurocor
European Technical Center
Temselaan 100
B-1853 Strombeek-Bever, Belgium
E-mail: webb.sf@pg.com

Zuccato, Ettore, Dr.
"Mario Negri" Institute for Pharmacological Research
Department of Environmental Health Sciences
Food Toxicology Unit
Via Eritrea 62
I-20157 Milan, Italy
E-mail: zuccato@marionegri.it

Zwiener, Christian, Dr.
Universität Karlsruhe
Engler-Bunte-Institut
Engler-Bunte-Ring 1
D-76131 Karlsruhe, Germany
E-mail: christian.zwiener@ciw.uni-karlsruhe.de

Chapter 1

Introduction: Pharmaceuticals in the Environment

K. Kümmerer

1.1
Historical Background

In the 1970s, for the first time, pharmaceuticals in the environment (namely hormones) were the subject of scientific interest and public awareness (Tabak and Brunch 1970; Norpoth et al. 1973). The conclusion most often reached was that the hormones are not easily biodegraded. During the 1980s, there has been only little interest in this topic. Other substances of environmental relevance such as heavy metals, polycyclic aromatic hydrocarbons, or chlorinated dioxins and furans as well as pesticides or detergents have been investigated very extensively during this period. Since the middle of the 1990s, awareness of pharmaceuticals in the environment has been growing. Parallel to this, the discussion of endocrine disrupting (sometimes called endocrine modulating) substances (EDS) and non-hormone pharmaceuticals, like lipid lowering agents and others, came into focus (Stan and Linkerhägner 1992). Since then, quite a lot of activities have been initiated relating to EDS, beginning in the USA, and for other pharmaceuticals mainly in Europe. Substances have been detected in sewage, the effluents of sewage treatment plants, surface water, manure and soil since the 1980s (Table 1.1). Most of those investigated so far were not easily biodegradable in test systems (see Chap. 4, 6, 7 and 8) and are only slowly eliminated in the environment – if at all.

1.2
Use

In 1990, about 50 000 drugs were registered in Germany, 2 700 of which accounted for 90% of total consumption and which, in turn, contained about 900 different active substances (figures for Italy see Chap. 3, for Austria see Sattelberger 1999). 250 antibiotic and antimycotic substances are in use in medicine and veterinary medicine in Germany. After application, many non-metabolised drugs are excreted by the patients and so reach wastewater. But husbandry, e.g. veterinary use or use as growth promoters in fattening as well as in aquaculture, also discharges drugs and their metabolites into the environment. Moreover, diagnostic agents and disinfectants after their administration reach wastewater and/or liquid manure, i.e. soil, sometimes in residual quantities. The substances may finally enter groundwater via soil after application of liquid manure or sewage sludge as fertilisers.

   The compounds in use can be classified according to their effects, but also "crosswise" according to chemical structure. Besides the active substances, formulation adjuvants and in some instances pigments and dyes are drug components. Normally, they

Table 1.1. Concentration of different drugs ($\mu g \, l^{-1}$) as measured in wastewater, surface waters, groundwater and drinking water

Active substance/ Group	Waste-water	Surface water	Ground-water (GW), Drinking water (DW)	References
Analgesics/ Antirheumatic agents	2.4 20	Up to 0.5 Up to 0.5 Up to 0.5	0.006 (DW)	UBA (1997) Ternes et al. (1997) Heberer et al. (1997)
Antibiotics	Approx. 1 0.1–1.7 Up to 1	Up to 1.7 Up to 6[a] Up to 1		Hirsch et al. (1999) UBA (1997) Ternes et al. (1997) Richardson and Bowron (1985)
Lipid lowering agents	1.7 up to 1	0.55	0.17 (DW) 7.5 (GW) 0.07 (DW)	Stan et al. (1994) Ternes et al. (1997) Heberer et al. (1997) Heberer et al. (1997)
Psychopharmacological agents	<1 Up to 6.1			UBA (1997) Ternes et al. (1997)
Cytostatic agents	Up to 5	Up to 0.02 Up to 4[a]		Aherne et al. (1990) Kümmerer et al. (1997) Steger-Hartmann et al. (1997) Kümmerer (1998)
X-ray contrast media		9[a] Up to 3.1[a] 0.01–0.15	Up to 0.07	Steger-Hartmann et al. (1998) Hirsch et al. (2000)

[a] STP-effluent (diluted by surface water).

are classified according to their therapeutic purpose (e.g. antibiotics, analgesics, antineoplastics, anti-inflammatory substances, antibiotics, antihistaminic agents, contrast media, etc.). Classification according to chemical structure is used mainly for subgroups of the active substances, e.g. β-lactams, cephalosporines, penicillins or quinolones and others within the group of antibiotics. A closely related chemical structure is accompanied by an identical or at least similar mode of action.

1.3
Legislation

Drugs and disinfectants are, like other chemicals such as biocides and pesticides, applied specifically because of their biological effect. Disinfectants in particular are often highly complex products or mixtures of active substances also used in hospitals, households, industry and husbandry. Within the registration process for chemicals (new substances), data referring to fate and effects of the compounds in the environment are necessary (e.g. EU 1996). In the USA, according to legislation, an environmental assessment is a prerequisite for their registration by the Federal Drug Administration (see Chap. 12 ff.). For the registration of pharmaceuticals, information on their environmental impact has only been requested in the last few years. A tiered approach is applied; the necessary information depends on amounts produced. Within the last few years, compound restrictions were only necessary for one, namely taxol. Taxol is used as an antineoplastic compound. It is isolated from the bark of the yew tree. As a result from its production, these plants were endangered. For all other cases, only a basic data set was necessary for registration. The FDA stated in 1995 that its environmental reviews had shown that the requirement could be eliminated in almost all cases. One reason might be the threshold used to trigger further investigations (Chap. 12). In the EU, too, there is no special legislation referring to the environmental impact for already existing, i.e. already registered substances.

Under European law, only "... if appropriate, special precautionary measures for the elimination and removal of unused products or waste material originating therefrom" need to be specified for drugs intended for human use. Article 4.6 of this directive says that the application for the *new* registration of a drug must be accompanied "... if applicable, by reasons for any precautionary or safety measures to be taken during storage of the product, its administration to patients and for the disposal of waste products, together with details on any potential risk which the product constitutes for the environment". There are no special investigations requested (EG 1993). Since 1995, this gap should have been closed for new substances intended for use in medicine (EG 1993), but there are no procedures established on how to gain the necessary information and data. Only drafts describing possible procedures have existed since 1994 (EU 1995). However, the implementing provisions and hence the scope of the necessary data for evaluating environmental fate have as of yet not been finalised or adopted (EU 1995). So far the EU is only demanding data on the environmental impact for new registrations of drugs used in veterinary medicine (Chap. 13 and 14). To appraise the environmental properties of active substances already on the market ("existing substances"), an environmental review has still not been laid down. Apart from a few notable exceptions, the necessary data is also unavailable from the manufacturers. This means that the risk for humans and the environment resulting from the discharge of active substances into the environment cannot be estimated at present.

For new substances used in veterinary medicine, environmental data has been required for registration since 1998 (see Chap. 13 and 14). Almost all compounds used today in medicine and veterinary medicine are so-called "existing substances"; i.e. they have been registered according to the old legislation. Therefore, the poor situation in respect to data on the environmental fate and effects of pharmaceuticals is not surprising.

1.4
Occurrence: Evidence of Drugs in the Aquatic Environment

Some investigations to prove the existence of drugs in sewage treatment plant (STP) effluents were carried out in the middle of the 1980s, mainly in Great Britain (Richardson and Bowron 1985; Aherne et al. 1990). The concentrations in the surface waters and the STP effluents were in the ng l^{-1} to µg l^{-1} range (Table 1.1). In Germany, first reports of a lipid lowering agent were reported in 1992 (Stan et al. 1994). Meanwhile, there is evidence of other drugs in STP effluents, surface water, groundwater and even drinking water (Table 1.1). An overview of the occurrence of some groups of pharmaceuticals in German STP effluents was given only recently (Ternes 1998), a detailed overview of the present international status of knowledge by Halling-Sørensen et al. (1998).

Evidence of a wide variety of different active substances in the aquatic environment as well as in liquid manure and in the soil also shows that the active substances are at least not completely eliminated in sewage treatment or biodegraded in the environment.

1.5
Fate

Diffuse input into the environment is the normal case. Because of the good manufacturing practice applied within production and the often high cost of the active substances, emissions from manufacturing are regarded as low. Locally high emissions are possible only in the case of accidents. To the author's best knowledge, no data is available about emissions during transport and storage (Chap. 10). Point sources for emissions are likely to be only of minor importance.

After application, most drugs are excreted partly non-metabolised. Some, such as X-ray contrast media, are excreted completely unchanged. Pharmaceuticals, diagnostic aids as well as disinfectants used in medicine enter municipal sewage and sewage treatment plants. Outdated medications or their remnants are sometimes disposed of down household drains, presumably 20–40% in Germany. If the drugs are not eliminated in sewage treatment plants, they may enter the aquatic environment and eventually reach drinking water (Fig. 1.1). Drugs used in animal husbandry, e.g. for veterinary purposes or as growth promoters (particularly in large-scale animal farming) as well as in aquaculture and their metabolites are also discharged into the environment through liquid manure and (waste)water. The substances may finally enter groundwater via soil after application of liquid manure or sewage sludge used as fertilisers (Fig. 1.1).

Drugs used in veterinary medicine and as growth promoters in livestock are excreted by animals and emitted into the soil with their manure. They also can be part of the runoff from soils after heavy rain which then passes into surface water. Drugs used in aquaculture are passed directly into surface water. For some compounds used in aquaculture, data about occurrence, fate and effects are published. The research into occurrence, fate and effects of veterinary pharmaceuticals and growth promoters is just beginning.

According to EU legislation, since 1994 the disposal of unused remnants by household waste has been permitted. In the case of Austria it is reported that about 25% are disposed of by household waste (Sattelberger 1999). Pharmaceuticals have been detected in the effluent from a landfill (Holm et al. 1995).

1.6
Effects

The active ingredients of medications have been selected or designed due to and because of their activity against organisms. In respect to their purpose one has to expect the following properties that are crucial for their environmental impact:

- effective against bacteria
- effective against fungi
- effective against higher organisms
- sometimes persistent

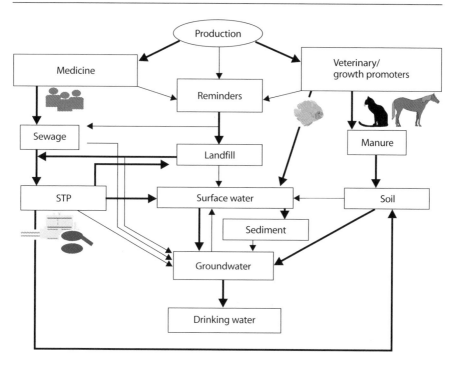

Fig. 1.1. Sources, distribution and sinks of pharmaceuticals in the environment

Only little information is available on the effects of the active substances on organisms in the aquatic and terrestrial environment. Effects of some compounds on environmental organisms have been found not only in high concentrations, i.e. in the g per litre range, but also in low concentrations in chronic tests, e.g. towards *Daphnia*, algae and bacteria (Holten Lützhøft et al. 1999; Backhaus and Grimme 1999; Al-Ahmad et al. 1999; Halling-Sørensen 2000; Kümmerer et al. 2000).

1.7
Risk

The risk of adverse effects for humans by ingestion of pharmaceuticals by drinking water seems to be negligible. The maximum possible intake within a life span (2 litres drinking water per day over 70 years) are far below the dosages used within therapy (Christensen 1998; Kümmerer and Al-Ahmad 1998). But the problem of how to extrapolate data from high dosage (short term ingestion within a therapy) to low dosage long term ingestion, i.e. "medication" via drinking water remains an unsolved issue. Furthermore, up to now the risk assessments have been conducted for single substances only and not for mixtures (see Chap. 12). Some of the compounds are cancerogenic, mutagenic or reproductive toxic (CMR compounds). There are no procedures to assess the risks connected to their emission into the environment. The following groups of drugs and diagnostic aids besides the CMR compounds may deserve special attention (Chap. 4):

- cytostatic agents, because of their frequently evident carcinogenic, mutagenic or embryotoxic properties,
- antibiotic agents and disinfectants, because of their potential for forming resistance and their bacterial toxicity, with the potential to disturb environmental bacterial consortia and processes, i.e. the elemental cycles,
- chlorophenols, chlorine-releasing reagents such as sodium hypochlorite, dichloroisocyanuric acid and others used as disinfectants and as bleaching agents or diagnostics like organic iodised X-ray contrast media, because they contribute to the adsorbable organic halogen compounds (AOX), and
- heavy metals, such as disinfectants and preservatives containing mercury, cytostatic agents containing platinum or contrast media containing gadolinium.

Other groups of drugs, for instance analgesics or sedatives, are also of interest for reasons of environmental hygiene because of the amounts used.

Besides toxicity, the element of persistence is of particular importance for the assessment of the environmental significance of substances (Klöpffer 1989). Persistent compounds increase the potential of long-term and hence varied effects as well as of multiple contamination of the ecosystem the longer the exposure lasts (Kümmerer and Held 1997). This cannot be tested in advance with the presently available test systems (Cairns and Mount 1990). Often standard tests are used for effect assessment and biodegradability testing (e.g. according to OECD series 200 and 300) developed for bulk chemicals. It is unclear to what extent the test systems have to be modified in order to obtain reliable results.

In the case of antimicrobials, resistant bacteria may be selected in the tanks of sewage treatment plants (STPs) or in other environmental compartments such as soil by recalcitrant antimicrobials. This may be one source of the growing number of pathogenic bacteria resistant to antibiotics in hospitals and the increase of severe nosocomial infections. In hospital effluent concentrations of antibiotics have been calculated as well as measured for single compounds that are in the range favouring the selection of resistant bacteria. The effluents are diluted by municipal sewage, but antibiotics from households are also present. The concentrations estimated for antibiotics in municipal sewage are for some groups, which act via similar or identical mechanisms, in a range that favours the selection of resistant bacteria. The extent to which this occurs and the significance thereof is unclear. In addition, active metabolites and disinfectants are also present.

Some procedures for risk assessment are in use. But it is far from clear which procedures, constraints and assessment factors should be used for pharmaceuticals (see Chap. 12–14).

1.8
Conclusion

It has to be stated that, in respect to what we should know for a sound risk assessment, too little data is available up to now. The input, occurrence, fate and effects of drugs in the environment is widely unknown (Römke et al. 1996; Halling-Sørensen et al. 1998; Daughton and Ternes 1999; Kümmerer 2001). There is an urgent need to reduce the gaps in our knowledge. The most important issues are addressed in Chap. 19.

References

Aherne GW, Hardcastle A, Nield AH (1990) Cytotoxic drugs and the aquatic environment. Estimation of bleomycin in river and water samples. J Pharm Pharmacol 42:741–742

Al-Ahmad A, Daschner FD, Kümmerer K (1999) Biodegradability of cefotiam, ciprofloxacin, meropenem, penicillin G, sulfametohoxazole and inhibition of wastewater bacteria. Arch Environ Cont Toxicol 37:158–163

Backhaus T, Grimme LH (1999) The toxicity of antibiotic agents to the luminescent bacterium *Vibrio fischeri*. Chemosphere 38:3291–3301

Cairns J Jr, Mount DI (1990) Aquatic toxicology. Environ Sci Technol 24:154–161

Christensen FM (1998) Pharmaceuticals in the environment – a human risk? Reg Tox Pharm 28:212–221

Daughton CG, Ternes TA (1999) Pharmaceuticals and personal care products in the environment. Agents of subtle change? Environ Health Persp 107(Supplement):907–938

EG (1993) Document 93/93/EWG(July 14th 1993) Official Journal of the European Community, No. L 214/22 (24.8.93)

EU (1995) Assessment of potential risks to the environment posed by medical products for human use (excluding products containing live genetically modified organisms). Direction General III, No. 5504/94 Draft 6, version 4, Brüssel, 5th January 1995

EU (1996) Technical Guidance Document (TGD) in Support of Commission Directive 93/67/EEC on Risk Assessment for New Notified Substances and Commission Regulation (EC) no 1488/94 on Risk Assessment for Existing Substances

Halling-Sørensen B (2000) Algal toxicity of antibacterial agents used in intensive fish farming. Chemosphere 40:731–739

Halling-Sørensen B, Nilesen N, Lanzky PF, Ingerslev F, Holten Lützhøft H-C, Jørgensen SS (1998) Occurrence, fate and effects of pharmaceutical substances in the environment – a review. Chemosphere 36:357–393

Heberer T, Schmidt-Bäumler K, Stan H-J (1997) Vorkommen und Bestimmung von Arzneimittelrückständen im Berliner Oberflächen- und Grundwasser. Fachgruppe Wasserchemie der GDCh, Jahrestagung, Lindau Mai 1997, Proceedings, S 103–106

Hirsch R, Ternes T, Haberer K, Kratz KL (1999) Occurrence of antibiotics in the aquatic environment. Sci Total Environ 225:109–118

Hirsch R, Ternes TA, Lindart A, Haberer K, Wilken R-D (2000) A sensitive method for the determination of iodine containing diagnostic agents in aqueous matrices using LC-electrospray-tandem-MS detection. Fresenius J Anal Chem 366:835–841

Holm JV, Rugge K, Bjerg PL, Christensen TH (1995) Occurrence and distribution of pharmaceutical organic compounds in the ground water down gradient of a landfill (Grinsted Denmark). Environ Sci Tech 29:1415–1420

Holten Lützhøft H-C, Halling-Sørensen B, Jørgensen SE (1999) Algal toxicity of antibacterial agents applied in Danish fish farming. Arch Environ Contami Toxicol 36:1–6

Klöpffer W (1989) Persistenz und Abbaubarkeit in der Beurteilung des Umweltverhaltens anthropogener Chemikalien. UWSF-Z Umweltchem Ökotox 1:43–51

Kümmerer K (1998) Eintrag von Pharmaka, Diagnostika und Desinfektionsmitteln aus Krankenhäusern in Abwasser und Gewässer. Habilitationsschrift, Universität Freiburg

Kümmerer K (2001) Emission of drugs, diagnostic agents, disinfectants and other compounds by hospitals into waste water – a review. Chemospere, accepted

Kümmerer K, Al-Ahmad A (1998) The cancer risk for humans related to cyclophoshamide and ifosfamide excretions emitted into surface water via hospital effluents. Cancer Det Prev 22, Suppl 1: 254

Kümmerer K, Held M (1997) Die Umweltwissenschaften im Kontext von Zeit – Begriffe unter dem Aspekt der Zeit. UWSF-Z Umweltchem Ökotox 9:169–178

Kümmerer K, Steger-Hartmann T, Meyer M (1997) Biodegradability of the anti-tumour agent ifosfamide and its occurrence in hospital effluents and sewage. Wat Res 31:2705–2710

Kümmerer K, Al-Ahmad A, Mersch-Sundermann V (2000) Biodegradability of some antibiotics, elimination of their genotoxicity and affection of waste water bacteria in a simple test. Chemosphere 40:701–710

Norpoth K, Nehrkorn A, Kirchner M, Holsen H, Teipel H (1973) Investigations on the problem of solubilityand stability of steroid ovulation inhibitors in water, waste water and activated sludge. Zbl Hyg I Abt Orig B 156:500–511

Richardson ML, Bowron JM (1985) The fate of pharmaceutical chemicals in the aquatic environment. J Pharm Pharmacol 37:1–12

Römbke J, Knacker T, Stahlschmidt-Allner P (1996) Umweltprobleme durch Arzneimittel. Forschungsbericht 106 04 121, Umweltbundesamt Forschungsbericht 96–060

Sattelberger S (1999) Arzneimittelrückstände in der Umwelt – Bestandsaufnahme und Problemstellung. Report of the Austrian Environmental Protection Agency, Vienna

Stan H-J, Linkerhägner M (1992) Indentifizierung von 2-(4-Chlorphenoxy)-2-methylpropionsäure im Grundwasser mittels Kapillargaschromatographie mit Atomemissionsdetektion und Massenspektrometrie. Vom Wasser 79:85–88

Stan H-J, Heberer T, Linkerhägner M (1994) Vorkommen von Clofibrinsäure im Gewässersystem – Ist der humanmedizinische Gebrauch Urasche für die Kontamination von Oberflächen-, Grund- und Trinkwasser? Vom Wasser 83:57–68

Steger-Hartmann T, Kümmerer K, Hartmann A (1997) Biological degradation of cyclophosphamide and its occurrence in sewage water. Ecotoxicol Environ Saf 36:174–179

Steger-Hartmann T, Länge R, Schweinfurth H (1998) Umweltverhalten und ökotoxikologische Bewertung von iodhaltigen Röntgenkontrastmitteln. Vom Wasser 91:185–194

Tabak HH, Bunch RL (1970) Steroid hormones as water pollutants. In: Developments in Industrial Microbiology. Washington, pp 367–376

Ternes T (1998) Occurrence of drugs in German sewage treatment plants and rivers. Wat Res 32:3245–3260

Ternes TA, Schuppert B, Hirsch R, Stumpf M, Haberer K (1997) Vorkommen von Pharmaka und Antiseptika in der aquatischen Umwelt. Fachgruppe Wasserchemie der GDCh, Jahrestagung, Lindau Mai 1997, Kurzfassungen, S 98–102

UBA (1997) Annual Report of the German Environmental Protection Agency, Berlin

Part I

Emission, Occurrence, Fate and Effects

Effects on Pharmaceuticals in the Environment – an Overview and Principle Considerations

P. Pfluger · D. R. Dietrich

For the 2 684 and more than 3 000 pharmaceutical compounds registered in Germany (Rote Liste 2000) and Great Britain (Ayscough et al. 2000), respectively, the predominant proportion of the available information is characterised by data from preclinical and clinical studies. These data and respective peer- and non-peer reviewed literature can either be retrieved from the pharmaceutical companies themselves or in a more concentrated fashion from on-line databases, e.g. Toxnet (http://www.sis.nlm.nih.gov/ToxSearch.cfm), which includes information from databases such as HSDB, Genetox, Toxline etc., and from literature databases, e.g. MedLine, Biosis and Embase. Little information can be found, however, on the fate, transport and effects of these pharmaceuticals once they have been released into the environment (direct disposal and/or indirect disposal via sewage treatment plants, STPs). This paucity of data raises several questions: do the pharmaceuticals reach the environment and in what quantity? What are the known and potential acute, subchronic and chronic adverse effects of these compounds in exposed environmental species and the ecosystem as a whole?

2.1
Occurrence of Pharmaceuticals in the Environment

Due to a lack of concern regarding the occurrence and effects of pharmaceuticals in the environment, no data appears in the literature until the middle of the 1970s. Then, one of the first reports concerned with pharmaceuticals in the environment was published by Garrison et al. (1976). Using GC/MS technology, they reported the presence of clofibric acid in the effluent of the Big Blue River sewage treatment plant in Kansas City, USA. Up to 2 μg l^{-1} clofibric acid were determined in raw and treated sewage waters. These concentrations were corroborated shortly thereafter by Hignite and Azarnoff (1977), who reported the presence of clofibric acid and salicylic acid at concentrations of up to 10 μg l^{-1} and 96 μg l^{-1} in sewage effluent. In view of the more recent analyses of sewage treatment effluents, which concurrently find the latter compounds in a concentration range approximately one order of magnitude lower (Stan et al. 1994; Heberer and Stan 1996; Heberer et al. 1997; Ternes 1998; Ternes et al. 1999a), the concentrations reported by Hignite and Azarnoff appear to be a little high. Indeed, the analyses of pharmaceuticals in environmental samples are apparently not a matter of triviality, but rather demand the highest attention as to sample preparation and treatment (Ternes et al. 1998). Due to the improved analytical techniques available as of the 1990s, the number of pharmaceuticals detected in environmental samples, mostly in sewage treatment effluents and rivers but also in ground- and drinking water (Heberer et al. 1997; Heberer et al. 1998), increased almost exponentially.

One of the major problems associated with the values obtained from the analyses of environmental samples is that the total influx of pharmaceuticals and the actual retention of the respective compounds in the sewage treatment plants are still difficult to quantify. The quantification of pharmaceuticals in raw sewage water as well as the calculation of retention in the sewage treatment plants would provide a better basis for environmental risk assessment. Presently the total influx of pharmaceuticals into sewage treatment plants can only be estimated using average patient dosing data and prescription information, as information regarding production amounts of pharmaceuticals in Germany and other European countries is not open to the public. One approach to classify and quantify the total amounts of prescribed pharmaceuticals in Germany was carried out by Schwabe and Paffrath (1996). They multiplied the average amount of daily doses with the (available) number of prescribed daily doses per year. However, the calculated weight in tonnes per year underestimated the real amount, as it did not include veterinary pharmaceuticals and human pharmaceuticals prescribed in hospitals or sold over the counter (OTC products). Henschel et al. (1997) estimated the use of a number of pharmaceuticals in Germany and came to the conclusion that, e.g. between 95 and 315 tonnes of salicylic acid reached the sewage treatment plants in 1994. Indeed, of the pharmaceuticals which predominate in the analyses of environmental samples as well as the lists compiled from prescription data, most belong to the class of analgesics (NSAIDs), antibiotics, hypotensives, antiasthmatics, diuretics and psycholeptics (Halling-Sørensen et al. 1998; Hartmann et al. 1998; Ternes 1998; Ternes et al. 1999a; Hirsch et al. 1999; Stuer-Lauridsen et al. 2000).

Pharmaceuticals are released into raw sewage and subsequently into the aquatic environment either as non-metabolised parent compounds or entirely as metabolites. As mammalian metabolism of the parent compound and excretion as well as the biodegradability of the parent compound or its primary metabolites are compound specific, the sewage treatment plant retention and environmental fate of pharmaceuticals has be to investigated on a case-by-case basis, as outlined in the recent review by Ayscough et al. (2000).

The need for the additional detection of metabolites is exemplified by clofibric acid. The active substance, clofibrate, could not be detected in sewage effluent and river water. Clofibric acid, however, its major metabolite, was found in significant amounts in the same study (Ternes 1998). Other commonly detected metabolites include salicylic acid, the major metabolite of the analgesic acetylsalicylic acid (Hignite and Azarnoff 1977; Ternes 1998), or dehydrated erythromycin, major metabolite of the antibiotic erythromycin (Hirsch et al. 1999). Most of the current information was obtained by a relatively small number of researchers, e.g. Kümmerer et al. (see Chap. 4, 7, and 19), Richardson and Bowron (Richardson and Bowron 1985), Ternes et al. (Ternes 1998; Ternes et al. 1998; Ternes et al. 1999a; Ternes et al. 1999b; Stumpf et al. 1996a,b).

Although the formidable advancement in analytical techniques provides better detection of parent compounds and metabolites, the greatest problem posed by pharmaceuticals in the environment lies in the fact that practically nothing is known about the environmental hazard of either the parent compounds or metabolites, as discussed below.

2.2
Environmental Effects of Pharmaceuticals on Organisms and Ecosystems

In view of the trace amounts of pharmaceuticals and their metabolites found in the environment, the question may be asked, whether it is sensible and feasible to assess potential adverse effects in exposed organisms and ecosystems. The problem, however, lies in the fact that these compounds are released from a point source (STP) and always occur as mixtures. In addition, the constant release, albeit at varying levels of concentration, provides for a chronic rather than an acute exposure scenario in the respective species and ecosystem exposed. Indeed, a recent review of the published literature on potential adverse effects of pharmaceuticals in aquatic organisms (Dietrich et al. 1998b) highlighted the paucity of data for single compounds while demonstrating the absolute lack of data on the effects of mixtures. Most of the information available on compounds such as β-blockers (metoprolol, propanolol), lipid regulators (clofibrate, bezafibrate), NSAIDs (diclofenac, ibuprofen, indomethacin, naproxen) and antibiotics (roxithromycin, trimethoprim, sulfamethoxazol) dealt with the medical use of these substances, i.e. preclinical (experimental data from rodents) and clinical studies and patient case studies. At best, data was available for *Daphnia magna* 48 hour immobilisation tests or zebrafish (*Danio rerio*) embryotoxicity tests (Henschel et al. 1997; Dietrich et al. 1998b), making any form of environmental risk assessment a questionable affair. Most currently available data on the effects of pharmaceuticals in the environment were obtained using standard test systems/procedures, e.g. algal growth inhibition tests (OECD 1984a), the *Daphnia magna* acute and chronic toxicity test (OECD 1984b) or embryotoxicity tests with zebrafish (DRETA, *Danio rerio* embryo teratogenesis assay; Dietrich et al. 1998c; Dietrich and Prietz 1999) and the African clawed frog *Xenopus laevis* (FETAX, frog embryo teratogenesis assay *Xenopus*, (ASTM 1991). An excellent overview on the present information was recently produced in the form of the Technical Report P390 by the British Environment Agency (Ayscough et al. 2000). The question must be raised, however, whether the standard acute test systems are of any value for the assessment of potential adverse effects in organisms chronically exposed to lowest concentrations of pharmaceuticals and/or their metabolites.

2.2.1
Risk Assessment

As discussed above, any form of environmental risk assessment must contain the element of probable causality. A test system and its specific parameters and endpoints are useful for risk assessment purposes only if there is a reasonable chance that they could also occur in the organism(s) or ecosystem(s) of interest. In other words, it is not very meaningful to employ a microbial growth inhibition test to assess the "ecotoxicity" of 17α-ethinyloestradiol, when all along it is clear that endocrinological endpoints and assays would be much more reasonable, relevant and sensitive. For example, the limits of classical ecotoxicology tests were revealed by a study of Henschel et al. (1997). Four pharmaceuticals and their respective metabolites were tested with different standard and non-standard ecotoxicology tests. The most sensitive tests were the non-standard tests, e.g. the BF-2 fish cell line (cytotoxicity and proliferation inhibition of fish cells). These tests all included relevant end points for the tested pharmaceuticals. All the classical standard tests, however, underestimated the toxicity of the four compounds. Hence, the choice of a relevant toxicity test is of great importance. The "right" test should include end points that detect effects associated with the specific mode of action of the chosen pharmaceutical. Most of the specific information regarding the mode of action, possible promising parameters as well as potential adverse (side) effects can be gleaned from the mammalian studies that have already been carried out for pharmaceutical registration and patient case studies. It is not suggested that the mammalian data can be directly extrapolated to the environmental situation; however, as a first point of entry for environmental risk assessment and experimental planning, these can be very helpful (Dietrich et al. 1998a,b,c; Dietrich and Prietz 1999).

2.2.2
Use of Pharmaceuticals, Mode of Action and/or Adverse Side Effects in Mammals as a Basis for Studying the Potential Environmental Impacts

When using mammalian data as a starting base, it is surprising to note that a high proportion of the pharmaceuticals on the market present with side effects (Rittmannsberger 1990), including immunosuppression, endocrine activity, deregulation of neural activity, etc. In many cases these side effects occur only in a very small subset of patients or following prolonged exposure to the compound in question. Extrapolating to the environment, however, would entail a completely different scenario: as mixtures of pharmaceuticals and/or their metabolites will be the predominant form of exposure for the organisms, all single compounds would have to be evaluated for their activity in a given endpoint, e.g. immunosuppression, vitellogenin induction and oestrogen receptor binding. Assuming additivity of the single activities, equivalent factors can be calculated and a Toxicity Equivalent Factor (TEF) approach implemented as has been the case for PCBs, Dioxin, Furans, etc. (Safe 1992, 1998). However, in order to do so, a prerequisite is to have the necessary basic understanding of the organisms and their normal physiological functions. For example, modulations of the immune system by pharmaceuticals have so far not been studied in aquatic organisms, more than likely due to a lack of proper understanding of the immune system, and consequently specific endpoints have not been established. One exception may be the case of antibiotics. Some of these substances have been in use in aquaculture to control for bacterial infections and as growth promoters (Moffitt 1991, 1998). As these antibiotics are of great economic importance in fish farming, their immunomodulating properties on fish were also partly studied (Lunden et al. 1998, 1999; Tafalla et al. 1999). Oxytetracycline, oxolinic acid and florfenicol, have demonstrated to produce a slight immunosuppression; however, whether this automatically implies that the organisms were more prone to pathogens and parasites has so far not been proven. More information on antibiotics is presented in Chap. 7 and Chap. 15.

In contrast to the insufficient information on immunomodulation, a wealth of data is currently published on adverse effects of xenobiotics, including pharmaceuticals on the androgenic or oestrogenic system, specifically of aquatic species. Starting with descriptions of hormone-like effects of structurally different compounds in the 1940s, the innovative publications of McLachlan directed the attention of the scientific community, the government and the public to this topic (McLachlan 1980, 1985, 1993; McLachlan et al. 1984, 1987; McLachlan and Newbold 1987; McLachlan and Korach 1995). Subsequently, varying and sometimes contradictory information became available dealing with different aspects of endocrine modulation. Today, the mode of action of the hormone-mimicking compounds is one of the best-understood fields in ecotoxicology. Their overall environmental impact, however, remains to be evaluated. More information on this topic is presented in Chap. 6.

2.2.3
Carbamazepine: An Example for Investigative Environmental Toxicology Using Mammalian Data

A good example to illustrate the imbalance between analytical and toxicological data is carbamazepine (Fig. 2.1), a widely prescribed antiepileptic drug, which is ubiquitously present in the aquatic environment. Median values of 2.1 μg l^{-1} in German STP effluents and 0.25 μg l^{-1} in German rivers have been reported (Ternes 1998; Ternes et al. 1999a). Removal in sewage treatment plants was found to be extremely low (7%), while the estimated prescription amount for 1995 in Germany was calculated to be 80 t (Schwabe and Paffrath 1996; Ternes 1998).

A recent literature review demonstrated a complete lack of ecotoxicological data for carbamazepine (Dietrich et al. 1998b). The analysis of the mammalian data in the literature suggested teratogenic effects and a possible antiandrogenic (oestrogenic) effect of carbamazepine. Juvenile rats treated for three months with carbamazepine presented with reduced prostate weight and decreased numbers of sperm (Dietrich et al. 1998b). Hence, a study was commissioned to investigate the potential toxicity and oestrogenic activity of carbamazepine in aquatic organisms (Pfluger et al. 2000). Both *Daphnia magna* immobilisation and zebrafish (*D. rerio*) and amphibian (*X. laevis*) embryotoxicity tests revealed a very moderate toxicity (teratogenicity and mortality in the 74–138 mg l^{-1} range. Furthermore, none of the expected oestrogenic effects (vitellogenin induction, increased ER expression, ER binding) could also be observed.

In addition to the above adverse effects in the mammalian studies, patient case studies indicated a possible immunosuppressive effect of carbamazepine, e.g. decreased IgA and IgM levels and increased natural killer-cell activity and phagocytosis (Garzon et al. 1986; Pacifici et al. 1991, 1992; Andrade-Mena et al. 1994; Andrade-Mena 1996). However, the results of the patient and rodent studies cannot be directly transferred to other organisms. Fish, for example, appear to lack IgA. Therefore, additional basic research on the immune system of fish has to be carried out before the potential immunosuppressive activities of carbamazepine can be properly evaluated.

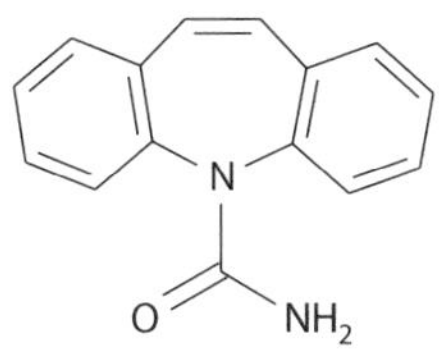

Fig. 2.1. Carbamazepine

2.3
A Final Perspective

Most of the available literature on pharmaceuticals in the environment deals with the analytical detection of these compounds in the aquatic environment. For a very few of these chemicals, the environmental fate is known. Data on the effects of these compounds in environmentally relevant organisms are, however, rare. This lack of information should be completed for many of the substances detected in environmental samples. Nevertheless, it should be stressed that the currently available standardised ecotoxicological tests are not sufficient, as they can underestimate the potential hazards of a given compound. Specific tests, tailored to include the compound-specific mode of action of a given pharmaceutical, have to be carried out to provide a better basis for environmental risk assessment. In conclusion, ecotoxicology must change its position from the current conservative to a more mechanistically oriented point of view.

References

Andrade-Mena CE (1996) Immunodepression induced by carbamazepine administration is mediated by CD 8+ spleen T cells. Int J Tissue React 18(2–3):81–85

Andrade-Mena CE, Sardo-Olmedo JA, Ramirez-Lizardo EJ (1994) Effects of carbamazepine on murine humoral and cellular immune responses. Epilepsia 35(1):205–208

ASTM (1991) Standard guide for conducting the frog embryo teratogenesis assay-*Xenopus* (FETAX). E 1439-91. American Society for Testing and Materials, Philadelphia, USA, pp 1–11

Ayscough NJ, Fawell J, Franklin G, Young W (2000) Review of human pharmaceuticals in the environment. Environment Agency, Bristol (Technical report P390)

Dietrich D, Knoll S, Schmid T, Rumpf S (1998a) Literaturrecherche zum Zusammenhang von Umweltschadstoffen und Schädigungen von Salmoniden im Liechtensteiner-, Werdenberger- und Rheintaler-Binnenkanal. Amt für Umweltschutz, St Gallen, Schweiz

Dietrich D, Schreiber H, Rumpf S (1998b) Literaturrecherche zu Pharmaka im aquatischen Milieu. Environmental Toxicology, University of Konstanz, Konstanz

Dietrich DR, Prietz A (1999) Fish embryotoxicity and teratogenicity of pharmaceuticals, detergents and pesticides regularly detected in sewage treatment plant effluents and surface waters. Toxicol Sci 48(1-S):151

Dietrich DR, Prietz A, Kiamos MA (1998c) *Danio rerio* embryotoxicity and teratogenicity assay (DRETA) for detecting waterborne embryo-toxicants and teratogens. Toxicol Sci 42(1-S):259

Garrison AW, Pope JD, Allen FR (1976) GC/MS analysis of organic compounds in domestic wastewaters. In: Keith CH (ed) Identification and analysis of organic pollutants in water. Ann Arbor Science,Ann Arbor

Garzon P, Gonzalez-Cornejo S, Hernandez-Hernandez G, Aguirre-Portillo L, Almodovar-Cuevas C, Navarro-Ruiz A (1986) Effects of antiepileptic drugs on concentration of serum proteins and immunoglobulins of epileptic patients. Gen Pharmacol 17(1):49–55

Halling-Sørensen B, Nielsen SN, Lanzky PF, Ingerslev F, Lützøhft HCH, Jorgensen SE (1998) Occurrence, fate and effects of pharmaceutical substances in the environment. A review. Chemosphere 36(2):357–393

Hartmann A, Alder AC, Koller T, Widmer RM (1998) Identification of fluoroquinone antibiotics as the main source of umu-C genotoxicity in native hospital wastewater. Environ Toxicol Chem 17(3):377–382

Heberer T, Stan HJ (1996) Vorkommen von polaren organischen Kontaminanten im Berliner Trinkwasser. Vom Wasser 86:19–31

Heberer T, Dünnbier U, Reilich C, Stan HJ (1997) Detection of drugs and drug metabolites in ground water samples of a drinking water treatment plant. Fresenius Environ Bull 6:438–443

Heberer T, Schmidt-Baumler K, Stan HJ (1998) Occurrence and distribution of organic contaminants in the aquatic system in Berlin. Part I: Drug residues and other polar contaminants in Berlin surface and groundwater. Acta Hydroch Hydrob 26:272–278

Henschel KP, Wenzel A, Diedrich M, Fliedner A (1997) Environmental hazard assessment of pharmaceuticals. Regul Toxicol Pharmacol 25(3):220–225

Hignite C, Azarnoff DL (1977) Drugs and drug metabolites as environmental contaminants: chlorophenoxyisobutyrate and salicylic acid in sewage water effluent. Life Sci 20(2):337–341

Hirsch R, Ternes TA, Haberer K, Kratz KL (1999) Occurrence of antibiotics in the aquatic environment. Sci Total Environ 225:109–118

Lunden T, Miettinen S, Lonnstrom LG, Lilius EM, Bylund G (1998) Influence of oxytetracycline and oxolinic acid on the immune response of rainbow trout (*Oncorhynchus mykiss*). Fish and Shellfish Immunol 8(3):217–230

Lunden T, Miettinen S, Lonnstrom LG, Lilius EM, Bylund G (1999) Effect of florfenicol on the immune response of rainbow trout (*Oncorhynchus mykiss*). Vet Immunol Immunopathol 67(4):317–25

McLachlan JA (1980) Estrogens in the environment. Elsevier, New York

McLachlan JA (1985) Estrogens in the environment II. Influences on development. Elsevier, New York

McLachlan JA (1993) Functional toxicology: a new approach to detect biologically active xenobiotics. Environ Health Perspect 101:386–387

McLachlan JA, Korach KS (1995) Symposium on estrogens in the environment III: Global health implications. Environ Health Perspect 103(Suppl 7):3–178

McLachlan JA, Newbold RR (1987) Estrogens and development. Environ Health Perspect 75:25–27

McLachlan JA, Korach KS, Newbold RR, Degen GH (1984) Diethylstilbestrol and other estrogens in the environment. Fundam Appl Toxicol 4:686–691

McLachlan JA, Pratt RM, Markert CL (1987) Developmental toxicology: mechanisms and risk. Cold Spring Harbor Laboratory, Cold Spring Harbor (Banbury Report)

Moffitt CM (1991) Oral and injectable applications of erythromycin in salmonid fish culture. Vet Hum Toxicol 33(Suppl 1):49–53

Moffitt CM (1998) Field trials of investigational new animal drugs. Vet Hum Toxicol 40(Suppl 2):48–52

OECD (1984a) *Alga*, Growth inhibition test. OECD Guidelines For Testing of Chemicals 201

OECD (1984b) *Daphnia sp.*, Acute immobilisation test and reproduction test. OECD Guidelines For Testing of Chemicals 202

Pacifici R, Paris L, Di Carlo S, Pichini S, Zuccaro P (1991) Immunologic aspects of carbamazepine treatment in epileptic patients. Epilepsia 32(1):122–127

Pacifici R, Di Carlo S, Bacosi A, Pichini S, Zuccaro P (1992) Immunomodulating properties of carbamazepine in mice. Int J Immunopharmacol 14(4):605–611

Pfluger P, Prietz A, Wasserrab B, Koster C, Knörzer B, Dietrich DR (2000) Untersuchungen zur aquatischen Toxizität und zur endokrinen Aktivität von Carbamazepin. EUREGIO Ökotoxikologie Service Labor, Universität Konstanz, Konstanz

Richardson ML, Bowron JM (1985) The fate of pharmaceutical chemicals in the environment. J Pharm Pharmacol 37:1–12

Rittmannsberger H (1990) Carbamazepine in the treatment of psychiatric diseases: effects and side effects. Wien Med Wochenschr 140(15):398–404

Rote Liste (2000) Bundesverband der pharmazeutischen Industrie e.V.

Safe SH (1992) Development, validation and limitations of toxic equivalent factors. Chemosphere 25(1–2):61–64

Safe SH (1998) Hazard and risk assessment of chemical mixtures using the toxic equivalency factor approach. Environ Health Perspect 106(Suppl 4):1051–1058

Schwabe U, Paffrath D (1996) Arzneiverordnungsreport '96. Aktuelle Daten, Kosten, Trends und Kommentare. Gustav Fischer Verlag, Stuttgart, Jena (Drug prescription report '96 current data, costs, trends and comments)

Stan HJ, Heberer T, Linkerhägner M (1994) Vorkommen von Clofibrinsäure im aquatischen System – Führt die therapeutische Anwendung zu einer Belastung von Oberflächen-, Grund- und Trinkwasser? Vom Wasser 83:57–68

Stuer-Lauridsen F, Birkved M, Hansen LP, Lützhøft H, Halling-Sørensen B (2000) Environmental risk assessment of human pharmaceuticals in Denmark after normal therapeutic use. Chemosphere 40:783–793

Stumpf M, Ternes TA, Haberer K, Baumann W (1996a) Nachweis von natürlichen und synthetischen Östrogenen in Kläranlagen und Fliessgewässern. Vom Wasser 87:251–261

Stumpf M, Ternes TA, Haberer K, Seel P, Baumann W (1996b) Nachweis von Arzneimittelrückständen in Kläranlagen und Fließgewässern. Vom Wasser 86:291–303

Tafalla C, Novoa B, Alvarez JM, Figueras A (1999) In vivo and in vitro effect of oxytetracycline treatment on the immune response of turbot, *Scophthalmus maximus* (L.). J Fish Dis 22(4):271–276

Ternes TA (1998) Occurrence of drugs in German sewage treatment plants and rivers. Wat Res 32(11):3245–3260

Ternes TA, Hirsch R, Mueller J, Haberer K (1998) Methods for the determination of neutral drugs as well as betablockers and beta2-sympathomimetics in aqueous matrices using GC/MS and LC/MS/MS. Fresenius J Anal Chem 362(3):329–340

Ternes TA, Hirsch RW, Stumpf M, Eggert T, Schuppert BF, Haberer K (1999a) Nachweis und Screening von Arzneimittelrückständen, Diagnostika und Antiseptika in der aquatischen Umwelt. ESWE-Institut für Wasserforschung und Wassertechnologie GmbH, Wiesbaden

Ternes TA, Stumpf M, Müller J, Haberer K, Wilken RD, Servos M (1999b) Behaviour and occurrence of estrogens in municipal sewage treatment plants. I. Investigations in Germany, Canada and Brazil. Sci Total Environ 225:81–90

Chapter 3

Environmental Loads and Detection of Pharmaceuticals in Italy

E. Zuccato · R. Bagnati · F. Fioretti · M. Natangelo · D. Calamari · R. Fanelli

3.1
Introduction

Since pharmaceuticals are anthropogenic substances, some of which enter the environment in considerable amounts and with potential toxic effects (Halling-Sørensen et al. 1998), substantial efforts have been made to assess the risk for ecosystems and humans (Henschel et al. 1997).

The rationale for risk assessment is as follows: *(a)* thousands of tons of human and veterinary drugs are produced and used in humans and animals throughout the world; *(b)* drugs and their metabolites reach the environment in substantial amounts through urinary and faecal excretion and the improper disposal of expired medications, which may contaminate ecosystems; *(c)* humans might be exposed to drug residues accumulating through the food chain or in drinking water; *(d)* drug molecules are specifically designed to penetrate biological membranes and reach target systems (enzymes, receptors etc.), thus increasing the probability of unwanted side effects on ecosystems; *(e)* data is scant about the environmental presence and persistence of drugs and the possible associated risks to ecosystems and man.

The present study was designed to contribute to the evaluation of human and veterinary drugs as environmental pollutants by estimating their theoretical environmental loads and measuring their concentrations in waters in Italy.

3.2
Experimental

Since no data on the input into the environment of human and veterinary drugs are available for Italy, we decided to assess their presence in the environment by directly measuring a group of pharmacologically active substances in selected environmental media. We identified the substances to be measured by two complementary approaches, in order to include as many major contaminants as possible.

First, we calculated the theoretical environmental load for major human and veterinary medicinal products in Italy, on the basis of lists of active substances with a theoretically high potential for environmental contamination. Second, we reviewed the reports in the literature about concentrations of pharmacologically active substances measured in environmental media in Europe and United States, then selected a further group of substances of potential concern for Italy.

3.2.1
Environmental Loads of Drugs for Human Use

The "leading medicinal products list" from the International Marketing Service (Italy) was used to identify the main 100 medicinal products for human use, by sales (number of units) in 1997 in Italy. Sales volumes of medicinal products were converted first to sales tons of active principles (by multiplying by the mean content of active principles in each product), and then to tons of active principles excreted as parent compound after therapeutic administration to humans (using published excretion rates; see Table 3.1). This preliminary evaluation only considered pharmaceuticals when excreted, at least in part, as parent compound.

Table 3.1 lists the 13 main active principles selected by this procedure, with their estimated environmental load in tons per year. The list includes drugs used in therapy in the range of grams, which are excreted in tenths of tons (i.e. antibiotics, ranitidine), and drugs administered in the range of milligrams, and are therefore excreted in hundreds of kilograms (digoxin, lisinopril, amyloride).

3.2.2
Environmental Loads of Drugs for Veterinary Use

Since no official data are available for Italy, sales of drugs for veterinary use were grossly estimated using unofficial data from AISA (Associazione Nazionale dell'Industria della Salute Animale). According to this association, which represents the major pharmaceutical firms in Italy, the overall sales of drugs for veterinary use in 1997 were 1/30 of those for human use, for all classes except antibiotics and antiparasitics, where the overall sales for veterinary and human use were comparable. In view of the lack of controlled data, we decided to include only a few of the most representative molecules in these two classes of drugs in the panel of substances to be analysed; namely amoxicillin, lincomycin (already included in the previous list), ivermectin and oxytetracycline. For the time being, growth promoters are not included in this list, since we do not know which molecules are used most in Italy, and to what extent.

3.2.3
Presence and Persistence of Drugs as Environmental Contaminants

Through a MEDLINE search and examination of the reference lists of all articles identified, we selected 106 papers published in international journals reporting concentrations in environmental media ($n = 32$), biodegradability ($n = 27$) and environmental toxicity ($n = 47$) of medicinal products. These 106 papers cited 101 pharmacologically active substances, which we then used in a further search for their pharmacokinetics (metabolic fate and excretion) and chemical characteristics of environmental relevance (solubility, pK_a, $\log K_{ow}$). Annual sales volumes were available for some of these substances and a theoretical environmental load was calculated on a nation-wide basis. Table 3.2 reports, as an example, a representative list of pharmacological substances measured in drinking water, seas, lakes and rivers; with the range of concentrations, place of measurement, and references. Table 3.3 indicates the persistence of pharmacological substances in the environment.

Table 3.1. Environmental load of selected drugs for human use in Italy (figures are calculated considering only excretion in humans; they do not include improper disposal and veterinary use)

Active substance	Sales (t yr^{-1} in Italy1997)[a]	Excretion as parent compound (%)[b]	Environmental load (t yr^{-1} in Italy1997)
Amiloride	0.69	Almost complete in urine (overall estimate 90%)	0.62
Amoxycillin	99.40	In urine: 60% after oral administration (overall estimate 60%)	59.64
Atenolol	8.38	90% in urine (overall estimate 90%)	7.54
Captopril	6.74	40–50% in urine (overall estimate 45%)	3.03
Ceftazidime	7.90	80–90% in urine (overall estimate 85%)	6.71
Ceftriaxone	16.31	40–65% in urine, part in feces (overall estimate 70%)	11.42
Digoxin	0.071	50–70% in urine (overall estimate 60%)	0.043
Furosemide	3.88	Almost complete in urine (overall estimate 90%)	3.49
Hydrochlorthiazide	1.52	Almost complete in urine (overall estimate 90%)	1.37
Lincomycin	10.21	50% in urine (overall estimate 50%)	5.11
Lisinopril	0.87	Almost complete in urine (overall estimate 90%)	0.79
Ranitidine	26.14	In urine: 30% after oral and 70% after parenteral administration (overall estimate 40%)	10.46
Sobrerol	55.23	In urine: 13% after intravenous and 24% after oral administration (overall estimate 15%)	8.28

[a] International Marketing Service. Leading medicinal products in Italy, 1997.
[b] Data review done for the JRC, Ispra, by the Mario Negri Institute, Milan, under study contract 2718. References: Martindale. The Extra Pharmacopeia. Thirtieth Edition. James EF Reynolds Ed. The Pharmaceutical Press. London 1993. PDR Generics (Physician Desk Reference). Medical Economics, Montvale, New Jersey 1995. British Medical Formulary. Number 32. British Medical Association and Royal Pharmaceutical Society of Great Britain. September 1996. Therapeutic Drugs. Sir Colin Dollery Ed. Churchill Livingstone. Edinburg 1991.

All information was subsequently organised in a data base in Italian on disk ("Banca dati farmacoambiente"), which accordingly reports sales volumes and theoretical environmental loads for Italy, chemical characteristics, metabolic fate, concentrations measured, persistence and environmental toxicity of about 101 pharmacologically active substances. The data base is available at the home page of the "Fondazione Lombardia per l'Ambiente" at the following URL: http://wwwflanet@flanet.org/ricerca/conclusi/farmacidb.zip.

Table 3.2. Pharmacological substances in drinking water, sea, lakes and rivers

	Active substance	Levels	Place	References
Drinking water	Bezafibrate	N.d.–27 ng l^{-1}	D	Stumpf et al. (1996)
	Bleomycin	5–13 ng l^{-1}	UK	Aherne et al. (1990)
	Clofibrate (clofibric acid)	Up to 170 ng l^{-1}	D	Stan et al. (1994); Heberer et al. (1995); Stumpf et al. (1996); Heberer and Stan (1997)
	Diazepam	10 ng l^{-1}	UK	Richardson and Bowron (1985)
	Diclofenac	1–6 ng l^{-1}	D	Stumpf et al. (1996)
	Ethinyloestradiol	N.d.–4 ng l^{-1}	UK	Aherne and Briggs (1989)
Water reservoirs	Ethinyloestradiol	1–3 ng l^{-1}	UK	Aherne and Briggs (1989)
	Norethisterone	N.d.–10 ng l^{-1}	UK	Aherne and Briggs (1989)
Sea	Clofibrate (clofibric acid)	0.5–7.8 ng l^{-1}	North Sea	Buser and Muller (1998)
Lakes	Clofibrate (clofibric acid)	1–9 ng l^{-1}	CH	Buser and Muller (1998)
	Bezafibrate	Up to 380 ng l^{-1}	D	Stumpf et al. (1996)
Rivers	Clofibrate (clofibric acid)	40 ng l^{-1} 30 ng l^{-1} Up to 180 ng l^{-1}	UK I D	Richardson and Bowron (1985) Heberer and Stan (1997) Heberer et al. (1995); Stumpf et al. (1996); Heberer and Stan (1997); Buser and Muller (1998)
	Dextropropoxyphene	1 µg l^{-1}	UK	Richardson and Bowron (1985)
	Diazepam	10 ng l^{-1}	UK	Richardson and Bowron (1985)
	Diclofenac	Up to 489 ng l^{-1}	D	Stumpf et al. (1996)
	Erythromycin	1 µg l^{-1}	UK	Richardson and Bowron (1985)
	Ethinyloestradiol	2–5 ng l^{-1}	UK	Aherne and Briggs (1989)
	Fenofibric acid	N.d.–172 ng l^{-1}		Stumpf et al. (1996)
	Gemfibrozil	N.d.–0.19 µg l^{-1}	D	Stumpf et al. (1996)
	Ibuprofen	Up to 139 ng l^{-1}	D	Stumpf et al. (1996)
	Indomethacin	Up to 121 ng l^{-1}	D	Stumpf et al. (1996)
	Norethisterone	N.d.–17 ng l^{-1}	UK	Aherne et al. (1985); Aherne and Briggs (1989)
	Sulfamethoxazole	1 µg l^{-1}	UK	Richardson and Bowron (1985)
	Tetracycline	1 µg l^{-1}	UK	Richardson and Bowron (1985)

Table 3.3. Environmental persistence, given as $t_{1/2}$, of pharmacologically active substances, measured in the environment or in laboratory conditions

Persistence	Substance	Reference
<1 day	Aspirin	Richardson and Bowron (1985)
	Diclofenac	Buser et al. (1998)
	Ephedrine	Richardson and Bowron (1985)
	Furazolidone	Husevag et al. (1991); Samuelsen et al. (1991); Lunestad et al. (1993); Ervik et al. (1994)
	Ibuprofen	Richardson and Bowron (1985)
	Paracetamol	Richardson and Bowron (1985)
	Penicillin	Galvachin and Katz (1994)
	Theobromine	Richardson and Bowron (1985)
	Theophylline	Richardson and Bowron (1985)
	Florfenicole	Hektoen et al. (1995)
1–19 days	Ivermectin	Lumaret et al. (1993); Halley et al. (1989); Bull et al. (1984)
	Norethisterone	Aherne and Briggs (1989)
	5-Fluorouracil	Kümmerer and Al-Ahmad (1997)
	Bacitracin	Galvachin and Katz (1994)
	Bambermycin	Galvachin and Katz (1994)
20–100 days	Cytarabine	Kümmerer and Al-Ahmad (1997)
	Gemcitarabine	Kümmerer and Al-Ahmad (1997)
	Mitoxantrone	Al-Ahmad et al. (1997)
	Monensin	Donoho (1984)
	Streptomycin	Galvachin and Katz (1994)
	Sulfadiazine	Hektoen et al. (1995)
	Treosulfan	Al-Ahmad et al. (1997)
	Trimethoprim	Hektoen et al. (1995)
	Tylosin	Galvachin and Katz (1994)
	Ceftiofur	Gilbertson et al. (1990)
101–364 days	Flumequine	Lunestad et al. (1993); Hektoen et al. (1995)
	Oxolinic acid	Samuelsen et al. (1992); Hektoen et al. (1995)
	Oxytetracycline	Bjorklund et al. (1990); Hektoen et al. (1995); Husevag et al. (1991); Lunestad et al. (1993); Jacobsen and Berglind (1988)
	Sarafloxacin	Hektoen et al. (1995)

Table 3.3. *Continued*

Persistence	Substance	Reference
≥1 year	Amitriptyline	Richardson and Bowron (1985)
	Clofibrate	Richardson and Bowron (1985)
	Codeine	Richardson and Bowron (1985)
	Cyclophosphamide	Steger-Hartmann et al. (1996); Kümmerer et al. (1996)
	Diethylstilbestrol	Gregers-Hansen (1964)
	Dextropropoxyphene	Richardson and Bowron (1985)
	Erythromycin	Richardson and Bowron (1985); Galvachin and Katz (1994)
	Ifosfamide	Kümmerer et al. (1996); Steger-Hartmann et al. (1996)
	Meprobamate	Richardson and Bowron (1985)
	Methyldopa	Richardson and Bowron (1985)
	Metronidazole	Richardson and Bowron (1985)
	Naproxen	Richardson and Bowron (1985)
	Pentobarbital	Eckel et al. (1993)
	Sulfadimidine	Van Gool (1993)
	Sulfamethoxazole	Richardson and Bowron (1985)
	Sulfasalazine	Richardson and Bowron (1985)
	Tetracycline	Richardson and Bowron (1985)
	Tolbutamide	Richardson and Bowron (1985)

3.2.4
Selection of Pharmacological Substances to be Measured in the Environment

The described procedure led to the selection of a list of pharmacologically active substances (Table 3.4), selected by the complementary approaches described above in order to increase the probability of including all potential major environmental contaminants.

3.2.5
HPLC-Electrospray MS-MS Method for Measuring Pharmacological Substances in Environmental Media

To measure concentrations of the pharmacological substances listed in water, sediments and soil, we used the recently developed HPLC-electrospray tandem MS technique. Aqueous samples (one-litre portions of drinking water, river, lake or sea water) were first adsorbed on a solid phase extraction (SPE) column (Lichrolut EN from Merck, Darmstadt, Germany), previously washed and conditioned with methanol and ethyl acetate. Columns were subsequently washed, then eluted with 6 ml of methanol. The solvent was taken to dryness and the residues were redissolved in 0.1% formic acid in water (HPLC mobile phase), and 20 µl were injected into the HPLC-electrospray tandem MS system without any further purification. The HPLC column was a Merck-C_{18} bonded silica column (15 cm long, 3 mm internal diameter); elution solvents were for-

Table 3.4. Selection of pharmacological substances to be measured in environmental media (water, sediments, soil)

Selected by	Pharmaceutical	Therapeutic group
Approach 1	Amoxycillin	Antibacterial (penicillins)
	Atenolol	Cardiovascular (beta blocking agents)
	Captopril	Antihypertensive (converting enzyme blockers)
	Ceftazidime	Antibacterial (cephalosporins)
	Ceftriaxone	Antibacterial (cephalosporins)
	Furosemide	Diuretic (sulfonamides)
	Lincomycin	Antibacterial (lincosamides)
	Ranitidine	Anti-ulcer (H_2-antagonists)
	Sobrerol	Antiasthmatic (beta$_2$-agonists)
	Ivermectin	Anthelmintic (avermectines)
	Oxytetracycline	Antibacterial (tetracyclines)
Approach 2	Bezafibrate	Lipid-reducing agent (fibrates)
	Clofibrate (clofibric acid)	Lipid-reducing agent (fibrates)
	Diazepam	Psycholeptic, anxiolytic (benzodiazepines)
	Erythromycin	Antibacterial (macrolides)
	Ibuprofen	Antiinflammatory (propionic acid derivatives)
	Cyclophosphamide	Antineoplastic (alkylating agents)
	Methotrexate	Antineoplastic (antimetabolites)

mic acid 0.1% in water (solvent A) and acetonitrile (solvent B). The elution program was from 95% A to 98% B in 12 minutes and then isocratic at 98% B for 4 minutes. The electrospray triple quadrupole MS (PE Sciex API 3000) operated in the tandem MS mode (multiple reaction monitoring, MRM), with detection of only the positive ions, using the turbo ion spray source. The method has been set up and validated for aqueous samples; validation for sediments and soil samples is in progress.

3.3
Preliminary Results and Prospects

Samples of drinking water, water from rivers and lakes around Milan, and water from the Adriatic sea, were collected and extracted. Sediments and soil samples were collected from the same areas. So far only a part of the samples has been analysed, and in river water we have identified some antibiotics (lincomycin, erythromycin), atenolol and bezafibrate, with concentrations in the 10–100 ng l^{-1} range, and sobrerol, cyclophosphamide and diazepam in the order of 1 ng l^{-1}, but work is still in progress and the final results will be presented elsewhere.

Preliminary results seem, however, to confirm the validity of the approach. To assess the dimension of the problem of pharmaceuticals as environmental contaminants we can theoretically take two paths: first "systematically", i.e. collecting samples (i.e. water, sediments, vegetables), and trying to identify all the chemicals present in them by a panel of tests and analyses (with the possible risk of missing important molecules); second "by loads", i.e. trying first to identify the major contaminants on a theoretical basis, then setting up specific methods for measuring them in environmental samples.

However, identification of the main contaminants on a theoretical basis is not solely a matter of loads. To contaminate the environment in substantial amounts, a pharmaceutical substance first must be used in substantial amounts; second it has to be excreted at least partly unmetabolised, otherwise we have to search for metabolites; third it must persist in the environment long enough to exert an effect, or at least to be detected, otherwise we must search for the environmental degradation products. Last but not least, to be considered toxicologically relevant it must exert some adverse effect on the environment or (by entering the food chain) on man. Unfortunately, for most human pharmaceuticals some of this basic knowledge is still lacking. Furthermore, it seems inadequate to assess long-life exposure effects of trace pharmaceuticals for humans and for environmental organisms, by using toxicological data from clinical trials, or extrapolating from the use of these pharmaceuticals in human therapy (high dosages, short-medium use). In order to assess the risk associated with contamination of the environment by pharmaceuticals better, we have to consequently improve our knowledge, especially by studying their persistence in the environment, whether and how much the food chain is affected, and the toxic potential of lifelong exposure to the main pharmaceuticals on the market or awaiting registration.

Acknowledgements

This work was supported in part by "Fondazione Lombardia per l'Ambiente" (contract no. 3095, 1998–99).

References

Aherne GW, Briggs R (1989) The relevance of the presence of certain synthetic steroids in the aquatic environment. J Pharm Pharmacol 41:735–736

Aherne GW, English J, Marks V (1985) The role of immunoassay in the analysis of microcontaminants in water samples. Ecotoxicol Environ Saf 9:79–83

Aherne GW, Hardcastle A, Nield AH (1990) Cytotoxic drugs and the aquatic environment: estimation of bleomycin in river and water samples. J Pharm Pharmacol 42:741–42

Al-Ahmad A, Kümmerer K, Schon G (1997) Biodegradation and toxicity of the antineoplastics mitoxantron hydrochloride and treosulfane in the closed bottle test (OECD 301 D). Bull Environ Contam Toxicol 58:704–711

Bjorklund H, Bondestam J, Bylund G (1990) Residues of oxytetracycline in wild fish and sediments from fish farms. Aquaculture 86:359–367

Bull DJL, Ivie GW, MacConnell JG, Gruber VF, Ku CC, Arison BH, Stevenson JM, VenHeuvel WJA (1984) Fate of Avermectin B1a in soil and plants. J Agric Food Chem 32:94–102

Buser HR, Muller MD (1998) Occurrence of the pharmaceutical drug clofibric acid and the herbicide mecoprop in various swiss lakes and in the north sea. Environ Sci Technol 32:188–192

Buser HR, Poiger T, Muller MD (1998) Occurrence and fate of the pharmaceutical drug diclofenac in surface waters: rapid photodegradation in a Lake. Environ Sci Technol 32:3449–3456

Donoho AL (1984) Biochemical studies on the fate of monensin in animals and in the environment. J Animal Sci 58:1528–1539

Eckel WP, Ross B, Isensee R (1993) Pentobarbital found in ground water. Ground Water 31:801–804

Ervik A, Thorsen B, Eriksen V, Lunestad BT, Samuelsen OB (1994) Impact of administering antibacterial agents on wild fish and blue mussels *Mytilus edulis* in the vicinity of fish farms. Dis Aquat Org 18:45–51

Galvachin J, Katz SE (1994) The pesticide of fecal-borne antibiotics in soil. J AOAC Int 77:481–485

Gilbertson TJ, Hornish RE, Jaglan PS, Koshy T, Nappier JL, Stahl GL, Cazers AR, Nappier JM, Kubicek MF, Hoffman GA, Hamlow PJ (1990) Environmental fate of ceftiofur sodium, a cephalosporin antibiotic. Role of animal excreta in its decomposition. J Agric Food Chem 38:890–894

Gool S Van(1993) Mogelike effecten van antibioca-residuen in dierlijke mest op het milieu. Tijdschr Diergeneeskd 118:8–10

Gregers-Hansen B (1964) Decomposition of diethylstilbestrol in soil. Plant and Soil 22:50–58

Halley BA, Jacob TA, Lu AYH (1989) The environmental impact of the use of invermectin: environmental effects and fate. Chemosphere 18:1543–1563

Halling-Sørensen B, Nielsen SN, Lanzky PF, Ingerslev F, Holten Lützhøft HC, Jørgensen SE (1998) Occurrence, fate and effects of pharmaceutical substances in the environment. Chemosphere 36:357–393

Heberer TH, Stan HJ (1997) Determination of clofibric acid and N-(phenylsulfonyl)-sarcosine in sewage, river and drinking water. Intern J Environ Anal Chem 67:113–124

Heberer TH, Butz S, Stan HJ (1995) Analysis of phenoxycarboxylic acids and other acidic compounds in tap, ground, surface and sewage water at the low ngl–1 level. Intern J Environ Anal Chem 58:43–53

Hektoen H, Berge JA, Hormazabal V, Yndestad M (1995) Persistence of antibacterial agents in marine sediments. Aquaculture 133:175–184

Henschel K-P, Wenzel A, Diedrich M, Fliedner A (1997) Environmental hazard assessment of pharmaceuticals. Regul Toxicol Pharmacol 25:220–225

Husevag B, Lunestad BT, Johannessen PJ, Enger O, Samuelsen OB (1991) Simultaneous occurrence of *Vibrio salmonicida* and antibiotic-resistant bacteria in sediments at abandoned aquaculture sites. J Fish Dis 14:631–640

Jacobsen P, Berglind L (1988) Persistence of oxytetracycline in sediments from fish farms. Aquaculture 70:365–370

Kümmerer K, Al-Ahmad A (1997) Biodegradability of the anti-tumor agents 5-fluoro-uracil, cytarabine, and gemcitabine: impact of the chemical structure and synergistic toxicity with hospital effluent. Acta Hydrochim Hydrobiol 4:166–174

Kümmerer K, Steger-Hartmann T, Baranyai A, Burhaus I (1996) Test of biodegradation of cyclophosphamide and isophosphamide using the closed bottle test (OECD 301 D). Zentralblatt fur Hygiene und Umweltmedizin 198:215–225

Lumaret JP, Galante E, Lumbreras C, Mena J, Bertrand M, Bernal JL, Cooper JF, Kadiri N, Crowe D (1993) Field effects of ivermectin residues on dung beetles. J Applied Ecol 30:428–436

Lunestad BT, Hansen PK, Samuelsen OB, Ervik A (1993) Environmental effects of antibacterial agents from aquaculture. Proceeding of the Euroresidue II Conference, pp 460–464

Richardson ML, Bowron J (1985) The fate of pharmaceuticals in the aquatic environment. J Pharm Pharmacol 37:1–12

Samuelsen OB, Solheim E, Lunestad BT (1991) Fate and microbiological effects of furazolidone in marine aquaculture sediment. Sci Tot Environ 108:275–283

Samuelsen OB, Lunestad BT, Husevag B, Holleland T, Ervik A (1992) Residue of oxolinic acid in wild fauna following modification in fish farms. Dis Aquat Org 12:111–119

Stan HJ, Heberer T, Linkerhägner M (1994) Occurrence of clofibric acid in the aquatic system – Is the use in human medical care the source of the contamination of surface, ground and drinking water? Vom Wasser 83:57–68

Steger-Hartmann T, Kümmerer K, Schecker J (1996) Trace analysis of the antineoplastic ifosfamide and cyclophosphamide in sewage water by two-step solid-phase extraction and gas chromatography-mass spectrometry. J Cromatography A 726:179–184

Stumpf M, Ternes TA, Haberer K, Seel P, Baumann W (1996) Determination of pharmaceutics in sewage plants and river water. Vom Wasser 86:291–303

Emission and Biodegradability of Pharmaceuticals, Contrast Media, Disinfectants and AOX from Hospitals

K. Kümmerer

After administration, pharmaceuticals are excreted by patients into the aquatic environment via wastewater. Unused medications are sometimes disposed of in drains. The drugs may enter the aquatic environment and eventually reach drinking water, if they are not biodegraded or eliminated during sewage treatment. Additionally, antibiotics and disinfectants are suspected of disturbing the wastewater treatment process and the microbial ecology in surface waters. Furthermore, resistant bacteria may be selected in the aeration tanks of STPs by the present antibiotic substances.

In this chapter, the emission of some typical pharmaceuticals, diagnostics and disinfectants by hospitals as a main pathway for the introduction of these substances into the aquatic environment is discussed. Data mainly from German hospitals of different sizes and medical service spectra, as well as from some European hospitals, are presented for this purpose. In hospitals as well as in practices, a variety of substances such as pharmaceuticals, diagnostics and disinfectants is in use for medical purposes.

4.1
Cytostatic Agents

Cytostatic agents (Fig. 4.1) are used for cancer therapy. Of two important compounds, ifosfamide and cyclophosphamide, approximately 400 kg and 250 kg respectively, were used in Germany in 1996 (Kümmerer and Al-Ahmad 2001). The amounts of cytostatics used are far below the quantitative relevance of other drugs like antibiotics (approximately 400 t yr^{-1} in Germany for medical purpose) or analgesics. The anticipated annual average concentrations for the cytostatics in Germany are a few ng l^{-1} in the wastewater and presumably below 1 ng l^{-1} in surface water (Kümmerer 1998). Carcinogenicity, mutagenicity and fetotoxic properties are often well demonstrated (Skov et al. 1990). Seen under the aspect of potential effluence into the environment, cytotoxics are an important group of drugs in terms of their risk potential for humans and the environment.

It has been shown that the degradability is largely independent of the mode of action and the chemical structure of the cytostatic agents. Most of the active substances investigated proved to have a low biodegradability (e.g. Kümmerer et al. 1996; Al-Ahmad et al. 1997; Kümmerer and Al-Ahmad 1997; Steger-Hartmann et al. 1997; Al-Ahmad and Kümmerer 1998). The active substances are expected to pass unchanged through municipal sewage treatment plants and thus reach surface waters (Aherne et al. 1990; Kümmerer et al. 1997a; Steger-Hartmann et al. 1997) in so far as they are not eliminated by adsorption onto sewage sludge. To judge from the results, an elimination of the substances by adsorption (e.g. in activated sludge) may be expected only in a small

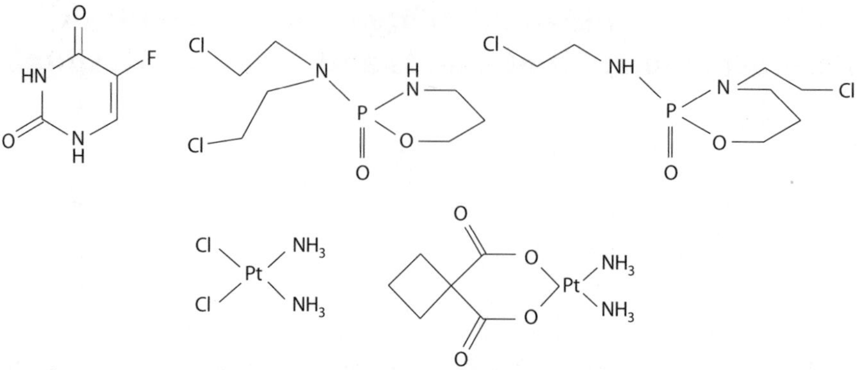

Fig. 4.1. Formula of some widely used cytostatics. *Top*: 5-fluorouracil, cyclophosphamide, ifosfamide; *bottom*: cis-platinum and carboplatinum (from *left* to *right*, respectively)

number of compounds such as mitoxantron and epirubicin (Kümmerer and Al-Ahmad 1999). However, due to their effective threshold in relation to bacteria, an impairment of the self-cleaning capacity of water or of the biological wastewater purification by cytostatic agents is not to be expected. Synergistic toxic effects of 5-fluorouracil with β-lactam antibiotics, cephalosporines, norfloxacin and other antibiotic agents against bacteria, as described in the medical literature, also occurred in the presence of wastewater from hospitals, because antibiotic agents are present in hospital effluents and, in lower concentrations, also in municipal wastewater. In preparations with hospital effluents, the IC_0 was far below 1 mg l^{-1} (Kümmerer and Al-Ahmad 1997) as it was >128 mg l^{-1} for 5 FU in tap water.

As the cytostatic substances occur in much higher concentrations in the patients' urine, a potential health hazard must be assumed for personnel entrusted with collecting the excretions of patients treated with antitumour agents. At the present state of knowledge, this risk is much greater than for the general population possibly ingesting these substances through the drinking water. For this reason, collecting patients' excretions is not recommended (Kümmerer and Al-Ahmad 1998).

With a laboratory lysimeter, the elimination of ifosfamide in a sanitary landfill was investigated. Up to 50% of the ifosfamide dissolved in the percolation water was eliminated under methanogenic conditions after 120 days (Schecker et al. 1998). Improvement of biodegradability by changing the chemical structure of a compound and retaining the active moiety is possible (Kümmerer et al. 2000a).

4.2
Antibiotics

In Europe, about 5 400 t of antibacterials are used in medicine (FEDESA 1997; Ungemach 2000). In Germany in 1998, approximately 412 t of antibiotics have been used for human applications, 103 t of these are in hospitals, which accounts for 25% of the total consumption. Between 1994 and 1996, the total consumption increased by about 30 tonnes (Erbe et al. 1997). The increase of the consumption in both hospitals and prescriptions by practitioners was approximately constant from 1996–1998 (Henninger et al. 2001). In view of the excretion rates, this would mean that the entire discharge volume of antibiotic agents into the wastewater is about 277 t from human medicine (Henninger et al. 2001). The expected concentrations of antibiotics in hospital effluents are of the same magnitude for some active substances and especially for groups of active substances, as for the semi-maximum inhibitory concentration (MIC_{50}) of pathogenic bacteria. Ciprofloxacin has been identified in a Swiss hospital as being the crucial source of the mutagenicity measured in hospital wastewater (Hartmann et al. 1998). The concentration measured was 3–89 g l^{-1}. The amoxicillin concentration measured in the wastewater of a big German hospital during a day course was 28 and 82.7 µg l^{-1} (Henninger et al. 2001). Amounts of antibiotics emitted into municipal wastewater in total correspond to a mean antibiotics concentration of approaching 71 µg l^{-1}, whereof 38 µg l^{-1} are due to penicillins (Henninger et al. 2001).

In the effluents of Swiss STPs, Alder et al. (2000) found up to 0.8 µg l^{-1} and predicted influent concentrations between 0.01–2.9 µg l^{-1}. For ciprofloxacin, for example, they detected up to 0.2 µg l^{-1} in 24 h mixed samples in the secondary effluent. Hirsch et al. (1999) found up to 6 µg l^{-1} of an degradation product of erythromycin (erythromycin-H_2O) in STP effluent and up to 1.7 µg l^{-1} of this compound in surface water. The development of resistance in biological films, i.e. in areas of high bacterial density, e.g. of sewage pipes or in activated sludge, therefore has to be taken into consideration. β-lactams were not detected. Some β-lactams may hydrolyse until they reach the STP and surface water (Al-Ahmad et al. 1999; Wiethan et al. 2000).

Tetracyclines, for example, are hardly discharged into the wastewater because of their high metabolic rate; moreover, they form relatively stable complexes with calcium ions.

Antibiotics are also used in farming and aquaculture for prevention, for therapy and as antimicrobially active substances to improve nutrient uptake in the gastrointestinal tract (growth promoters). Consumption in prevention and therapy is largely determined by modern animal breeding and fattening methods and conditions. By far the largest quantities of antibiotic agents are used in poultry and pig fattening. 5 000 t were used in husbandry (FEDESA 1997; Ungemach 2000) in 1996. Rough estimates say that in Germany 54 tonnes were used in poultry breeding and fattening and 135 tonnes in pig breeding and fattening in 1994 (Erbe et al. 1997). These figures are only rough estimates and are highly unreliable, due to inadequate data. In husbandry about one third is used for veterinary treatment, i.e. therapeutically and for prophylactic reasons, two thirds were used as growth promoters, i.e. 28 t for pigs and 30 t for poultry (Ungemach 2000). Only about 1% of the total quantity is used for other species (cattle, calves, geese, etc.). The consumption of growth promoters, which, according to literature, may be twice as high, has not been taken into account in these figures. Moreover, antibiotic agents are also used in aquaculture (fish farming) and for pets.

Active substances from important groups of antibiotics were of low biodegradability in simple tests (Al-Ahmad et al. 1999; Kümmerer et al. 2000b; Halling-Sørensen et al. 2000). 15–17% elimination were of non-biotic origin in this simple batch test. In a STP simulation, about 65% of ciprofloxacin were eliminated by sorption, while 30% were detected in the effluent (Kümmerer et al. 2000b). β-lactams were eliminated by up to 70–90%.

The results are in agreement with the low biodegradability determined for antibiotics in soil (Hübener et al. 1992; Marengo et al. 1997; Weerasinghe and Towner 1997). Ciprofloxacin was eliminated by adsorption in a test vessel which also contained sediment (Bayer 1991). Due to adsorption in activated sludge, the occurrence of resistance and disturbance of the biological processes as well as of the sludge reconditioning, in STPs, in soil or in sediments, cannot be excluded. Although fluorquinolone carboxylic acids in aqueous solutions are photolysed (Burhenne et al. 1997a,b), this mechanism of elimination is of no significance for wastewater ingredients on the way to and in the wastewater treatment facility. Turbidity, water shading, and water depth, as well as the seasonal changes in sunlight exposure, have a substantial impact on surface waters. Also, these substances may be adsorbed in sediments and hence be no longer amenable to photochemical degradation. Active substances discharged with liquid manure can be washed off from topsoil after rain. Furthermore, the direct discharge especially from poultry processing, meat processing, aquaculture and from pet animals (e.g. aquariums), is also possible and can contribute towards an increase in the total concentration of antibiotics in sewage and surface water.

In a simple simulation of surface water, ciprofloxacin and ceftazidime did not select resistant bacteria as far as they are detectable with classical microbiological methods (Wiethan et al. 2000). But only a few percent of bacteria present are detectable with these methods. As the bacterial density is low in surface waters, a weakening of the self-cleaning capacity of surface waters and a negative impact on aquatic communities caused by the discharge of antibiotic agents cannot be excluded if they are not eliminated in sewage treatment facilities. Only a small decrease in the number of individuals or species of bacteria can be highly significant for surface waters. At the present state of knowledge, the transfer of these substances from surface water via bank filtrate or soil passage into groundwater cannot be excluded.

4.3
Disinfectants

Large quantities of disinfectants are used for surface, instrument and skin disinfecting, product ingredients almost inevitably reach the wastewater. Many of the active substances are at most trivially biodegradable, or are difficult to eliminate, especially quaternary ammonium compounds (QACs) (ECETOC 1993). They are likely to disturb the wastewater purification process (Augustin et al. 1982; Guhl and Gode 1989). QACs are mainly active towards gram positive bacteria. After a period of several weeks of selection and/or adaptation of bacteria in a test system, benzalkonium chloride (Fig. 4.2) was degraded (Al-Ahmad et al. 2000; Kümmerer et al. 2001). An inhibitory concentration of $IC_{50} = 10$ mg l^{-1} and $IC_{100} = 30$ mg l^{-1} has been found for non-adapted activated sludge, whereas the figure was $IC_{77} = 100$ mg l^{-1} (Bayer 1995) for adapted activated sludge.

QACs form hydrophobic ion pairs together with anionic surfactants, such as LAS and SDS. The ion pairing changes the physicochemical properties. The ionic surfactant character is masked, as a hydrophobic ion pair is formed. The fate and effects in the environment of ion pairs are different from those of individual components. The improved elimination of QACs in the presence of LAS (Gerike 1982) is probably not due to a better biodegradability of QAC in the presence of LAS, but to the higher hy-

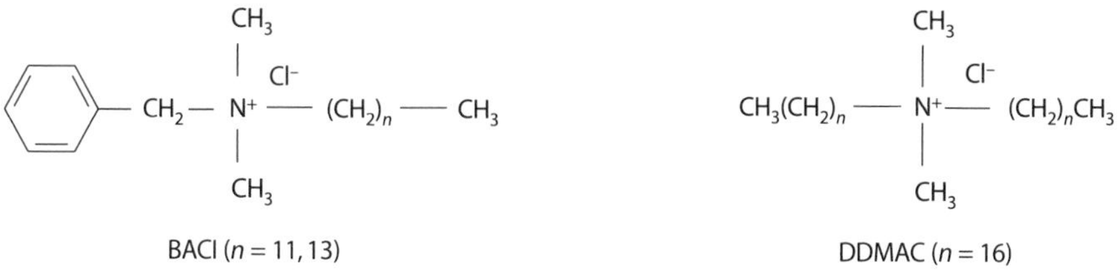

Fig. 4.2. Formula of two quaternary ammonia compounds (QAC) frequently used as disinfectants: benzalkonium chloride (*left*) and didecyldimethylammonium chloride (DDMAC) (*right*)

drophobicity of the ion pair and hence the elimination with the sludge. The nature of the inorganic counter ion influences the biodegradability (Janosz-Raiczyk 1992). The same results were obtained for organic ions such as the surfactants linear alkylbenzenesulfonate (LAS) and sodium dodecylsulfate (SDS). The biodegradability of the organic anions was even worse in the presence of the QACs than as pure compounds (Kümmerer 1998).

QACs are known to be effective against aquatic microorganisms, even in low concentrations (Tubbing and Admiraal 1991). An efficiency gap exists in relation to gram negative bacteria (Russel et al. 1992). The dose/efficiency curve of benzalkonium chloride is very steep. Inhibitory effects against denitrifying bacteria have been measured at concentrations as low as $1-2$ mg l^{-1} (Wagner and Kayser 1991). QAC concentrations of $4-5$ mg l^{-1} have been found in hospital effluents, with similar values being measured for benzalkonium chloride (Kümmerer et al. 1997b). Hingst et al. (1995) reported that by determining the maximum tolerated concentrations of pathogenic germs, a much higher prevalence of germs resistant against QACs was observed in samples from STP effluents. As a consequence of their low biodegradability, the Freiburg University Hospital has eliminated products containing benzalkonium chloride or other QACs for a number of years. Therefore, the QAC concentration in the effluent from this hospital was much lower than in the ones from hospitals of comparable size and medical service spectrum and even smaller hospitals (Kümmerer et al. 1997b).

4.4
Heavy Metals

4.4.1
Platinum

Platinum can be discharged into the various environmental compartments from a variety of sources (Lustig et al. 1997). One major source are cars equipped with catalytic converters. Hospital effluents contain platinum from excretions by patients treated with the cytostatic agents cis-platinum and carboplatinum (Fig. 4.1) (Kümmerer and Helmers 1997). After administration of the cytostatic agents, the platinum is excreted by the patients and so reaches the municipal sewer system.

The concentrations in 2 h mixed wastewater samples were between 20 and 3 580 ng l^{-1}, with a daily average between <10 and 660 ng l^{-1} for a hospital of maximum size. Absolute emissions are lower in hospitals with fewer care services and of smaller size.

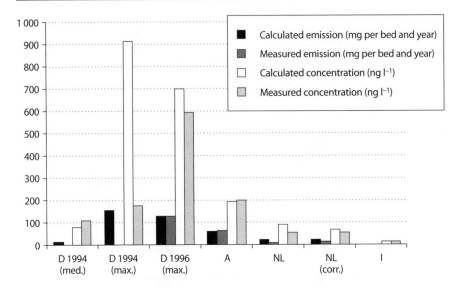

Fig. 4.3. Measured and calculated concentrations as well as specific amounts of platinum emitted by the European hospitals investigated (*max.*: hospital of maximum medical service spectrum; *med.*: hospital of medium medical service spectrum)

The specific emissions per year and bed differ less than the concentrations with values between 14 mg yr^{-1} bed^{-1} (low medical service spectrum) and 150 mg yr^{-1} bed^{-1} (maximum medical service spectrum).

In Germany in 1996, the total platinum emissions into the public sewage systems via hospitals were approximately 14.3 kg yr^{-1}, which corresponds to 12% of total emissions from cars and hospitals (Fig. 4.3). For the Netherlands and Austria, 6% and 3.3% were estimated respectively (Kümmerer et al. 1999). Emissions from other sources cannot be quantified (Helmers and Kümmerer 1999).

4.4.2
Mercury

In spite of successfully reduced emissions into the aquatic environment in the past, mercury continues to be one of the heavy metals whose discharged volume is still too high. The discharge of mercury from public health institutions is attributable to preservatives containing mercury usually found in diagnostic agents (e.g. Thiomersal®) and in disinfectants (Merbromin = Mercurochrom®, Nitromersol) as well as in diuretic agents such as mercurophyllin (Craig 1986).

The mercury concentrations measured in the central wastewater channel of European hospitals of different sizes were between 0.04 and 2.6 μg l^{-1} (Gartiser et al. 1994; Leppold 1997), corresponding to an annual load of approximately 220–250 g. As far as the skin disinfectant Mercurochrom® was concerned, it was shown that the administration of this agent at the Freiburg University Clinical Centre alone accounted for about 1–1.5% of the sludge contamination at the sewage treatment facility in 1996. Based on the volume of prescriptions collected by the national health insurance institutions in 1994, approximately 100 kg of mercury were used through Mercurochrom® in Germany, most of which is likely to have reached the wastewater during or after its application. Mercurochrom® was eventually replaced by mercury-free alternatives at the Freiburg University Clinical Centre (Kümmerer 1998).

Oxidising components of cleaning or disinfecting agents help to remobilise mercury in amalgam separators of dental treatment units (Kümmerer et al. 1997c). The remobilisation of mercury in amalgam separators with oxidising disinfecting components is expected to cause an additional mean mercury load of about 32.5 kg yr^{-1}. This appears to be little when compared with other sources and the quantities actually retained by mercury separators. The International Commission for the Protection of the River Rhine (IKSR) found in its interim report that "... the mercury values in 1993 (in surface waters) were still twice to four times the value of the target specification ... about 44% (of 1100 kg yr^{-1}) of the point-to-point emissions originate from municipal wastewater (approximately 440 kg yr^{-1}) ..." (IKSR 1994). The report of the International Commission for the Protection of the River Rhine expressly notes that further measures for reducing discharges from the municipal/public sector must be taken at the source, i.e. at the inlet site.

The mercury load remobilised from dental amalgam through oxidising disinfecting components in amalgam separators accounts for an average of 7.3% of the public wastewater, which could be lowered to 0.3% if disinfectants without oxidising properties were used (Kümmerer et al. 1997c). But part of the mercury emitted into the wastewater is also discharged together with the sludge; the proportion is unknown. From the medical point of view, the regular disinfecting of suction units of dental treatment units is unnecessary, although this is still done in many hospitals and private dental surgeries. Replacing disinfectants with cleaning agents without oxidising components could help to reduce the mercury emission into the aquatic environment to a substantial degree. In view of the substantial significance of mercury in terms of environmental hygiene and the high toxicity of methyl mercury, abiotically formed mainly in sediments or through different bacteria (Craig 1986), this measure is reasonable and highly efficient in terms of the efforts involved.

4.4.3
Gadolinium

Besides its application in medicine, gadolinium is also used in nuclear engineering and, together with other rare earth elements, in the production of colour monitors. Due to its high magnetic moment, gadolinium is used in magnetic resonance imaging in the form of organic complexes (Hammond 1995). Gadolinium complexes typically used in magnetic resonance imaging (MRI) are gadodiamid and gadopentat (Fig. 4.4). Following administration, the organic complexes are very quickly excreted (>95% within 24 h) unchanged (Nycomed 1995). The gadolinium complexes are emitted into public sewage systems and into surface waters via the hospital wastewater. They were shown to be non-biodegradable (Nycomed 1995). The bacterial toxicity is low (EC_{10} in the *Ps. putida* inhibitory test is 870 μg l^{-1}, Nycomed 1995). Nothing is known about the fate and effects in the environment. The concentrations measured in hospital effluents are in the range of a few μg l^{-1} to 100 μg l^{-1} (Kümmerer and Helmers 2000).

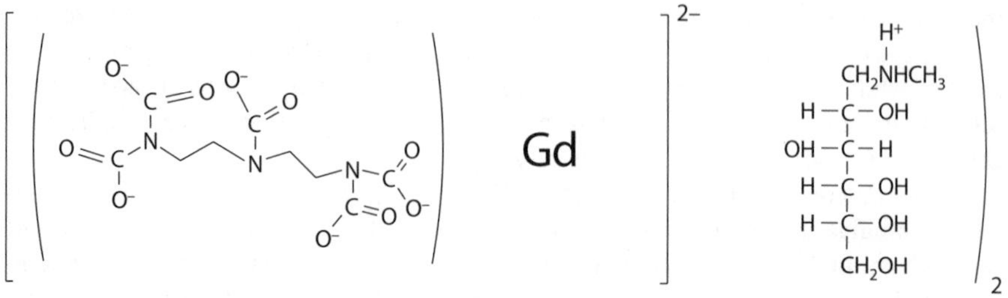

Fig. 4.4. (DTPA)Gd-dimeglumine (Diethylenetriaminepentaacetate-Gd(III)-bis-(D-(-)-1-methylamino-1-desoxy-D-glucite) used as contrast aid in magnetic resonance imaging

Falter and Wilken (1998) have measured between 0.3 and 1.9 mg kg^{-1} in water works sludge. Vivian (1986) found 0.6–2 mg kg^{-1} in sewage sludge, in own measurements 1.3 ±0.05 mg kg^{-1} ($n = 4$) of dry substance were found. From the good correspondence of these data it may be assumed that there is no substantial enrichment in sewage sludge. The natural background concentration of gadolinium in rivers is about 0.001 μg l^{-1}, peak concentrations of as much as 1.1 μg l^{-1} in the effluent from STPs are possible (Bau and Dulski 1996). Increased concentrations have been found in rivers in regions with high population density. Concentrations of 0.2 μg l^{-1} have been measured in rivers influenced by STPs discharge (Bau and Dulski 1996). With 0.12–0.3 μg l^{-1}, the estimated average gadolinium concentration by contrast media in surface waters in Germany is within this range. This suggests that the concentrations well above the natural background are partly due to the emission of contrast media containing gadolinium (Kümmerer and Helmers 2000). Emissions by hospitals and practitioners account for some of this alleged anomaly (Table 4.1).

Bau and Dulski (1996) suspect that the gadolinium complexes are stable enough to pass through municipal sewage treatment facilities. With a stability constant of K = 10^{28} the stability of Fe(III)-EDTA complexes is very much greater than those of the appropriate gadolinium complexes (K = 10^{23}) (Falter and Wilken 1998).

However, since iron(III) salts are used as flocculation agents, gadolinium could be supplanted by Fe(III) from these complexes with the effect that toxic Gd(III) is released. In the future it is expected that some of the Gd containing contrast aids can be replaced by others containing micro particles of highly paramagnetic iron oxides that are enclosed by a polymeric organic membrane.

4.5
AOX (Adsorbable Organic Halogen Compounds)

The major mass carriers for the AOX are most likely solvents, disinfectants, cleaners and drugs containing chlorine, as well as iodised X-ray contrast media (Fig. 4.5). Studies conducted at a number of German hospitals have shown that the AOX concentration in mixed daily samples, taken at the discharge points into the public sewage system, is in the range from 0.13–0.94 mg l^{-1} (mean 0.43 mg l^{-1}). The AOX contamination in wastewater part flows from individual sectors of hospitals can be substantially higher (Gartiser et al. 1994). In 24 h mixing samples from European hospitals, AOX concentra-

Table 4.1. Emission of gadolinium in Germany

Basis of calculation (data from)	Total use for MRI in Germany (kg yr^{-1})	Emissions by hospitals (kg yr^{-1})	Predicted environmental concentration (μg l^{-1})	Predicted environmental concentration attributable to hospitals (μg l^{-1})
Local data Freiburg		132		0.3
Local data Berlin	1 355	741	3.1	1.7
Federal Statistical Agency	1 160	484	2.6	1.1

Fig. 4.5. Basic structure of iodised X-ray contrast media (R = NHR', COONR"R'''; COOH in case of ionic contrast media)

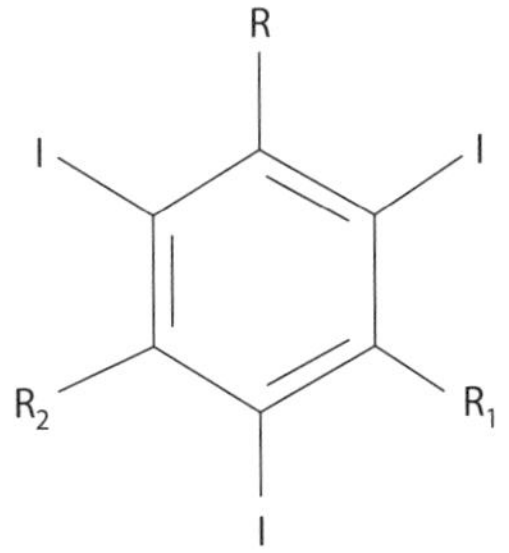

tions varied from 1.1–7.76 mg l^{-1} (Haiß et al. 1998). In some laboratory effluents, the AOX concentration measured was even higher (0.05–14.2 mg l^{-1}, mean 2.73 mg l^{-1}, Kümmerer et al. 1998). The AOX concentrations determined in laboratory effluents were high in five laboratories and very low in four other laboratories. The strong scatter of the measured values also showed in a high standard deviation. The lowest concentrations were measured in the wastewater from kitchens and laundries (0.015 mg l^{-1}). At night the concentrations in the central sewage system were often insignificantly lower, whereas they were at times even higher at night than during the day in the effluent from medical sectors: in effluents from medical sectors 0.12–1.71 mg l^{-1}, mean 0.95 mg l^{-1}, in the total effluents mean 1.11 mg l^{-1}; minimum 0.07 mg l^{-1}, maximum 2.64 mg l^{-1}. In samples taken during weekends, the concentrations in the effluents from all the sectors investigated were below 0.2 mg l^{-1}, in most instances between 0.06 and 0.10 mg l^{-1}. In the case of the highest concentration measured in the effluents from a laboratory (14.2 mg l^{-1}), the AOX concentration dropped to 1.8 mg l^{-1} after improvements in the disposal practice and handling of halogenised solvents.

In general, the maximum contribution of drugs to the AOX is not above 11% (Kümmerer et al. 1998). Beyond that, it is also known that the AOX concentration in the urine of persons not treated with drugs is very low, 0.001 mg l^{-1} (Koppe and Stozek 1993) to 0.2 mg l^{-1} (Schulz and Hahn 1997). Due to the dilution effect, no substantial contribution from hospitals consequently expected.

Chloramine T and other agents form elementary chlorine, which is responsible for the disinfecting effect of these substances. Due to the potential of organic halogen compounds being formed, additional wastewater pollution cannot be ruled out entirely. According to literature, the AOX formation through chloramine T is, however, substantially lower than through other elementary chlorine formers, such as sodium hypochlorite (Hahn et al. 1994). 4–6% of the latter are generating AOX (Schulz and Hahn 1997). This additional AOX pollution can be avoided by dispensing with chlorine-forming ingredients such as hypochlorite or 1,3-dichlorisocyanuric acid in cleaners and disinfectants, or in direct chlorine bleach. The disinfecting with active substances not splitting off elementary chlorine can also help to reduce AOX (Schulz and Hahn 1997). However, PVP-iodine-based disinfectants do not contribute to AOX.

Hospitals cannot be neglected as contributors to AOX in urban wastewater. The organic iodine compounds may account for about 50% of the AOX input into municipal wastewater. Brominated organic compounds are negligible for the AOX in the effluents from hospitals. Chlorinated or iodinated compounds play a much more important role for the AOX. A separate determination of AOCl, AOBr and AOI in partial effluent streams helps to identify possible sources of AOX emissions and to envisage emission reducing measures. More specifically, the times of AOX peak loads in a daily concentration profile can be identified and assigned to relevant activities and processes in hospitals (Haiß et al. 1998).

4.6
Iodised X-Ray Contrast Media

A surprisingly high proportion of AOI in the AOX was found in the municipal wastewater. Also, unlike the AOCl, it showed a pronounced weekly progression with minimal values on weekends (Oleksy-Frenzel et al. 1995). With reference to chloride, the proportion of AOI fluctuated between 23% and 53% of the total AOX. The proportion of AOI was particularly high when effluents from hospitals were discharged (Drewes and Jekel 1997). During the examination of the distribution of the molecular weight of the water ingredients detected with organic sum parameters, it was found that 80% of the organic substances in the AOI belong to the low molecular fraction (mol mass < 1000) (Oleksy-Frenzel et al. 1995). The molecular weights of most organic iodine X-ray contrast media are in the range from 700 and 900. This may be seen as an indicator that the AOI is mainly caused by iodised X-ray contrast media.

For all iodised X-ray contrast media (Fig. 4.5), which are in use today, the biological half-life for excretion is about 2 hours. Normally, X-ray contrast media are given to patients in radiology departments. Once the examination is completed, the patients normally leave the departments immediately and excrete the contrast medium either at the appropriate ward or (out-patients) at home (about 30% of all patients).

Especially in hospitals with major radiological departments, iodised X-ray contrast media make a substantial contribution towards AOX. They are not easily and completely biodegradable (Kalsch 1999; Steger-Hartmann et al. 1999). Surveys and comparisons with measurements have demonstrated that a large proportion of the AOX from hospital effluents is present as AOI (Ziegler et al. 1997; Erbe et al. 1998). The AOI is not necessarily the greatest contributor to the AOX in the effluents from hospitals. Instead, organic iodine compounds can account for about 50% of the AOX pollution (Haiß et al. 1998). Since iodised X-ray contrast media are not only used in hospitals but also in doctors' surgeries, a substantial proportion of iodine in the public sewage system could be diffusely discharged through X-ray contrast media.

Particularly when inexplicably high AOX values are measured, this could be an indication of a hospital with a radiological department, major radiological surgeries or maybe a manufacturer of X-ray contrast media being the discharger. Hirsch et al. (2000) detected iodised organic contrast media in the effluent of STPs in concentrations up to 3 µg l^{-1}. In surface water up to 0.3 µg l^{-1} were analysed, in tap water up to 0.07 µg l^{-1} were detected.

Compared with other drugs, a particularly low general and local toxicity is specified for X-ray contrast media, which are always given in high doses. Contrast media are not allowed to have any intrinsic pharmacodynamic effects. This may be seen as an indicator that their discharge into the aquatic environment is less problematic under the aspect of human toxicity. Nevertheless, they ought to be discharged in the smallest quantities possible due to their persistence and under the aspects of environmental hygiene and ecotoxicity. The issue of how to assess X-ray contrast media with their high persistence and mobility in water, in terms of environmental chemistry, ecotoxicology and environmental hygiene, needs to be investigated further.

References

Aherne GW, Hardcastle A, Nield AH (1990) Cytotoxic drugs and the aquatic environment. Estimation of bleomycin in river and water samples. J Pharm Pharmacol 42:741–742

Al-Ahmad A, Kümmerer K (1998) Biodegradation of the antineoplastics vindesine, vincristine and vinblastine, and toxicity against bacteria in the aquatic environment. Cancer Det Prev 22 (Suppl 1/1998):136

Al-Ahmad A, Kümmerer K, Schön G (1997) Biodegradation and toxicity of the antineoplastics mitoxantron hydrochloride and treosulfane in the closed bottle test. Bull Env Cont Toxicol 58:704–711

Al-Ahmad A, Daschner FD, Kümmerer K (1999) Biodegradability of cefotiam, ciprofloxacin, meropenem, penicillin G, and sulfametohoxazole and inhibition of waste water bacteria. Arch Environ Cont Toxicol 37:158–163

Al-Ahmad A, Wiedmann-Al-Ahmad M, Schön G, Daschner FD, Kümmerer K (2000) The role of *Acinetobacter* for biodegradability of quaternary ammonium compounds. Bull Env Cont Toxicol 64:764–770

Alder AC, McArdell CS, Giger W, Golet EM, Molnar E, Nipales NS (2000) Presentation held at the conference Antibiotics in the Environment. CWIEM East Anglian Region, 2 February 2000

Augustin H, Bauer U, Bessens E, Bestmann G, Botzenhart K, Dietz F, Genth H, Gerike P, Jung KD, Kettrup A, Robra K-H, Zullei N (1982) Mikrozide Wirkstoffe als belastende Verbindungen im Wasser. Vom Wasser 58:297–335

Bau M, Dulski P (1996) Anthropogenic origin of positive gadolinium anomalies in river waters. Earth Planet Sci Lett 143:245–255

Bayer AG (1991) Aerobic metabolism of ^{14}C-ciprofloxacin in an aquatic model ecosystem. Bayer PF-Report 3539, 29 July 1991

Bayer AG (1995) Preventol R50, Preventol R80 – summary of toxicity and ecotoxicity. Technical Information, January 1995

Burhenne J, Ludwig M, Nikoloudis P, Spiteller M (1997a) Photolytic degradation of fluoroquinolone carboxylic acids in aqueous solution. Primary photoproducts and half-lives. ESPR-Environ Sci Pollut Res 4:10–15

Burhenne J, Ludwig M, Spiteller M (1997b) Photolytic degradation of fluoroquinolone carboxylic acids in aqueous solution. Isolation and structural elucidation of polar photometabolites. ESPR-Environ Sci Pollut Res 4:61–71

Craig PJ (1986) Organomercury compounds in the environment. In: Craig PJ (ed) Organometallic components in the environment. Principles and reactions. Longman Group Ltd., Harlow

Drewes JE, Jekel M (1997) Untersuchungen zum Verhalten organischer Abwasserinhaltsstoffe bei der Wiederverwendung kommunaler Kläranlagenabläufe zur künstlichen Grundwasseranreicherung. gwf Wasser Abwasser 138:223–224

ECETOC (ed) (1993) DHTMAC – Aquatic and terrestrial hazard assessment, CAS No. 61789-80-9. European Center for Ecotoxicology and Toxicology of Chemicals, Brussels (Technical Report No. 53)

Erbe T, Kümmerer K, Daschner, FD (1997) Antibitotika in der aquatischen Umwelt. Erhebung des Antibiotikaverbrauchs für die Bereiche Krankenhaus, Praxis und Tierhaltung unter dem Aspekt der Resistenzentwicklung in der aquatischen Umwelt. Freiburg (internal report)

Erbe T, Kümmerer K, Gartiser S, Brinker L (1998) Röntgenkontrastmittel, Quelle für die AOX-Belastung durch Krankenhäuser. Fortschr Röntgenstr 169:420–423

Falter R, Wilken R-D (1998) Determination of rare earth elements by ICP-MS and ultrasonic nebulization in sludges of water treatment facilities. Vom Wasser 90:57–64

FEDESA (1997) European Federation of Animal Health, press release 6 September 1998

Gartiser S, Brinker L, Uhl A, Willmund R, Kümmerer K, Daschner F (1994) Untersuchung von Krankenhausabwasser am Beispiel des Universitätsklinikums Freiburg. Korresp Abw 49:1618–1624

Gerike P (1982) Bioelimination von kationischen Tensiden. Tenside Deterg 19:162–164

Guhl W, Gode P (1989) Störungen der Funktion biologischer Kläranlagen durch Chemikalien: Vergleich der Grenzkonzentration mit Ergebnissen im Sauerstoffzehrungstest. Vom Wasser 72:165–173

Hahn M, Liebau A, Rüttinger HH, Thamm R (1994) Electrochemical investigation of chloramine T. Anal Chim Act 289:35–42

Haiß A, Hubner P, Zipfel J, Kümmerer K (1998) AOX im Abwasser europäischer Kliniken. Vom Wasser 91:315–323

Halling-Sørensen B, Holten Lützhøft H-C, Andersen HR, Ingerslev F (2000) Environmental risk assessment of antibiotics: comparison of mecillinam, trimethoprim and ciprofloxacin. J Antimicrob Chemother 46(Suppl 1), in press

Hammond CR (1995) Gadolinium. In: Lide DR (ed) CRC Handbook of chemistry and physics, 78th edn. CRC Press Inc., Boca Raton, Florida

Hartmann A, Alder AC, Koller T, Widmer R (1998) Identification of fluorochinolone antibiotics as the main source of umuC genotoxicity in native hospital waste water. Environ Toxicol Chem 17:383–393

Henninger A, Herrel M, Strehl E, Kümmerer K (2001) Resistance caused by emission of antibiotics into waste water from hospitals and households? Predicted environmental concentrations vs. effect concentrations. submitted

Helmers E, Kümmerer K (1999) Anthrpogenic platinum fluxes: quantification of sources and sinks, and outlook. ESPR Environ Sci Pollut Res 6:29–36

Hingst V, Klippel KM, Sonntag H-G (1995) Untersuchungen zu Epidemiologie mikrobieller Biozidresistenzen. Zbl Hyg 197:232–251

Hirsch R, Ternes T, Haberer K, Kratz KL (1999) Occurrence of antibiotics in the aquatic environment. Sci Tot Environ 225:109–118

Hirsch R, Ternes TA, Lindart A, Haberer K, Wilken R-D (2000) A sentive method for the determination of iodine containing diagnostic agents in aqueous matrices using LC electro spray tandem MS-detection. Fres J Anal Chem 366:835–841

Hübener B, Dornberger K, Zielke R, Gräfe U (1992) Microbial degradation of cyclosporin A. UWSF-Z Umweltchem Ökotox 4:227–230

IKSR (1994) Vergleich der Gewässergüte des Rheins mit den Zielvorgaben 1990–1993 – Zwischenbilanz. Internationale Kommission zum Schutz des Rheins, Technisch-wissenschaftliches Sekretariat, Koblenz (Aktionsprogramm Rhein)

Janosz-Raiczyk M (1992) Biodegradation of alkyldipolyethoxybenylammonium chloride. Tenside Surf Det 29:436–441

Kalsch W (1999) Biodegradation of the iodinated X-ray contrast media diatrizote and iopromide. Sci Tot Environ 225:143–153

Koppe P, Stozek, A (1993) Kommunales Abwasser – Seine Inhaltsstoffe nach Herkunft, Zusammensetzung und Reaktionen im Reinigungsprozeß einschließlich Klärschlämme. Vulkan-Verlag, Essen

Kümmerer K (1998) Eintrag von Pharmaka, Diagnostika und Desinfektionsmitteln aus Krankenhäusern in die aquatische Umwelt. Habilitationschrift, Universität Freiburg

Kümmerer K, Al-Ahmad A (1997) Biodegradability of the anti-tumour agents 5-fluorouracil, cytarabine and gemcitabine: impact of the chemical structure and synergistic toxicity with hospital effluents. Acta hydrochim hydrobiol 25:166–172

Kümmerer K, Al-Ahmad A (1998) The cancer risk for humans related to cyclophoshamide and ifosfamide excretions emitted into surface water via hospital effluents. Cancer Det Prev 22, Suppl 1:254

Kümmerer K, Al-Ahmad A (1999) Epirubicinhydrochlorid in der aquatischen Umwelt – Biologische Abbaubarkeit und Wirkung auf aquatische Bakterien. 7. Nordwestdeutscher Zytostatika-Workshop. Hamburg-Harburg 29.–31.1. 1999 (Proceedings: 10–11)

Kümmerer K, Helmers E (1997) Hospitals as a source of gadolinium in the aquatic environment. Environ Sci Technol 34:573–577

Kümmerer K, Al-Ahmad A, Steger-Hartmann T (1996) Verhalten des Zytostatikums Epirubicin-Hydrochlorid in der aquatischen Umwelt – Erste Ergebnisse. Umweltmed Forsch Prax 1:133–137

Kümmerer K, Steger-Hartmann T, Meyer M (1997a) Biodegradability of the anti-tumour agent ifosfamide and its occurrence in hospital effluents and sewage. Wat Res 31:2705–2710

Kümmerer K, Eitel A, Braun U, Hubner P, Daschner F, Mascart G, Milandri M, Reinthaler F, Verhuef J (1997b) Analysis of benzalkonium chloride in the effluent from European hospitals by solid-phase extraction and HPLC with post-column ion-pairing for fluorescence detection. J Chromatogr A 774:281–286

Kümmerer K, Wallenhorst T, Kielbassa A (1997c) Mercury emissions from dental chairs and their reduction. Chemosphere 35:827–833

Kümmerer K, Erbe T, Gartiser S, Brinker L (1998) AOX-Emissions from hospitals into municipal waste water. Chemosphere 36:2437–2445

Kümmerer K, Helmers E, Hubner P, Mascart G, Milandri M, Reinthaler F, Zwakenberg M (1999) European hospitals as a source for platinum in the environment: emissions with effluents – concentrations, amounts and comparison with other sources. Sci Tot Environ 225:155–165

Kümmerer K, Al-Ahmad A, Bertram B, Wießler M (2000a) Biodegradability of antineoplastic compounds in screening tests: improvement by glucosidation and influence of stereo-chemistry. Chemosphere 40:767–773

Kümmerer K, Al-Ahmad A, Mersch-Sundermann V (2000b) Biodegradability of some antibiotics, elimination of their genotoxicity and affection of waste water bacteria in a simple test. Chemosphere 40:701–710

Kümmerer K, Al-Ahmad A, Henninger A (2001) Affection of bacterial populations by benzalkonium chloride monitored by means of chemotaxonomy in a batch test system using high bacterial density. Wat, accepted

Leppold J (1997) Bestimmung von chemischem Sauerstoffbedarf und Schwermetallen im Abwasser europäischer Kliniken. Diploma thesis. University for Applied Sciences, Albstadt-Sigmaringen

Lustig S, Schierl R, Alt F, Helmers E, Kümmerer K (1997) Statusbericht: Deposition und Verteilung anthropogen emittierten Platins in den Umweltkompartimenten in Bezug auf den Menschen und sein Nahrungsnetz. UWSF-Z Umweltchem Ökotox 9:149–151

Marengo JR, Kok RA, Velagaleti R, Stamm JM (1997) Aerobic degradation of ^{14}C-sarafloxacin hydrochloride in soil. Environ Toxicol Chem 16:462–471

Nycomed (1995) Environmental Data Sheet Omniscan®, Ismaning bei München

Oleksy-Frenzel J, Wischnack S, Jekel M (1995) Bestimmung der oganischen Gruppenparameter AOCl, AOBr und AOJ in Kommunalabwasser. Vom Wasser 85:59–68

Russell AD, Hugo WB, Ayliffe GAJ (1992) Principles and Practice of Disinfection, Preservation and Sterilization, 2nd edn. Blackwell Scientific Publications, Oxford

Schecker J, Al-Ahmad A, Bauer MJ, Zellmann H, Kümmerer K (1998) Elimination des Zytostatikums Ifosfamid während der simulierten Zersetzung von Hausmüll im Labormaßstab. UWSF-Z Umweltchem Ökotox 10:339–344

Schulz S, Hahn HH (1997) Der Kanal als Reaktor – Untersuchungen zur AOX-Bildung durch Wirkstoffe in Reinigungsmitteln. gwf Wasser Abwasser 138:109–120

Skov T, Lynge E, Maarup B, Olsen J, Roth M, Withereik H (1990) Risks for physicians handling antineoplastic drugs. Lancet 336:1446

Steger-Hartmann T, Kümmerer K, Hartmann A (1997) Biological degradation of cyclophosphamide and its occurrence in sewage water. Ecotoxicol Environ Saf 36:174–179

Steger-Hartmann T, Länge R, Schweinfurth H (1999) Environmental risk assessment for the widely used iodinated X-ray contrast agent iopromide (Ultravist). Ecotoxicol Environ Saf 42:274–281

Tubbing, DMJ, Admiraal W (1991) Inhibition of bacterial and phytoplanktonic metabolic activity in the lower river Rhine by ditallowdimethylammonium chloride. Appl Environ Microbiol 57:3616–3622

Ungemach FR (2000) Figures on quantities of antibacterials used for different purposes in the EU countries and interpretation. Acta Vet Scand, submitted

Vivian CMG (1986) Rare earth element content of sewage sludges dumped at sea in Liverpool Bay. UK Environ Techn Lett 7:593–596

Wagner R, Kayser G (1991) Laboruntersuchungen zum Einfluß von mikrobiziden Stoffen in Verbindung mit wasch- und reinigungsmittelrelevanten Substanzen sowie von Tensidabbauprodukten auf die Nitrifikation. Projekt Wasser-Abfall-Boden, Baden-Württemberg, Förderkennzeichen 88 068, Stuttgart and Karlsruhe

Weerasinghe CA, Towner D (1997) Aerobic biodegradation of virginiamycin in soil. Environ Toxicol Chem 16:1873–1876

Wiethan J, Al-Ahmad A, Henninger A, Kümmerer K (2000) Simulation des Selektionsdrucks der Antibiotika Ciprofloxacin und Ceftazidim in Oberflächengewässern Blank mittels klassischer Methoden. Vom Wasser 95:107–118

Ziegler M, Schulze Karal C, Steiof M, Rüden H (1997) Reduzierung der AOX-Fracht von Krankenhäusern durch Minimierung des Eintrags iodorganischer Röntgenkontrastmittel. Korresp Abw 44:1404–1408

Chapter 5

Emissions from Clinical-Chemical Laboratories

P. Hubner

5.1
Introduction

The benefits of medical laboratory analysis for the early identification and timely treatment of diseases, diagnoses and their verification, for forecast assessments and the monitoring of therapies, avoidance of infection risks (e.g. AIDS, hepatitis C, blood group and antibody analysis) and many others are undisputed. Today, laboratory investigations play a crucial part in as much as 64% of all diagnoses.

Every year, many different determinants and many different parameters are analysed in varying degrees. The automated in vitro diagnosis in medical/diagnostic routine laboratories of hospitals with 400–600 beds (central medical care) generates liquid residues with an average volume of about 2–100 $m^3 a^{-1}$. The proportion of reaction concentrates in this volume is on average 3–8 $m^3 a^{-1}$. They tend to be heavily contaminated with patient material such as blood, serum, urine, etc., and with test reagents carrying different environmental risk potentials (Hubner and Erbe 1998; Hubner 1999; Hubner et al. 2000).

5.2
Issues

Liquid residues from automatic analysers in medical/diagnostic routine laboratories are largely discharged into the public sewer system. Only a small fraction is disposed of as hazardous waste requiring special attention. The runoff from analysers is normally discharged into the public sewer system even if the manufacturers of the devices have already provided for an ecologically sensible twin-flow split, i.e. reaction concentrate heavily polluted with test reagents and patient material as well as slightly polluted rinsing/washing water. Rinsing and washing water accounts for most of the wastewater from clinical-chemical analysers. At the present state of development it can be discharged directly into the public sewer system.

The liquid reaction residues from the automatic analysers and/or of those found in the various test kits of in vitro diagnostics contain a multitude of chemicals with a wide range of different environmental effects that ought to be viewed in a critical light in terms of their ecotoxicity and mutagenicity. Analyses of laboratory wastewaters have also shown that the partial flow from this functional area can constitute a focal point of pollution in the wastewater area of medical facilities, although the actual chemical load may be comparatively small (Lange, no year; Murr 1992; Gartiser et al. 1996).

5.3
Ecological Aspects of Instrument Runoffs and Test Reagents

Even if given a promise of utmost confidentiality, most manufacturers of automatic analysers and test reagents for medical-diagnostic routine laboratories are not prepared to divulge ecologically meaningful data and information such as outline formulas for the composition of the test reagents, controls, calibrators, etc., which would allow the analyst to calculate or at least to estimate the approximately realistic composition of the flow-off ingredients classed as critical, especially the heavily polluted reaction concentrates. This data could, in turn, be used to determine the mean daily concentration and the daily/annual loads if the water consumption and/or the wastewater volume of the laboratory and of the hospital is known. Quantities and liquid volumes alone are no valid criteria for the ecological harmfulness of the ingredient substances or of the liquid reaction mixtures. What is needed, rather, is an accurate knowledge of the ecotoxicological potential, i.e. data on biodegradability, ecotoxicity, mutagenicity and the persistence of the ingredients contained in the flow-offs from the analysers.

Only a few manufacturers provide details on critical (ingredient) substances in a (semi-)quantitative form. However, these specifications normally provide no full details on the active ingredients/agents or additives such as preservatives, stabilisers, detergents, etc., or on the chromogens used in many clinical-chemical reactions. As a rule, environmentally relevant data and information is not available, and the details given by the manufacturers tend to include only those substances/substance groups for which information with environmental relevance is already partly available.

From an ecological point of view, the liquid residues from automatic analysers or from the different test reagents also contain substances that must be viewed critically in terms of ecotoxicological criteria, such as mutagenic effects, persistence, biodegradability, bioaccumulation and compatibility in technical sewage treatment and clarification. The classification or evaluation of the chemical ingredients tends to fail mainly because the EU safety data sheets, manufacturers' product sheets, and special ecotoxicological databases provide no or only very rudimentary information and data with regard to the ecotoxicological profile.

Table 5.1 shows that the reaction concentrates of the automatic analysers in the photobacteria test (G_L) and in the *Daphnia* test (G_D) vs. drinking water must be classed as highly ecotoxic. Furthermore, there is a clear indication of mutagenic effects of the

Table 5.1. Ecotoxicity of liquid reaction mixtures from automatic analysers in the photobacteria test (G_L) and in the *Daphnia* test (G_D) vs. drinking water (Lange, no year; Murr 1992)

	Boehringer[a] Hitachi 911	Sysmex[a] M 2000	Mixed sample[a] reaction concentrates	Drinking water
G_L	320	3.840	5.120	2
G_D	1.740	16.820	22.370	1–2

[a] Mixed samples and instrument flow-offs show clearly mutagenic effects in the Ames test and the hamster cell test (Lange, no year; Murr 1992).

liquid reaction residues from automatic analysers heavily polluted with test reagents and human material (Lange, no year; Murr 1992; Gartiser et al. 1996; Hubner et al. 2000). Zahn-Wellens tests (OECD 1992; EN 29888 1993) have meanwhile demonstrated the non-elimination of mutagenicity through microbial degradation within 28 days for parts of the reaction mixture (Hubner et al. 2000). The same holds for the inherent biological degradability of the reaction concentrates (Hubner and Erbe 1998; Hubner et al. 2000).

The test reagents used for in vitro diagnostics constitute a chemical mix (virtually unchanged in liquid reaction residues) from a wide variety of different chemical substances/substance groups with an equally wide range of environmental risk potential. A small selection of these test reagents is listed below (see Table 5.2). These are chlorinated and non-chlorinated organics such as substituted toluidine, 4-chlorophenol, 2-chloro-4-nitrophenyl-β, 2-chloro-4-nitrophenol, diethanolamine, 2-hydroxybenzylalcohol, o-cresolphthaleine-complex, 8-hydroxychinoline, 5-chloro-2-methyl-4-thiazol-3 (preservative) etc., buffer solutions such as triethanolamine, imidazolacetate and tris buffers etc., but also dye reagents such as coomassie blue ferrocin or brilliant blue.

Table 5.2. Manufacturers' specifications on the masses of ingredients classed as critical, for the automatic analyser Hitachi 717 E (Dept. Clinical Chemistry)

Test parameters	Ingredients	Higher order chemical substance group	Mass per 100 test (mg)	Mass per year (mg)
Albumin (ALB)	Bromine in bromine cresol green	Halog. arom. comp.	1.69	153.05
Bilirubin total (T-BIL)	Chlorine in dichloro-phenyldiazonium salt	Halog. org. comp.	2.13	314.54
Bilirubin direct (D-BIL)	Sodium nitrite	WGK 2	1.11	109.96
Cholesterol (CHOL)	Chlorine in dichloro-phenol; Phenol	Halog. arom. comp., WGK 3; Arom. comp., WGK 2	11.43 11.46	[a] [a]
Creatinine (CREA)	Bromine in tribrom-hydr. benzoic acid; Cyanide in K-hexa-cyanoferrate	Halog. arom. comp. Complex cyanides	52.02 0.02	23 708.12 9.12
Total protein (TP)	Copper in copper sulphate	Heavy metal comp., WGK 2	19.33	4 902.09
Glucose (GLUC)	Phenol	Aromat. comp., WGK 2	31.08	16 323.84
Uric acid (UA)	Bromine in tribrom-hydr. benzoic acid; Cyanide in K-hexa-cyanoferrate	Halog. arom. comp. Complex cyanides	1 554.00 1.55	254 016.80 253.36
Triglycerides (TRIG)	Chlorine in p-chlorophenol; Cyanide in K-hexa-cyanoferrate	Halog. arom. comp., WGK 2; Complex cyanides	106.05 1.09	[a] [a]

[a] Parameter determined with other analysers.

Test reagents also include ingredients such as inorganic salts, some containing heavy metals, quaternary ammonium salts, magnesium sulfate, ammonium sulfate, ammonium heptamolybdate, potassium iodide, sodium hypochlorite (cleaning agents), copper sulfate, calcium chloride, sodium acid (preserving agent), potassium hexacyanoferrate(II) and many others. But the chemical mix also features organic salts such as lithium picrate, magnesium acetate, potassium sodium tartrate, cyclohexyl-aminopropansulfate, 4-nitrophenyl-phosphate, dichlorophenyl-diazonium salt, S-butyrylthiochloniodide etc., inorganic acids and alkalines such as sulfuric acid, hydrochloric acid, sodium hydroxide solution, lithium hydroxide and organic acids such as 5,5'-dithio-bis-2-nitrobenzoic acid, N-(2-acetamido)-imino-diacetic acid, ethylenediaminetetraacetic acid, triolein etc. In addition, other ingredients are enzymes such as glucose-dehydrogenase, glucose-6-phosphate-dehydrogenase or peroxidase.

A mutagenic and/or carcinogenic potential is known from a number of these (active) ingredients, with such potentials suspected in a much greater number. Also, useful information and data on ecotoxicity and biodegradability are available in only very few cases. As a rule, the assessment using environmentally relevant data privided in EU safety data sheets or water hazard classes in databases can be made only if the test reagents have already been classified for the environmental sector in accordance with European and international specifications and standards. If these reagents are subsumed under the Drugs Law (which is found occasionally on the national level), there is no obligation for identification or labelling in terms of environmental relevance. In the former case there is at least an initial indication of the pollutant potential of the liquid residues from analysers, with the qualifying restriction that the EU safety data sheets for the test reagents requiring identification and labelling normally include no immediately useful notices with respect to environmental relevance.

With reference to the realistic water consumption of a medium-sized hospital (500 regular beds) of approximately 100 000 $m^3 a^{-1}$, the active ingredient bromine in tribromine hydroxy-benzoic acid (used for determining uric acid, Table 5.2), for instance, results in a concentration of 2.5 $\mu g\, l^{-1}$. Dilution by the factor 100 therefore results in a concentration of approximately 25 $ng\, l^{-1}$ in the communal sewage system.

Every year many different determinants and many different parameters are analysed in varying degrees, with the test kits used for in vitro diagnostics being composed of a wide variety of different ingredients, both in their nature and in their quantity. A rough estimate shows that the concentration of ingredients such as chromogens, preservatives, inactive ingredients, etc., account on average for 2–30 $\mu g\, l^{-1}$ of the hospital wastewater, with the annual loads reaching the gram and kilogram range (Hubner and Erbe 1998; Hubner 1999; Hubner et al. 2000).

Most tests are normally carried out every year in the respective clinical chemistry departments. The concentrations and annual loads of the ingredients heavily polluted with test reagents and human material from automatic analysers therefore tend to be higher than from the analysers in the other departments. With reference to the total wastewater volume of a medium-sized hospital (see above), the flow-off concentrations from clinical-chemical analysers are moving more in the direction of the $mg\, l^{-1}$ range, and the masses per year are more in the kg range than in the gram range.

5.4
Summary and Outlook

The test reagents used for in vitro diagnostics constitute a chemical mix (virtually unchanged in liquid reaction residues) from a wide variety of different chemical substances/substance groups with an equally wide range of environmental risk potential. These include chromogens, inorganic and organic salts, acids and alkalines, stabilisers, preservatives, buffers, enzymes, coenzymes, heavy metals and detergents.

The reaction concentrations of analysers used in medical-diagnostic routine laboratories are to be classed as highly ecotoxic. There are also clear indications of a mutagenic effect in the Ames test, the hamster cell test and the SOS chromotest (genotoxicity test). Studies involving the biodegradability in the Zahn-Wellens test have also demonstrated that the mutagenic effect cannot be eliminated in some instrument flow-offs and that the biodegradability is limited.

As the breakdown of the reaction mixes from analysers in medical-diagnostic routine laboratories tested in the Zahn-Wellens test is only partially acceptable, some of the instrument flow-offs pose the risk of being discharged into surface waters and therefore enriching in the food chain. Mutagenicity studies involving the instrument flow-off also demonstrate that the flow-off from analysers in immunology departments show a particularly pronounced mutagenic effect and that the severe mutagenic effect is only sporadically eliminated by biological degradation. Further investigations need to be made in this field, also with a view to ecotoxicity, persistence, accumulation capability, etc.

From the ecological point of view, the decision whether the instrument flow-off is to be disposed of as special liquid waste or as wastewater is not so much determined by the liquid volume of the reaction concentrates heavily polluted with human material and chemicals, but rather by their ecotoxicological potential and persistence. The legal issue of whether the reaction mix trapped separately within the analysers is to be treated as normal waste and is therefore allowed to be discharged into the public sewage system needs to be clarified (definition of the "point of transfer" or of the "site of waste generation").

To account for the principle of due care and attention, the liquid residues from automatic analysers should be compulsorily separated into two partial flow offs labelled "low pollution level" and "high pollution level", with the former (at the present state of knowledge) being allowed to be discharged into the public sewage system. Liquid residues identified as "heavily polluted" should be disposed of as special chemical waste at least until further verified data on environmentally relevant aspects such as persistence, mutagenicity, ecotoxicity, biodegradability and compatibility in technical sewage treatment and clarification is available to a degree adequate to allow proper risk assessment.

The classification or evaluation of the chemical ingredients tends to fail mainly because the EU safety data sheets, manufacturers' product sheets, but also special ecotoxicological databases, provide no or only very rudimentary information and data on ecotoxicity, mutagenicity and biodegradability. Only a few manufacturers provide details on critical (ingredient) substances in a (semi-)quantitative form. However, these specifications normally provide no full details on the active ingredients/agents or additives such as preservatives, stabilisers, detergents, etc., or on the chromogens used in many clinical-chemical reactions. As a rule, environmentally relevant data and information is not available, and the details given by the manufacturers tend to include only those substances/substance groups for which information with environmental relevance is already partly available.

The quantitative detailing of the quantities or of the liquid volumes, but also the pollutant concentrations and loads determined by analysis or by balancing and other wastewater relevant (summation) parameters, can help to make risks more visible and manageable. However, numerical physical/analytical data can also be misleading because they reflect only one aspect. Without proper insights into ecotoxicity, mutagenicity, persistence, hormonal effects and biodegradability, they may lead to a false sense of security and the unjustified assumption of greater certainty.

References

EN 29888 (1993) Bestimmung der aeroben biologischen Abbaubarkeit organischer Stoffe im wässrigen Medium. Statischer Test (Zahn-Wellens Test). Europäisches Komitee für Normung, Brüssel. In: Deutsche Einheitsverfahren zur Wasser-, Abwasser- und Schlammuntersuchung. VCH Verlagsgesellschaft, Weinheim, New York, Basel, Cambridge

Gartiser S, Brinker L, Erbe T, Kümmerer K, Willmund R (1996) Belastung von Krankenhausabwasser mit gefährlichen Stoffen im Sinne § 7a WHG. Acta hydrochim hydrobiol 24(2):90–97

Hubner P (1999) Flüssige Rückstände aus medizinisch-diagnostischen Routinelaboratorien – Entstehungsorte, Bestimmungsparameter, Mengen und ökologische Bedeutung. In: Flöser V (Hrsg) Krankenhausabwasser: Beschaffenheit – Behandlung – Maßnahmen zur Reduzierung von Schadstoffen – Hygienische Aspekte. expert verlag GmbH, Renningen-Malmsheim (KONTAKT & STUDIUM der Technischen Akademie Esslingen, Band 593, S 97–117)

Hubner P, Erbe T (1998) Untersuchungen zur Abfallentsorgung – Verwertung und Vermeidung von Abfällen in klinisch-chemischen Laboratorien. Ministerium für Umwelt und Verkehr Baden-Württemberg, Stuttgart (Abschlußbericht)

Hubner P, Mersch-Sundermann V, Bulowski I, Nahkur E, Kümmerer K (2000) Mutagene Effekte und biologische Abbaubarkeit von flüssigen Reaktionsrückständen aus Analysatoren der in-vitro Diagnostik klinisch-chemischer Routinelaboratorien. Vom Wasser 95:293–306

Lange T (no year) Membranverfahren zur Vorbehandlung klinischer Laborabwässer. Diplomarbeit, FH Braunschweig-Wolfenbüttel, Fachbereich Versorgungstechnik

Murr S (1992) Ordnungsgemäße Entsorgung von flüssigen Abfällen aus klinisch-chemischen Analysatoren. Diplomarbeit, FH München, Fachbereich Physikalische Technik

OECD (1992) Guidelines for testing of chemicals. 302 B: Zahn-Wellens Test. Adopted by the Council on 17th July 1992. OECD, Paris

Chapter 6

Pharmaceuticals in the Environment: Focus on 17α–ethinyloestradiol

R. G. Kozak · I. D'Haese · W. Verstraete

6.1
Introduction

Until recently there has been little awareness about the side effects of pharmaceutical residues in wildlife and in humans. However, this is changing. Especially in the last two years, many reports identifying the presence of unwanted pharmaceutical drugs in environmental water have been published. Moreover, the increasing scarcity of water resources confronts society with the challenge of understanding the hazards that these pharmaceuticals and their main metabolites may pose. Methods to evaluate and decrease these hazards have become topics of intensive research.

The most used oestrogenic component of oral contraceptives, 17α-ethinyloestradiol (EE$_2$), finds its way to the environment mainly through sewage. Likewise the natural endogenous oestrogens, of which the most potent is 17β-oestradiol (E$_2$), EE$_2$ is metabolised in the human body before its excretion. It is mostly conjugated with glucuronides and sulfates (Carr and Griffin 1998). This conjugation, which inactivates the hormonal activity, increases the water solubility and therefore makes the conjugates more mobile in the environment than the free hormones. After 24 hours, only 3% of the oral dose of EE$_2$ (20–50 µg d^{-1}) remains in plasma and up to 60% is excreted in the urine (Carr and Griffin 1998). Free E$_2$ and EE$_2$ are practically non water-soluble and have a high sorption potential (logK_{oc}). The logK_{oc} relates to the logK_{ow} through linear correlation (Table 6.1). The natural hormone and the synthetic oestrogen are steroids; their structural formulas are presented in Fig. 6.1.

Oral contraceptives are among the pharmaceuticals most sold world-wide. On a global scale, they are estimated to be consumed by approximately 60 million women

Table 6.1. Physicochemical characteristics of the natural 17β-oestradiol (E$_2$) and the pharmaceutical 17α-ethinyloestradiol (EE$_2$)

	MW	Solubility[a] (mg l^{-1})	Melting point[b] (°C)	Rotation index[b] (αD)	Vapor Pressure[c] (Torr)	LogK_{ow}
E$_2$	272.4	12.96	178	+81°	2.25×10^{-10}	3.1[c]
EE$_2$	296.4	4.83	146	+1°	4.50×10^{-11}	4.2[d]

[a] Tabak et al. (1981).
[b] Fieser and Fieser (1959).
[c] Quoted by Williams et al. (1999).
[d] Quoted by Ternes et al. (1999b).

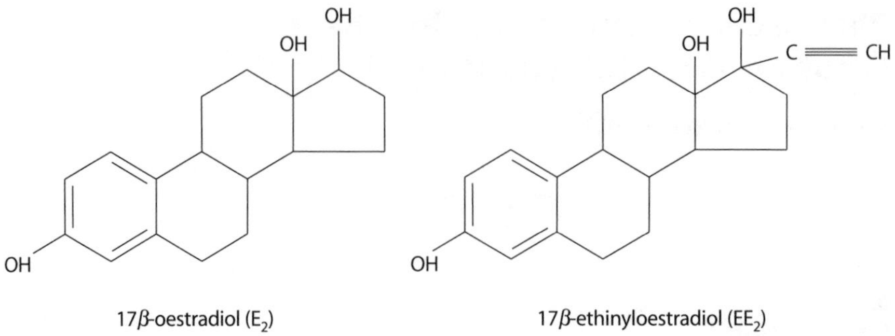

Fig. 6.1. Structural formulas of the principal human oestrogen: 17β-oestradiol (E$_2$) and the main synthetic pharmaceutical oestrogen: 17α-ethinyloestradiol (EE$_2$)

(Murad and Kuret 1991). Although E$_2$ is also used for pharmaceutical purposes, the extra oestrogen load due to the E$_2$ used therapeutically contributes less than 5% compared with the natural excretion (Christensen 1998).

Concentrations of E$_2$ and EE$_2$ have been reported in raw sewage, effluents of wastewater treatment plants and in surface water (Table 6.2). There is a broad range of concentrations recorded by different authors. This may be due to the different sampling locations and population densities, methodology, and conditions of sampling, such as time of the year and weather and analytical techniques. The different techniques utilised in the environmental detection of E$_2$ and EE$_2$ have different precision and sensitivities. In many cases, either E$_2$ or EE$_2$ or both of them are reported to be below the technical detection limits.

Since most of the oestrogens, either endogenous or pharmaceutical, are mainly excreted in conjugated forms, the presence of "free" oestrogen in the aquatic environment probably results from their deconjugation by bacteria in the environment (Desbrow et al. 1998; Tyler et al. 1998). This might be the case in wastewater treatment plants (Sattelberger et al. 1998; Ternes et al. 1999a). In that sense, Sattelberger et al. (1998) reported that the concentrations of EE$_2$ in the effluent were increased in relation to those of the influent in the wastewater treatment plant (WWTP) of Vienna, Austria. In the Netherlands, while E$_2$ and EE$_2$ were found in effluents and surface water, the hormone-glucuronides in the matching samples were not present in concentrations above the limits of detection (Belfroid et al. 1999). The same situation was reported in sewage effluent waters in Sweden by Larsson et al. (1999). Ternes et al. (1999b) confirmed the presence of glucuronidase activity in activated sludge, no lag phase was observed and the glucuronides were immediately cleaved. All these findings strongly suggest that the bacteria in the environment can render the inactive glucuronides into active hormones.

The exposure to environmental oestrogens might cause adverse health effects and both E$_2$ and EE$_2$, are classified as endocrine disrupters. According to one of the most complete definitions, proposed by Kavlock (1996) and adopted by the US Environmental Protection Agency (EPA) in 1997, an endocrine disrupter is "an exogenous agent that interferes with the synthesis, secretion, transport, binding, action, or elimination of natural hormones in the body that are responsible for the maintenance of homeo-

Table 6.2. Reported environmental concentrations of 17β-oestradiol (E$_2$) and 17α-ethinyloestradiol (EE$_2$)

Hormone	Concentration (ng l^{-1})	Type of sample, location	Reference
E$_2$	0–20	Raw sewage, USA	Tabak et al. (1981)
	48–148	Raw sewage, Israel	Shore et al. (1993): E$_1$+ E$_2$
	38–89	Influent, Austria	Sattelberger et al. (1998)
	0–20	Effluent, USA	Tabak et al. (1981)
	24–48	Effluent, Israel	Shore et al. (1993): E$_1$+ E$_2$
	max. 20	Effluent, Germany	Stumpf (1996)[a]
	1–10	Effluent, Germany	Kalbfus (1997)[c]
	3–48	Effluent, UK	Environment Agency (1997)[c]
	21–130	Effluent, Austria	Sattelberger et al. (1998)
	<0.6–12	Effluent, the Netherlands	Belfroid et al. (1999)
	1.1	Effluent, Sweden	Larsson et al. (1999)
	max. 64	Effluent, Canada	Ternes et al. (1999a)
	max. 3	Effluent, Germany	Ternes et al. (1999a)
	23–25	Lake water, Israel	Shore et al. (1993): E$_1$+ E$_2$
	<0.3–5.5	Surface water, the Netherlands	Belfroid et al. (1999)
EE$_2$	500–2 250	Raw sewage, USA	Tabak et al. (1981)
	4–13	Influent, Austria	Sattelberger et al. (1998)
	250–1 780	Effluent, USA	Tabak et al. (1981)
	0.3–0.5	Effluent, Germany	Kalbfus (1995)[b]
	max. 62	Effluent, Germany	Stumpf (1996)[a]
	0.2–7	Effluent, UK	Desbrow et al. (1998)
	14–22	Effluent, Austria	Sattelberger et al. (1998)
	<0.2–7.5	Effluent, the Netherlands	Belfroid et al. (1999)
	4.5	Effluent, Sweden	Larsson et al. (1999)
	max. 15	Effluent, Canada	Ternes et al. (1999a)
	max. 42	Effluent, Germany	Ternes et al. (1999a)
	<5 (n.d.)	River water, UK	Aherne et al. (1985)
	2–15	River water, UK	Aherne et al. (1989)[b]
	<5 (n.d.)	River water, Germany	Stumpf (1996)[a]
	<0.1–4.3	Surface water, the Netherlands	Belfroid et al. (1999)
	<5 (n.d.)	Potable supplies, UK	Aherne et al. (1985)

n.d.: non detectable, below detection limit.
[a] Data reviewed by Desbrow et al. (1998).
[b] Data reviewed by Halling-Sørensen et al. (1998).
[c] Data reviewed by Sattelberger et al. (1998).

stasis, reproduction, development, and/ or behaviour". Many scientific groups world-wide have stated the hypothesis that there might be an association, at least in part, between this increased exposure to oestrogens and the adverse trends in reproductive health, which has been observed during the last decades (Giwercman and Skakkebæk 1992; Carlsen et al. 1995; Colborn 1995; Patlak 1996; Van Waeleghem et al. 1996; Campbell and Hutchinson 1998). This is supported by evidences that exposure to high oestrogen concentrations during fetal development or childhood may lead to teratogenic or carcinogenic lesions in the reproductive system (Sharpe and Skakkebæk 1993). Furthermore, oestrogens are thought to be implicated in breast, ovarian and endometrium cancer, based on the facts that natural oestrogens promote cell prolif-eration and hypertrophy of female secondary organs (Soto et al. 1995). However, the human risk derived from the environmental uptake of EE_2 seems not to be significant according to Christensen (1998).

EE_2 has the potential to disrupt normal physiological functions not only in humans but also in wildlife. The sensitivity range of the different tested organisms towards the pharmaceutical oestrogens is broad. Besides, interspecies sensitivity, intraspecies sen-sitivity as well as the sensitivity variation during their life cycles have to be consid-ered. The experimental evidences raise concerns that due to the extreme potency of this synthetic oestrogen, it may be able to cause adverse biological effects, even at very low concentrations. Although the amounts of drugs found in the aquatic environment are several magnitudes lower compared to those applied in medicine (Ternes 1998), the potential adverse effects on aquatic organisms can not be neglected without care-ful studies. As a matter of fact, EE_2 is considered to be a potential hazard to fish and aquatic organisms, even in the range of 0.1–10 ng l^{-1} (Routledge et al. 1998; Larsson et al. 1999).

There is increasing evidence that actual treatments of sewage are not sufficient to eliminate E_2 and EE_2, at least to an extent in which their biological activity would be of no concern. Consequently, the amounts not eliminated in the sewage treatment enter the aquatic environment through sewage effluents. In this context, sewage treatment plants serve as important point sources, especially for surface water in densely popu-lated urban areas (Stan and Heberer 1997).

The general objective of this work was to increase the understanding of the pro-cesses related to environmental fate and degradation of EE_2 in comparison to the natu-ral E_2. Specifically, its purpose is to evaluate their biodegradation by three types of microbiological communities: mineral drinking water, surface water and activated sludge from a municipal wastewater treatment plant. This new information should contribute to obtaining better insight into the fate and behaviour of these micropol-lutants that are reported to be omnipresent in the environment and may constitute a risk.

6.2
Materials and Methods

6.2.1
Chemicals, Glass Material and Water

17β-oestradiol (E_2) and 17α-ethinyloestradiol (EE_2) were obtained from Sigma-Aldrich (Bornem, Belgium), minimum purity: 98% (HPLC tested). Glass material was used whenever possible to avoid adsorption. All glassware was rinsed with a solution of HNO_3 (minimum 65%, reagent p.a., VEL, Leuven, Belgium), 1/10 v/v, and with MilliQ water. Unless indicated, all media, dilutions and solutions were prepared in MilliQ water (Millipore, Molsheim, France).

6.2.2
Colony Counts

The spread plate technique was utilised to assess the colony counts (CFU ml^{-1}). A 0.1 ml-sample, in triplicate, was plated in pre-dried agar plates. All agar media as well as the physiological solution (NaCl 0.85% w/v), for the decimal dilutions, were prepared in MilliQ water and autoclaved for 20 min at 121 °C. All incubations were done at 28 ±2 °C. Bacto R2A Agar (Difco, Detroit, USA) was used for drinking mineral water and Nutrient Agar (Oxoid, Nepean, USA) was used for general counting in surface water and in activated sludge.

6.2.3
Analytical Methods

Biochemical Oxygen Demand (BOD). BOD-measurements were performed with the OxiTop$^{®}$-system, based on piezoresistive electronic pressure. As a source of biomass, activated sludge from the recycle tank of a domestic wastewater treatment plant (Ossemeersen, Gent, Belgium) was administered to a final concentration of 0.2 g suspended solids per litre. E_2 and EE_2 were dosed to a final concentration of 60 mg l^{-1}. The inorganic nutrients were supplemented according to ISO 9888 and the pH was adjusted to 7.4 at the beginning of the test. All samples were processed in duplicates. Samples were incubated in brown bottles at 20 °C, containing a chemical nitrification inhibitor (Nitrification Inhibitor Formula 2533, Hach Company, Loveland, USA) and pellets of NaOH were used to trap CO_2. Every 5 days, the bottles were opened to refresh air and the NaOH was changed.

Radioimmuno Assay (RIA). Two commercial radioimmuno assays (RIA) kits (Diagnostic System Laboratories, Houston, USA), were used to quantify 17β-oestradiol (DSL-3900) and 17α-ethinyloestradiol (DSL-9500). According to the specifications given by the producers, the cross-reactivity of oestradiol antiserum, was 6.90% for oestrone, 0.27% for 17β-oestradiol-3-glucuronide, <0.1% for oestrone-sulfate, <0.1% for oestrone-3-glucuronide and <0.1% for oestriol. The tracer consisted of ^{125}I labelled E_2 or EE_2 (<5 μCi) and radioactivity was measured in a gamma counter (127 gammamaster LKB Wallac, Turku, Finland) for 1 minute. Results were corrected by subtracting the non specific bound (NSB). Since the kits have been designed for serum samples, water samples were diluted 1:10 in serum containing no hormone (zero standard serum, Diagnostic System Laboratories, Houston, USA, DSL-39101 and DSL-9501 for E_2 and EE_2 respectively). The lowest E_2 standard has a concentration of 1.5 ng l^{-1} and 10 ng l^{-1} for EE_2. These were considered to be the detection limits. Therefore, detection limits for the water samples (diluted 1:10 in serum) were calculated as 15 ng l^{-1} and 100 ng l^{-1} for E_2 and EE_2, respectively. Activated sludge samples were centrifuged at 4 000 g for 15 min at 4 °C. E_2 and EE_2 concentrations were measured in the supernatant. Drinking and surface water samples were directly measured. Samples were stored in 2 ml-aliquots in RIA glass tubes (Vel, Leuven, Belgium) and stored at –70 °C until measurement. When needed, samples were diluted with MilliQ until they reached the desired concentration which fit within the standard curve range. Samples were measured in triplicates.

Yeast Screen (YES). Oestrogenic activity was determined by an assay based on a recombinant *Saccharomyces cerevisiae* containing the human oestrogen receptor (Glaxo Group Research Ltd., United Kingdom) as described by Routledge and Sumpter (1996). Methodological modifications were done in order to test aquatic samples according to Tanghe et al. (1999), where double strength medium was prepared and added 1:1 to the aquatic samples. The assay was carried out under sterile conditions in a 96-well optically flat bottom microtiter plate (Novolab, Geraardsbergen, Belgium). Values were corrected for the turbidity caused by the yeast growth according to the following formula proposed by Sohoni and Sumpter (1998):

$$\text{Corrected value} = \text{absorbance sample (540 nm)} - [\text{absorbance sample (630 nm)} - \text{absorbance blank (630 nm)}]$$

Samples and standards were measured four times.

6.2.4
Biodegradation Experiments: Biological Material and Experimental Design

Mineral Water. Chaudfontaine (Chaudfontaine, Belgium) mineral water was used as a source of oligotrophic microorganisms. The water contained about 90 large CFU ml^{-1} and more than 300 small CFU ml^{-1}. To obtain a final concentration of 1 µg l^{-1}, 10 ml of EE$_2$ and E$_2$ stock solutions with MilliQ were administered to the glass bottles (1 l). A treatment of E$_2$ or EE$_2$ plus glycine (1 mg l^{-1}) (Fluka, Bornem, Belgium) and controls of sterile mineral water (autoclaved for 20 min at 121 °C) was also included. Incubations were done in the dark at 28 ±2 °C for 48 days. Each treatment and control was performed in 3 different bottles.

Surface Water. Surface water was collected in May from a canal in Gent City (Coupure). Water temperature was 17 °C and pH 8.35. The water was thoroughly mixed, filtered through a 100 µm-pore clothe filter and immediately used. E$_2$ and EE$_2$ were administrated to 250 ml-Pyrex glass Erlenmeyer flasks by the addition of 100 µl of stock solutions prepared in acetone (Aldrich, Bornem, Belgium). After complete evaporation of the solvent, the flasks were filled with 100 ml of surface water, distilled water or sterile surface water (autoclaved for 20 min at 121 °C) for treatments and controls, respectively, to obtain final concentrations of 1, 10 or 100 µg l^{-1}. Incubations were done in the dark, at 28 ±2 °C or at 18 ±4 °C in rotary shakers operating at 125 rpm, for 33 days. Every treatment and control was performed in three different flasks.

6.2.5
Activated Sludge: Zahn-Wellens Test (ISO 9888)

The Zahn-Wellens test (ISO 9888) is a standardised batch static test that examines aerobic biodegradability of organic compounds, soluble under the conditions of the test. This test is equivalent to the OECD 302B test (Pagga 1997). Due to the low solubility of E_2 and EE_2, the compounds were weighted and directly added to obtain a theoretical final concentration of approximately 50 mg l^{-1} total organic carbon (TOC), corresponding to about 60 mg l^{-1} of E_2 or EE_2. This was done according to the ISO 10634 norm (Guidance for the preparation and treatment of poorly water-soluble compounds for the subsequent evaluation of their biodegradability in an aqueous medium). Ethylene glycol (Sigma, Bornem, Belgium), a known biodegradable compound under the test conditions, was used to assess the activity of the sludge. A solution was prepared according to the specifications of the norm to obtain a theoretical final concentration of 50 mg l^{-1} TOC. Activated sludge was obtained from the recycle tank of a domestic wastewater treatment plant (Ossemeersen, Gent, Belgium). The final concentration was 0.2 g l^{-1} suspended solids (10^9 CFU ml^{-1}) and the added volume of activated sludge was about 10% of the final volume. The flasks were incubated in the dark in a temperature-controlled room at 28 ±2 °C on a rotary shaker at about 130 rpm. The shaking ensured sufficient mixing of the activated sludge as well as adequate oxygen supply to maintain aerobic conditions. Each hormone was tested in three different flasks.

6.2.6
Toxicity Evaluation: Nitrox

Toxicity measurements with an enriched nitrifying culture were performed according to Gernaey et al. (1997). A fast dissolved oxygen electrode (EH-CONDUCTA 905-S) was used to monitor dissolved oxygen consumption caused by bacterial respiration, and allyl thiourea (ATU) was used as a selective nitrification inhibitor. To adapt the technique to non water-soluble compounds, 48 h incubations at 28 °C were done before measurements. Concentrations above 10 mg l^{-1} of E_2 or EE_2 were directly added. While for concentrations below 10 mg l^{-1} concentrated solutions were prepared in acetone and the solvent was completely evaporated before the addition of the nitrifying sludge, which was diluted 1:2 with 0.01 M phosphate buffer, 0.137 M NaCl, pH 7.4. NH_4^+ was added once a day, as NH_4Cl to obtain a final concentration of 1 mg N g^{-1} volatile suspended solids. Controls of nitrifying sludge under the same incubation conditions, with and without the addition and posterior evaporation of acetone were also included. The toxicity of the samples was calculated according to the formula, proposed by Gernaey et al. (1997).

6.2.7
Statistical Analyses

Statistics analyses were performed, whenever indicated, with Excel (Microsoft). Significantly different means were discriminated using a single-factor analysis of variance, ANOVA. Unless otherwise indicated, data are expressed as mean ±standard error ($X \pm SE$).

6.3
Results

Biodegradation of E_2 and EE_2 appear to be essential for environmental hygiene. To evaluate the persistence of E_2 and EE_2 in natural waters containing oligotrophic bacteria, the steroids were dosed to drinking mineral water bottles and incubated in the dark, at 28 °C. In a second treatment, glycine (gly) was supplemented ($1 \, mg \, l^{-1}$) in addition to E_2 or EE_2 as an extra source of carbon and nitrogen to evaluate whether the degradation of the hormones could be enhanced by the addition of a biodegradable carbon source at a higher concentration. The concentrations were monitored in time with radioimmuno assay (RIA) optimised to measure environmental water samples. The results of the RIA measurements of E_2 and EE_2 are presented in Table 6.3. After long incubation periods, such as 48 days, even if the concentrations showed a slight tendency to decline, both hormones were quite persistent in mineral water. This suggests that no significant biodegradation occurred under these conditions. Neither physicochemical degradation nor adsorption was observed, as shown in the controls that were autoclaved prior to the addition of the hormones. Neither the removal of E_2, nor that of EE_2, was apparently influenced by the addition of a readily degradable substrate, such as glycine. The biological removal of E_2 seems to occur in surface water when the hormone was artificially supplemented, as shown in Fig. 6.2. Yet after 33 days of incubation, the samples still showed oestrogenic activity, measured with the recombinant yeast screen (YES). However, the activity seemed to be significantly reduced with respect to the initial figures for both E_2 and EE_2. The decrease in oestrogenic activity was about 65% for the surface water supplemented with E_2 and about 56% for that supplemented with EE_2. After 33 days the final values of oestrogenic activity due to E_2 or EE_2 supplementation were not significantly different from one another. However, the shapes of the curves were quite different. The oestrogenic activity in the vessels supplemented with E_2 diminished as fast as after 2 days, and then seemed to reach a steady phase, in a second order decay. The curve of EE_2 presented a more defined lag phase. This lag phase seemed to extend approximately 15 days, after which the oestrogenic activity due to EE_2 supplementation decreased. The difference in the curve shapes may indicate that the microbial community present in this surface water exhibits different capacities to degrade E_2 and EE_2. The fast decline for E_2 is most likely not due to sorption since this effect was not observed for EE_2, which even has a higher sorption potential.

It has been shown that the concentration can influence the biodegradation rates in a significant way (Pfaender and Bartholomew 1982). Moreover, taking into account that the environmental concentrations of E_2 and EE_2 are so low, the estimation of micro-

Table 6.3. Measured concentrations of 17β-oestradiol (E_2) and 17α-ethinyloestradiol (EE_2) dosed at 1000 ng l^{-1} to drinking mineral water bottles and incubated for 0, 6 and 48 days, in the dark at 28 °C. Treatments included the addition of the hormones (E_2, EE_2), the hormone and glycine, at 1 mg l^{-1} (E_2 + gly, EE_2 + gly,) and controls of autoclaved mineral water (autoclaved + E_2, autoclaved + EE_2). Data are expressed as means $\pm SE$ ($n = 3$)

Time (d)	Concentration (ng l^{-1})					
	E_2	EE_2	E_2 + gly	EE_2 + gly	Autoclaved + E_2	Autoclaved + EE_2
0	272 ±22	158 ±11	310 ±40	155 ±12	315 ±35	148 ±20
6	212 ±13	166 ±16	282 ±34	135 ±19	320 ±30	130 ±18
48	206 ±13	110 ±15	240 ±39	187 ±18	240 ±39	153 ±19

biological thresholds towards them is a relevant issue. Different concentrations of E_2 were supplemented to surface water and the oestrogenic activity was measured and expressed in E_2 concentration by using a standard curve (Table 6.4). The profiles of

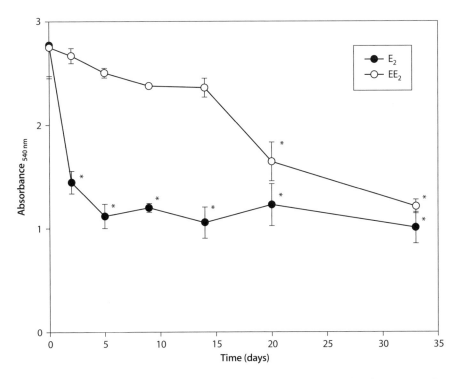

Fig. 6.2. Oestrogenic activity, measured by the recombinant yeast screen assay of surface water supplemented with 1 µg l^{-1} of 17β-oestradiol (E_2) or 17α-ethinyloestradiol (EE_2) over a period of 33 days. Values correspond to the mean $\pm SE$ ($n = 3$). * Significantly different from day 0 (ANOVA, $p < 0.05$)

Table 6.4. Biodegradation of 17β-oestradiol (E_2), supplemented at 1, 10, and 100 µg l^{-1}, by surface water. Incubation was done over 33 days in the dark at 28 °C. Oestrogenic activity was measured with the recombinant yeast screen assay and expressed as E_2 concentration. Data are expressed as means $\pm SE$ ($n = 3$). Values followed by the letter a, b, c are significantly different from the value of the correspondent concentration at day 0, 2 and 9 respectively, ANOVA ($p < 0.001$)

Time (d)	E_2 (µg l^{-1})		
	1	10	100
0	0.98 ±0.10	11.78 ±1.51	112.56 ±15.00
2	0.49 ±0.04	1.28 ±0.06[a]	5.28 ±0.20[a]
9	0.22 ±0.01[a]	0.78 ±0.06[a]	7.41 ±0.25[a]
20	0.18 ±0.01[a]	0.62 ±0.06[a]	0.83 ±0.16[a, b, c]
33	0.17 ±0.01[a]	0.16 ±0.02[a, b, c]	0.11 ±0.02[a, b, c]

the tested concentrations of E_2 present different slopes; the higher the concentration, the higher the decay of the oestrogenic activity. Indistinctly of the supplemented concentration, a decrease in the oestrogenic activity was observed. The results in Table 6.4 suggest that microorganisms naturally present in surface water are able to decrease E_2 concentration even at concentrations of 1 µg l^{-1} of E_2. The fact that the values after 33 days of incubation are not significantly different no matter what the initial concentration was indicates the possibility that at a certain level, the degradation ceases. Hence, the postulated lower biological threshold towards E_2 in surface water seems to be in the order of 0.1 µg l^{-1}.

The Zahn-Wellens test (ISO 9888) is a standardised batch test that examines aerobic biodegradability of organic compounds, as the only carbon source in a mineral medium inoculated with activated sludge from a municipal source. This test is equivalent to the OECD 302B test (Pagga 1997). The biological removal by activated sludge of E_2 at high concentration, in part dissolved and in part in suspension, was evident under the Zahn-Wellens method. This is shown by the decrease of the concentration in solution (Table 6.5) and the higher oxygen uptake compared to the controls (Fig. 6.3). The residual E_2-concentration in solution after 19 days of incubation amounted 1.3 mg l^{-1}, which is much higher than the residual 0.1 µg l^{-1} obtained in the surface water experiment. The higher E_2 dose (above solubility limit) resulting in a combination of several processes such as solubilisation, adsorption and degradation together with the shorter incubation time in the Zahn-Wellens test might be responsible for the difference in residual concentration compared to the surface water experiment. After pre-exposure of the activated sludge to E_2, the plateau of the oxygen uptake curve was reached more quickly, indicating that the adaptation of microbiology to the hormone increased its degradation. Moreover, the natural E_2 was much more efficient than the synthetic EE_2 to support bacterial growth (data not shown). No physicochemical removal of E_2 was observed since no elimination of E_2 was noted in the control where no biomass was added.

According to the ISO 9888, an adsorption to the sludge less than 20% can be considered as "low". E_2 and, especially, EE_2 were strongly adsorbed on the sludge. The maximum adsorption of E_2 to the sludge was estimated to be about 28% and that of EE_2 was about 68% after 3 hours of incubation. These figures were calculated from the ratio between the concentrations of the hormones with and without sludge, measured by RIA (Table 6.5, e.g. $(4.7 - 3.4) / 4.7 \times 100 = 28\%$), and assuming that the differences in concentration were completely due to adsorption, i.e. no degradation. The solubil-

Table 6.5. Concentration of 17β-oestradiol (E_2) and 17α-ethinyloestradiol (EE_2) in solution, measured by radioimmuno assay (RIA), in the ISO 9888/Zahn-Wellens test after 0, 11 and 19 days of incubation. Controls of E_2 and EE_2 without activated sludge are also shown. Data are expressed as means ±SE ($n = 3$)

Time (d)	Concentration (mg l^{-1})		Control E_2 (no sludge)	Control EE_2 (no sludge)
	E_2	EE_2		
0 (3h)	3.4 ±0.5	1.1 ±0.2	4.7 ±0.5	3.5 ±0.4
11	1.4 ±0.2	1.2 ±0.2	4.1 ±0.5	3.2 ±0.6
19	1.3 ±0.2	1.5 ±0.3	5.2 ±0.8	3.4 ±0.3

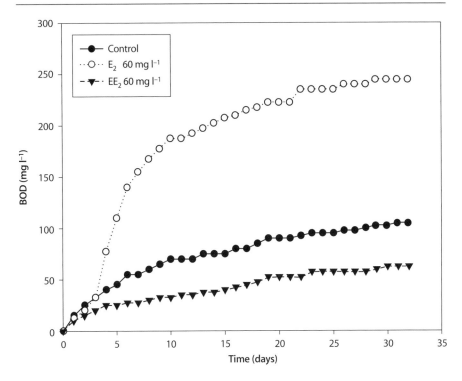

Fig. 6.3. Biochemical oxygen demand (BOD) of activated sludge (control) and activated sludge supplemented with 60 mg l^{-1} of 17β-oestradiol (E$_2$) or 17α-ethinyloestradiol (EE$_2$) in the ISO 9888/Zahn-Wellens test conditions over 32 days, at 20 °C. The values represent the average of duplicates

ity limit for E$_2$ is 12 mg l^{-1} (Table 6.1), which is far below the spiked concentration. Yet, only 3.4 mg l^{-1} E$_2$ was measured after 3 h in the soluble phase. Several processes such as solubilisation and adsorption may create a sensitive equilibrium below the solubility limit.

In the case of EE$_2$, no biological removal leading to its decrease in solution occurred under the Zahn-Wellens test conditions (Table 6.5). Furthermore, under the same conditions, the oxygen uptake curve of the activated sludge supplemented with 60 mg l^{-1} EE$_2$ was below that of the control (Fig. 6.3). These results suggest that under these conditions and supplemented at these high concentrations, EE$_2$ might be toxic for the activated sludge. To evaluate the possible toxicity of EE$_2$, a test involving nitrifying inhibition was carried out. Nitrifiers play a fundamental role in wastewater treatment plants, oxidising NH$_4^+$ into NO$_2^-$ and the latter into NO$_3^-$, and they are known to be a sensitive group of microorganisms towards toxicants. Different concentrations of EE$_2$ were incubated with nitrifying sludge, and after 48 hours the respiration was measured, and the inhibition was calculated. When 60 mg l^{-1} EE$_2$ were tested, a significant inhibition in nitrifying oxygen uptake was observed (Fig. 6.4). Moreover, the toxic effect of EE$_2$ seemed to be dose dependent for concentrations above 10 mg l^{-1}. On the contrary, the oxygen uptake of the nitrifying sludge was not decreased by E$_2$, even when it was supplemented at 60 mg l^{-1}. The effect of EE$_2$ on the nitrifying sludge activity was

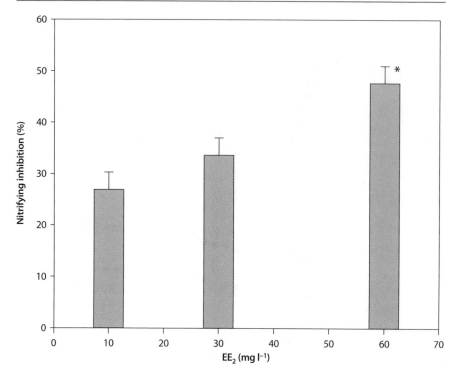

Fig. 6.4. Inhibition of nitrifying sludge oxygen uptake incubated, in the dark 48 hours at 28 °C, with different concentrations of EE_2. Values correspond to the mean $\pm SE$ ($n = 3$). * Significantly different from the control with no EE_2 supplementation (ANOVA, $p < 0.05$)

also tested in concentrations of 1 mg l^{-1}, 10 μg l^{-1} and the more environmentally relevant 1 μg l^{-1}. No differences in oxygen uptake with respect to those of the controls were observed, suggesting that under these conditions, concentrations below 10 mg l^{-1} are not significantly inhibitory for the nitrifying sludge.

6.4
Discussion

The results presented in this work show that two different assays are compatible and have high sensitivity to measure E_2 and EE_2; both the RIA and the YES can be used as useful tools to measure these micropollutants in environmental waters.

No biodegradation of E_2 or EE_2 (Table 6.3) occurred in natural mineral drinking water, even after long incubation periods. This fact indicates that the microbiological community naturally present, although expected to be adapted to grow on very low organic carbon concentrations, was not able to cope with these substrates. Therefore, if an eventual contamination of drinking water by E_2 or EE_2 occurred, the steroids can be expected to be persistent under these conditions. It has to be pointed out that up to now, both the reported environmental concentrations in drinking water (Aherne et al. 1985) as well as the predicted environmental ones (Christensen 1998), are in the range of below detection limit to 1.2 ng l^{-1}. Since the steroids were persistent at higher concentrations, the removal of these low levels in drinking water appears quite unlikely.

In surface water, the curve of the oestrogenic activity due to EE_2 supplementation over time presented a more defined lag phase compared to that of the natural E_2 (Fig. 6.2). Initial lag phases are believed to occur when bacteria are introduced in a closed medium where the cells must adapt their enzymatic set to that which is the most appropriate to their environment at that moment (Masschelein 1992). The absence of a lag phase in the E_2 curve might suggest that the microbiology present in the surface water was already adapted to E_2 or could more easily cope with it. The difference in the shapes of the curves may indicate that the microbial community present in this surface water exhibits different capacities to degrade E_2 or EE_2. In that sense, the ratio between EE_2 and E_2 in surface water is higher than the theoretical ratio based on human secretion rates of natural and synthetic oestrogens, indicating a faster degradation of the natural oestrogen (Larsson et al. 1999) not only in wastewater treatment plants but also in surface waters. Moreover, the fact that some oestrogenic activity is still present after 33 days of incubation suggest that the removal of E_2 and EE_2, or that of their oestrogenic metabolites, is not complete under these conditions. Since the laboratory conditions were not very different from those of the environment (neither other compounds nor microbiology was added), this might also be the case under environmental circumstances.

Because many bacteria can readily grow even on the traces of dissolved organic carbon (DOC) present in distilled water, the existence of lower threshold concentrations is very difficult to be demonstrated (Schmidt and Alexander 1985). The lower microbiological threshold towards E_2 appears to be established in the order of 0.1 μg l^{-1} for surface water.

An important adsorption on to the sludge, of E_2 and EE_2, was observed in the Zahn-Wellens test. The maximum adsorption of E_2 on the sludge was estimated to be 28% whereas that of EE_2 was even higher, 68% (Table 6.5). The log octanol/water partition coefficients are quite high for these hormones (Table 6.1). Tabak and Bunch (1970) discussed the evidence of initial adsorption of E_2 and EE_2 on the sludge mass in their experiments, but did not provide any figures. This high sorption potential on the sludge may probably contribute to the removal of these hormones in wastewater treatment plants. If that is the case, the use of sludge as fertiliser may cause the potential contamination of soils and groundwater (Ternes et al. 1999a). Moreover, this has to be considered for experimental planning and evaluation and also as a main factor in modelling the fate of the hormones in the environment. Currently, it is very difficult to obtain physicochemical data and standardised biodegradation tests suitable for poorly water-soluble compounds with important adsorption to the sludge. Therefore, many assumptions and extrapolations have to be made in order to model the fate of E_2 and EE_2; it becomes difficult to calculate the predicted environmental concentrations (PEC). Especially due to the relevance of modelling in the decision-making processes leading to norms and regulations, these are important issues and require further investigations.

Because these steroids present high sorption potentials, concentrations in the surface water are estimated to be rather minor compared to those in riverbed sediments, which might act as sinks for E_2 and EE_2. Since anaerobic conditions usually prevail there, the study of the anaerobic breakdown seems to be important, especially in the context of long term accumulations. Furthermore, much of the sediment dwelling fauna may become exposed to high levels of oestrogens. Thus, it is important to include these groups of species in toxicological studies.

Taken as a whole, the results of the measurement of the concentrations in solution (Table 6.3), the oxygen uptake (Fig. 6.3) and the support of cell growth indicate that the removal of E_2 by activated sludge at high concentrations is evident. Microbiology in activated sludge is able to degrade E_2; the identity of the specific microorganisms involved in its removal still needs to be known. Working with lower concentrations of E_2 but with approximately the same sludge concentration, 0.26 g l^{-1} suspended solids compared to 0.2 g l^{-1} of the ISO 9888, Ternes et al. (1999b) reported that after a period of 1–3 hours, more than 95% of the spiked concentration of E_2 (both at 1 µg l^{-1} or at 1 mg l^{-1}) had vanished in their experiments. They concluded that almost all the added E_2 had been quantitatively oxidised to oestrone (E_1), which was then eliminated in an approximated time linear dependent way, with no observed further degradation products.

Physicochemical degradation of E_2 does not seem to occur in natural mineral drinking water, surface water or in activated sludge experiments. Except for photolytic effects that were not included in the experiments, biodegradation appears to be the main route of degradation of E_2 in surface water and in activated sludge.

The microbial removal of EE_2 is not so evident (Table 6.5, Fig. 6.2 and 6.3). Our data corroborate other indications from the literature, which also pointed out that the synthetic oestrogen exhibits greater overall resistance to microbial degradation than the natural E_2. (Tabak et al. 1981; Ternes et al. 1999a,b). The high EE_2/E_2 ratio in the environment compared to that of the excretions also supports that finding. Therefore, environmental aspects of EE_2 need to be rigorously addressed, in particular those related to the stimulation of its biodegradation/remediation in the environment.

Toxicity of EE_2 regarding activated sludge does not seem to be of direct concern, since only high concentrations of the steroid exhibited these effects in nitrifying sludge. Yet it is still remarkable that EE_2 triggers effects at mg l^{-1} levels to these quite essential microbial species.

Considering the fact that the reproductive system in the majority of species remains largely uncharacterised, it is very difficult to evaluate the effect that these low environmental concentrations of E_2 or EE_2 may cause, and it is even more difficult to assess a no observed effect concentration (NOEC).

The overall fate and destination of E_2 and EE_2 are summarised in Fig. 6.5. The fact that sewage treatment plants might act as point sources of non-easily biodegradable hormones and pharmaceuticals in fresh water, among them contraceptives, requires additional study. Methods to further remove these compounds at the treatment plants and to monitor their removal efficiency is needed. The search for more "environmentally compatible" pharmaceuticals is another important field of investigation in which a multidisciplinary approach is required.

Acknowledgements

We thank Dr. Tom Tanghe for his valuable suggestions and critical comments during this work. We also thank Professor J. M. Kaufman and L. Verdonck for their kind advice with the RIA.

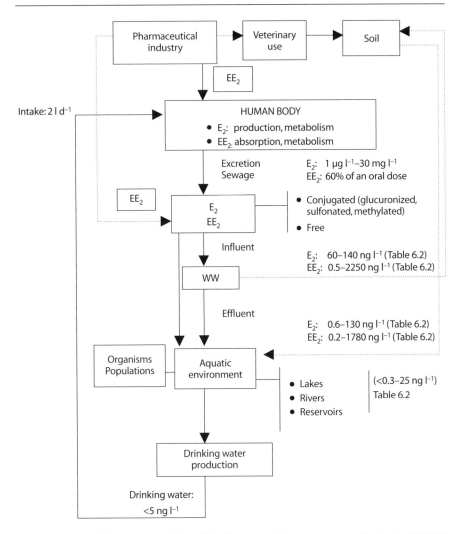

Fig. 6.5. Scheme of the environmental fate of the pharmaceutical oestrogen: 17α-ethinyloestradiol (EE$_2$) and the natural oestrogen: 17β-oestradiol (E$_2$)

References

Aherne GW, English J, Marks V (1985) The role of immunoassay in the analysis of microcontaminants in water samples. Ecotoxicology and Environmental Safety 9:79–83

Belfroid AC, Van der Horst A, Vethaak AD, Schäfer AJ, Rijs GBJ, Wegener J, Cofino WP (1999) Analysis and occurrence of estrogenic hormones and their glucuronides in surface water and waste water in The Netherlands. Sci Total Environ 225:101–108

Campbell PM, Hutchinson TH (1998) Wildlife and endocrine disrupters: requirements for hazard identification. Annual Review. Environmental Toxicology and Chemistry 17:127–135

Carlsen E, Giwercman A, Keiding N, Skakkebæk NE (1995) Declining semen quality and increasing incidence of testicular cancer: is there a common cause? Environmental Health Perspectives 103:137–139

Carr BR, Griffin JE (1998) Fertility controls and its complications. In: Wilson JD, Foster DW, Kronenberg HM, Reed LP (eds) Williams Textbook of Endocrinology. W.B. Saunders Company, Philadelphia, pp 901–925

Christensen FM (1998) Pharmaceuticals in the environment: a human risk. Regulatory Toxicology and Pharmacology 28:212–221

Colborn T (1995) Environmental Estrogens: health implications for human and wildlife. Environmental Health Perspectives 103:135–136

Desbrow C, Routledge EJ, Brighty GC, Sumpter JP, Waldock M (1998) Identification of estrogenic chemicals in STW effluent. 1. Chemical fractionation and in vitro biological screening. Environmental Science and Technology 32:1549–1558

Fieser LF, Fieser M (1959) Estrogens. In: Steroids. Reynold Publishing Corporation, New York, pp 444–502

Gernaey K, Verschuere L, Luyten L, Verstraete W (1997) Fast and sensitive acute toxicity detection with an enrichment nitrifying culture. Water Environmental Research 69:1163–1169

Giwercman A, Skakkebæk NE (1992) The human testis – an organ at risk? International Journal of Andrology 15:373–375

Halling-Sørensen B, Nors Nielsen S, Lanzky PF, Ingerslev F, Holten Lützhøft HC, Jørgensen SE (1998) Occurrence, fate and effects of pharmaceutical substances in the environment– A Review. Chemosphere 36:357–393

ISO (1995) Water quality – Guidance for the preparation and treatment of poorly water soluble compounds for the subsequent evaluation of their biodegradability in an aqueous medium (ISO 10634)

ISO (1997) Water quality – Evaluation of aerobic biodegradability of organic compounds in aqueous medium – Static test (Zahn-Wellens method, ISO 9888)

Kavlock RJ (1996) Research needs for risk assessment of health and environmental effects of endocrine disrupters: A review of the U.S. EPA-sponsored workshop. Environmental Health Perspectives 4:715–740

Larsson DGJ, Adolfsson-Erici M, Parkkonen J, Pettersson M, Berg AH, Olsson PE, Förlin L (1999) Ethinyloestradiol – an undesired fish contraceptive? Aquatic Toxicology 45:91–92

Masschelein WJ (1992) Unit processes in drinking water treatment. Marcel Dekker Inc., New York, pp 365–395

Murad F, Kuret JA (1991) Estrógenos y Progestágenos. In: Goodman Gilman A, Rall TW, Nies AS, Taylor P (eds) Goodman and Gilman's. The pharmacological basis of therapeutic (in Spanish). Editorial Medica Panamericana, Buenos Aires, pp 1340–1366

Pagga U (1997) Standardised tests on biodegradability. In: SETAC Europe (ed) Biodegradation kinetics: generation and use data for regulatory decision making. SETAC Europe, Brussels, pp 69–80

Patlak M (1996) A testing deadline for endocrine disrupters. Environmental Science and Technology 30:540A-544A

Pfaender FK, Bartholomew GW (1982) Measurements of aquatic biodegradation rates by determining heterotrophic uptake by radiolabelled pollutants. Applied and Environmental Microbiology 44:159–164

Routledge EJ, Sumpter JP (1996) Estrogenic activity of surfactants and some of their degradation products assessed using a recombinant yeast screen. Environmental Toxicology and Chemistry 15:241–248

Routledge EJ, Sheahan D, Desbrow C, Brighty GC, Waldock M, Sumpter JP (1998) Identification of estrogenic chemicals in STW effluent: 2. In vivo responses in trout and roach. Environmental Science and Technology 32:1559–1565

Sattelberger R, Hartler W, Lorbeer G, Scharf S (1998) Steroidhormone in der aquatischen Umwelt – Erste Untersuchungsergebnisse aus Österreich. In: Kroiß H (ed) Hormonell aktive Substanzen in der Umwelt. Riegelnik, Wien (Wiener Mitteilungen 153, pp 59–70)

Schmidt SK, Alexander M (1985) Effects of dissolved organic carbon and second substrates on the biodegradation of organic compounds at low concentrations. Appl Environ Microbiol 49:822–827

Sharpe RM, Skakkebæk NE (1993) Are oestrogens involved in falling sperm, counts and disorders of the male reproductive tract? Lancet 341:1392–1395

Shore LS, gurevitz M, Shemesh M (1993) Estrogen as an environmental pollutant. Bulletin of Environmental Contamination and Toxicology 51:361–366

Sohoni P, Sumpter JP (1998) Several environmental oestrogens are also anti-androgens. Journal of Endocrinology 158:327–339

Soto AM, Sonnenschein C, Chung KL, Fernandez MF, Olea N, Olea Serrano F (1995) The E-SCREEN assay as a tool to identify estrogens: an update on estrogenic environmental pollutants. Environmental Health Perspectives 103:113–122

Stan HJ, Heberer T (1997) Pharmaceuticals in the aquatic environment. Analysis Magazine 25:M20–M23

Tabak HH, Bunch RL (1970) Steroid hormones as water pollutants I: Metabolism of natural and synthetic ovulation inhibiting hormones by microorganisms of activated sludge and primary settled sewage. Developments in Industrial Microbiology 11:367–376

Tabak HH, Bloomhuff RN, Bunch RL (1981) Steroid hormones as water pollutants II: Studies on the persistence and stability of natural urinary and synthetic ovulation inhibiting hormones in untreated and treated waste-waters. Developments in Industrial Microbiology 22:497–519

Tanghe T, Devriese G, Verstraete W (1999) Nonylphenol and estrogenic activity in aquatic environmental samples. Journal of Environmental Quality 28:702–709

Ternes TA (1998) Occurrence of drugs in German sewage treatment plants and rivers. Wat Res 0:1–6

Ternes TA, Stumpf M, Mueller J, Haberer K, Wilken RD, Servos M (1999a) Behaviour and occurrence of estrogens in municipal sewage treatment plants. I. Investigations in Germany, Canada and Brazil. Science of the Total Environment 225:80–91

Ternes TA, Kreckel P, Mueller J (1999b) Behaviour and occurrence of estrogens in municipal sewage treatment plants – II. Aerobic batch experiments with activated sludge. Sci Tot Environ 225:91–99

Tyler C, Jobling RS, Sumpter JP (1998) Endocrine disrupting in wildlife: a critical review of the evidence. Critical Reviews in Toxicology 28:319–361

Waeleghem K Van, Clercq N De, Vermeulen L, Schoonjans F, Comhaire FH (1996) Deterioration of sperm quality in young healthy Belgian men. Human Reproduction 11:325–329

Williams RJ, Jürgens MD, Johnson AC (1999) Initial predictions of the concentrations and distribution of 17β-oestradiol, oestrone and ethinyl oestradiol in 3 English rivers. Wat Res 33:1663–1667

Chapter 7

What Do We Know about Antibiotics in the Environment?

T. Kümpel · R. Alexy · K. Kümmerer

7.1
Introduction

Antibiotics are extensively used in human and veterinary medicine as well as in aquaculture to prevent or to treat microbial infections and in livestock production to promote the growth of animals. As biocidal substances are designed with the aim of causing a biological effect, they may affect water and soil dwelling organisms when reaching the environment. However, little is known on the occurrence and fate of antibiotics in the environment and their impact on the ecosystem.

An intensive literature search was performed in order to obtain information on antimicrobials with regard to their ecotoxicity. The literature investigation was performed with the help of several medicinal, chemical, agricultural and environmental databases. "Antibiotics" was combined with keywords such as adsorption, soil, sludge, sediment, biodegradation, photodegradation, fate, surface water, groundwater, sewage, and environment.

7.2
Emission and Occurrence of Antibiotics in the Environment

Antibiotics are applied in human medicine in large quantities for the treatment of diseases. After administration, these substances or their metabolites are excreted into wastewater and reach the sewage treatment plant (STP). If they are not eliminated during the purification process they pass the sewage system and may end up in the environment, mainly in the water compartment.

Antibacterial substances applied in the veterinary field are exposed to the environment when manure is spread on fields. These antibiotics may end up in soil or sediment, if not degraded, or in groundwater due to runoff from soils.

For the treatment and prevention of infections in intensive fish farming antimicrobial agents are distributed directly to the water resulting in high local concentrations in the water compartment and the adjoining sediments.

Although antibiotics were applied in large quantities over a period of some decades, the existence of these substances in the environment received very little attention until recently. Only a few investigations reported findings of antimicrobial substances in different environmental compartments as detailed in the following sections.

7.2.1
Wastewater, Surface Water and Groundwater

A few commonly used antibiotics were detected in wastewaters of pharmaceutical producing sites or hospitals in high concentrations, sufficiently potent to cause adverse effects on wastewater bacteria (Qiting and Xiheng 1998; Hartmann et al. 1998, 1999; Wiethan et al. 1999). Loads of antibacterials in communal wastewater are lower, as the highly polluted wastewater of hospitals is mixed with wastewater containing lower amounts. However, some of the extensively applied antibiotics were also detected in communal wastewater (Hirsch et al. 1999).

The detection of antibacterial agents in surface water has to be considered as problematic, indicating that little or no degradation of the substances found took place during sewage purification. A variety of antibiotics were already detected in different studies in surface water in concentrations up to 1 µg l^{-1} (Richardson and Bowron 1985; Hirsch et al. 1999; Ternes 1998; Watts et al. 1983; Pearson and Inglis 1993).

Findings of antibiotics in groundwater are rare. Local emissions from fields fertilised with animal slurry might be a source of antibiotics in groundwater due to runoff from soil. However, the load of antibacterial agents in groundwater in rural areas with high concentrations of livestock proved to be small in an investigation performed by Hirsch et al. (1999). Antimicrobial residues were found in 2 groundwater samples out of 59 tested. Nevertheless, local emission of antibiotics may result in high concentrations even in groundwater, as demonstrated for groundwater downgradient of a landfill originating from a pharmaceutical production site (Holm et al. 1995).

7.2.2
Soil and Sediment

Residues of two antibiotics extensively used in livestock production were recently detected in soil fertilised with animal slurry, in concentrations which would demand further extensive ecotoxicological investigations for new pharmaceuticals according to the guideline EMEA/CVMP/055/96 (Hamscher et al. 2000).

High loads of antibiotics in sediments in concentrations potent enough to inhibit the growth of bacteria were reported for aquaculture. The fact that the exposure is of high local concentration has to be considered as critical. The substances used in fish farming can enter the sediments directly from the water without undergoing any kind of purification process. Some investigations demonstrated the presence of antibiotics extensively applied in fish farming in sediments beneath fish farms (Jacobsen and Berglind 1988; Coyne et al. 1994; Migliore et al. 1995).

7.3
Fate of Antibiotics in the Environment

As severe impacts on aquatic and terrestrial ecosystems caused by antimicrobials in the environment cannot be excluded, their elimination is of predominant importance.

Substances reaching the environment may undergo different reactions resulting in partial or complete elimination of the parent compound. Based on the degradation behaviour, biocides can be divided into the following groups:

- antibiotics and metabolites that are mineralised by microorganisms and therefore completely eliminated,
- antibiotics that are partly degraded and
- antibiotics that persist in the environment.

Elimination processes can be of biotic or abiotic nature. Biological degradation plays a key role in the environment, but also elimination due to photochemical or hydrolytical reactions takes place.

7.3.1
Biodegradation

Degradation studies of several antibacterials are demonstrated in literature. While some antibiotics used in human treatment seem to be well degradable in communal sewage treatment plants, others are poorly degradable or not degradable at all and therefore persist in the environment with the potential to affect the ecosystem (Ternes 1998; Richardson and Bowron 1985).

Microbial degradation in surface water is slower than in the sewage system due to a lower density of bacteria. Most antibiotics investigated so far proved to be stable in a test simulating surface water (Al-Ahmad et al. 1999; Kümmerer et al. 2000; Cerovec 2000; Wiethan et al. 1999).

Antibiotics occurring in soil and sediment proved to be quite persistent in laboratory testing and field studies. Substances extensively applied in fish farming had long half-lives in soil and sediment, as reported in several investigations (Marengo et al. 1997; Samuelsen et al. 1992, 1994; Hansen et al. 1992; Hektoen et al. 1995; Jacobsen and Berglind 1988; Capone et al. 1996). However, some substances were at least partly degradable (Gilbertson et al. 1990; Samuelsen et al. 1994, 1991; Donoho 1984; Capone et al. 1996).

7.3.2
Photodegradation and Hydrolysis

Although microorganisms play a key role in the degradation process in the environment, the disappearance of substances is not solely the result of biological activity of water or soil dwelling organisms. If a substance is sensitive towards light, photodecomposition may be of major significance in the elimination process, as reported in literature (Lunestad et al. 1995). Photodecomposition takes place mainly in surface water, since soil and sediment prevent a substance from undergoing photochemical degradation due to the lack of light in these matrices. Samuelsen (1989), for example, investigated the persistence of a substance sensitive towards light in sea water as well as in sediments. The antibacterial substance proved to be stable in sediments rather than in sea water. As no mechanism of decomposition is known for this antimicrobial except photodegradation (Oka et al. 1989) the substance remains in the sediment for a long period, as proved by Lunestad and Goksøyr (1990).

Another kind of abiotic elimination of substances is hydrolysis. Instability in water was demonstrated for some antibiotics (Halling-Sørensen 2000).

It has to be noted that the results of bio- or photodegradability studies depend on conditions, e.g. temperatures, composition of matrix etc., as demonstrated in the following examples: Gavalchin and Katz (1994) studied the degradability of 7 faecal-borne antibiotics in soil and showed the disappearance of 5 antibiotics after incubation at 30 °C, while only 2 antibacterials were eliminated when the samples were incubated at 4 °C.

The influence of the soil composition on elimination and half-life was demonstrated by Weerasinghe and Towner (1997), studying the aerobic biodegradability of an anti-microbial agent in different soils under laboratory conditions. The substance was found to degrade in each type of soil but half-lives varied within a range from 87 to 173 days.

Pouliquen et al. (1992) studied the elimination of an antibiotic in sea water. The half-lives of the substance under investigation varied due to differences in temperature, light intensity and flow rate from one test tank to another.

Substances that are readily biodegradable in one environment might be long-lived in another because of environmental factors (Alexander 1981).

7.3.3
Complex Formation and Adsorption

The disappearance of a substance during the test period does not indicate biological or photochemical degradation in each case. The tendency to bind to soil particles or the formation of complexes with ions present in several matrices is known for some antibiotics (Marengo et al. 1997; Plate 1991; Hektoen et al. 1995; Rabølle and Spliid 2000). Binding to particles or complex formation may cause a loss in detectability as well as a loss in antibacterial activity. The loss of antibacterial activity, for example, was proved for an aquaculture antimicrobial in sea water driven by the formation of complexes with magnesium and calcium present in marine water (Lunestad and Goksøyr 1990). This finding is interesting not solely from the degradation point of view, but also un-derlines the problematic nature of applying such potentially inactive antibiotics in aquaculture, especially in marine fish farming, as it clearly shows the necessity of us-ing considerably more antibiotics for treating fish in marine water.

7.4
Effects on the Environment

If a substance is not eliminated in any way it can reach the environment with the po-tential to adversely affect the aquatic and terrestrial organisms. Bacteria, fungi and micro algae are the organisms primarily affected, as these substances are solely designed with the intention of exerting an effect on microorganisms. In general, ef-fects of antibacterial agents on bacteria and micro algae are found to be 2 to 3 orders of magnitude below the toxic values for higher trophic levels (Wollenberger et al. 2000).

Since experimental parameters influence the results of a toxicity investigation some-times by orders of magnitude (Koller et al. 2000), the exact conditions of testing (e.g. temperature, pH value, time scale etc.) have to be stated in order to be capable of estimating the impacts on the environment. Therefore, the effects outlined below should just give an idea what may happen if an antibacterial is present in the environ-ment.

7.4.1
Wastewater and Sewage System

Antibiotics have the potential to affect the microbial community in sewage systems. The inhibition of wastewater bacteria may seriously affect organic matter degradation, therefore the effects of antibacterial agents on the microbial population are of great interest.

A reduction in the number of bacteria together with alterations of microbial populations were observed in a model sewage purification system when different commonly applied antibiotics were added in concentrations that may occur in hospital wastewater (Stanislawska 1979). These findings are in accordance with results of Kümmerer et al. (2000) and Al-Ahmad et al. (1999). As inhibitory concentrations in laboratory testing for a variety of antibiotics were found to be in the same order of magnitude as concentrations expected for hospital wastewater, effects on microbial populations of sewage systems could not be excluded for these substances.

Nitrification is an important step in wastewater purification, eliminating toxic ammonia. Several antibiotics proved to have low toxicity in relation to nitrifying bacteria in acute tests. These substances showed no effects upon nitrification in concentrations even higher than the environmentally expected concentrations (Tomlinson et al. 1966; Gomez et al. 1996). However, the time scale significantly influences the results. An antimicrobial was found to require high concentrations to inhibit the nitrification process in a short term test (2 to 4 hours) but a prolonged test period over 5 days showed effects one order of magnitude below the inhibitory concentrations of the acute test (Tomlinson et al. 1966).

A development of antibiotic resistance and selective effects on bacterial communities due to the permanent exposure to antibacterials in sewage systems are not yet proved (Wiethan et al. 2000). However, this topic needs further consideration and investigation. The problem of resistance development will not be discussed here further as it was not primarily focused on in the study.

7.4.2
Surface Water

Substances which are not or only partly degradable in the sewage treatment plant will reach surface water and affect organisms of different trophic levels. Toxicity tests with bacteria showed that chronic exposure to antibiotics is critical rather than acute exposure. Thomulka and McGee (1993) determined the toxicity of different antibiotics in relation to *Vibrio harveyi* in two bioassay methods. Almost no toxic effects were reported after short incubation times when luminescence was used as an endpoint. But in a long term assay using reproduction as an endpoint, a toxic effect could be detected for almost all substances, in environmentally relevant concentrations. These results are in accordance with the observations of Froehner et al. (2000). Comparing the results of short and long term bioassays with *Vibrio fischeri* demonstrated the risk of underestimating the severe effects of substances with delayed toxicity in acute tests. Similar findings concerning toxicity values were reported by Backhaus and Grimme (1999). In a long term bioluminescence inhibition test with *Vibrio fischeri*, effect values (EC_{10}) for two antibiotics were found in the range of concentrations expected in the environment.

Nitrifying bacteria in a model aquatic system with synthetic fresh water were significantly affected by an aquaculture antibiotic. The disruption of the nitrification process already occurred in concentrations likely to be found in fish treatment tanks and sediments (Klaver and Matthews 1994).

The results of the toxicity tests with bacteria indicate that direct toxic effects on natural bacterial communities can not be excluded, possibly with adverse influences on organic matter degradation.

Sensitivity of algae towards antibiotics varied widely. In an algal toxicity test *Selenastrum capricornutum* was found to be two to three orders of magnitude less sensitive against most antibiotics than micro algae *Microcystis aeruginosa*. Growth of *Microcystis aeruginosa* was inhibited in concentrations of less than 0.1 mg l^{-1} (Halling-Sørensen 2000). Similar observations were documented by Holten Lützhøft et al. (1999). The potential ecotoxicological effect of an antibacterial substance on *Chlorella* spp. and *Selenastrum capricornutum* in an acute toxicity test was outlined by Lanzky and Halling-Sørensen (1997). The results indicated that potential adverse effects of antibiotics on algae could not be excluded. As algae are the basis of the food chain, even slight decreases in the algal population may affect the balance in an aquatic system.

Organisms of higher trophic levels such as crustaceae are less likely to be seriously affected by antimicrobials since they are non-target organisms. Adverse impacts on these organisms are reported, but in most cases in environmentally irrelevant concentrations. Effect concentrations are often within a range from 10 to 100 mg l^{-1} or even more, as summarised by Holten Lützhøft et al. (1999). However, secondary effects due to changes in the natural balance are not negligible.

Reproductive effects and adverse impacts on early life stages of different organisms might be caused by the existence of antibiotics in the environment, which may result in dramatic effects on the population. A significantly depressed hatching rate of cysts of *Artemia* spp. and a high mortality of nauplii as well as toxic effects on reproduction of *Daphnia magna* demonstrated the serious impacts of antibiotics on these organisms (Migliore et al. 1993, 1997; Brambilla et al. 1994; Wollenberger et al. 2000). The potential of altering the pigmentation of *Artemia salina* nauplii resulting in a lower fitness of the individuals was proved for an antibiotic, underlining the toxic potential of antimicrobial agents (Brambilla et al. 1994). LC_{50} values below 100 mg l^{-1} for an antibacterial agent indicated a significant toxicity on *Culex pipiens molestus* larvae and *Daphnia magna* (Marcì et al. 1988). Based on the results, the authors outlined the possibility of considerable damage to the natural equilibrium, since the organisms under investigation constitute the nourishment of other aquatic animals, and therefore their disappearance affects other organisms as well.

Besides the impacts on the populations outlined above, the behaviour of aquatic organisms can also be affected. Phototaxis of *Daphnia magna*, for instance, was proved to be influenced by antibiotics (Dojmi di Delupis et al. 1992; Brambilla et al. 1994).

Antimicrobial agents are not likely to adversely affect fish. In all studies effects are either found in environmentally irrelevant concentrations, or no toxic effects were observed at all. Nevertheless, indirect effects can not be excluded, resulting from adverse alterations of the natural balance due to the impact of antimicrobials on lower trophic levels.

Toxicity tests with different fish species (*Acartia tonsa, Brachydanio rerio, Lebistes reticulatus, Salmo gairdneri, Salvelinus namaycush*) showed no toxicity of antibiotics against the species tested (Lanzky and Halling-Sørensen 1997; Canton and van Esch 1976; Marking et al. 1988). However, skeleton deformations are reported for an antimicrobial extensively applied in aquaculture, but in concentrations higher than that expected in the environment (Lunestad 1992).

7.4.3
Soil and Sediments

Several papers addressed the impacts of antibiotics on soil dwelling organisms. Antimicrobials may have qualitative and quantitative effects upon the resident microbial community of the sediment, which can affect the degradation of organic matter. Furthermore, direct toxic effects upon the resident organisms can not be excluded, as summarised by Nygaard et al. (1992).

The composition of the soil dwelling community proved to be affected by antimicrobial substances. Strong inhibitory effects on several bacteria as well as a reduction in hyphe length of active moulds in forest soil were observed when antibiotics were added in concentrations of 10 mg kg^{-1} soil (Colinas et al. 1994). Influences on the microbial composition in soil were also demonstrated by Hossian and Alexander (1984), in environmentally irrelevant concentrations. Growth of fungi seems to be favoured by the existence of antibiotics in soil as proved by Patten et al. (1980).

The situation in sediments beneath fish farms is critical due to high local concentrations of antimicrobials. A reduction in the number of bacteria was observed for some antimicrobial agents in concentrations relevant for fish farm sediments. Activity of organisms was affected as well. A temporary effect on sulfate reduction was observed when antibiotics were added to sediment, either due to growth inhibition of sulfate reducing bacteria or the fermenting and acetogenic bacteria supplying them with substrate (Hansen et al. 1992).

Antibiotics present in soil and sediment can lose their antimicrobial activity as a result of binding to sediment particles or complex formation with ions, which was demonstrated for a few substances. However, contradictory results concerning the loss of antibacterial activity due to binding or complex formation were found for one and the same substance (Lunestad and Goksøyr 1990; Björklund et al. 1991; Hansen et al. 1992; Hektoen et al. 1995). The reason for this could be the differences in sediment composition, which seems to play a key role in the effects of substances upon the resident population.

Non-target organisms living in soil were not found to be affected by antibiotics. Effects of two antibiotics in environmentally relevant concentrations on earthworms, springtails and enchytraeids were investigated. Both antibiotics showed no toxicity on the organisms under investigation exposed to antibiotics. Nevertheless, indirect effects due to changes in the microbial community could not be excluded (Baguer et al. 2000).

The potential of a pollutant to accumulate in organisms has to be considered as critical. Antibiotics, which are poorly water soluble, especially if the bioconcentration factor is between 500 and 1 000 or the octanol/water distribution coefficient exceeds the value of 3, tend to accumulate in organisms. The enrichment of substances in organisms was proved for some antibiotics (Migliore et al. 1993; Lunestad 1992).

7.5
Conclusion

Little is known on the occurrence and fate of antibiotics in the environment and the related risk posed on aquatic and terrestrial ecosystems. An environmental risk assessment can not be performed on the basis of these data. Further research is needed.

Since knowledge about antibiotics with regard to their ecotoxicity is very limited, a reduction in the use of antimicrobial agents should be encouraged as far as possible.

Acknowledgements

This work was supported by grants of the German Federal Environmental Agency, Berlin (UBA).

References

Al-Ahmad A, Daschner FD, Kümmerer K (1999) Biodegradability of cefotiam, ciprofloxacin, meropenem, penicillin G and sulfamethoxazole and inhibition of waste water bacteria. Arch Environ Contam Toxicol 37:158–163

Alexander M (1981) Biodegradation of chemicals of environmental concern. Science 211:132–211

Backhaus T, Grimme LH (1999) The toxicity of antibiotic agents to the luminescent bacterium *Vibrio fischeri*. Chemosphere 38:3291–3301

Baguer AJ, Jensen J, Krogh PH (2000) Effects of the antibiotics oxytetracycline and tylosin on soil fauna. Chemosphere 40:751–757

Björklund H, Råbergh CMI, Bylund G (1991) Residues of oxytetracycline in wild fish and sediments from fish farms. Aquaculture 86:359–367

Brambilla G, Civitareale C, Migliore L (1994) Experimental toxicity and analysis of bacitracin, flumequine and sulphadimethoxine in terrestrial and aquatic organisms as a predictive model for ecosystem damage. Quimica Analitica 13:573–577

Canton JH, Esch GJ van (1976) The short-term toxicity of some feed additives to different freshwater organisms. Bull Environ Contam Toxicol 15:720–725

Capone DG, Weston DP, Miller V, Shoemaker C (1996) Antibacterial residues in marine sediments and invertebrates following chemotherapy in aquaculture. Aquaculture 145:55–75

Cerovec C (2000) Entwicklung und Anwendung von HPLC Methoden für die Analyse von Antibiotika in verschiedenen Testsystemen. Diplomarbeit, Fachhochschule und Berufskollegs NTA, Isny im Allgäu

Colinas C, Ingham E, Molina R (1994) Population responses of target and non-target forest soil organisms to selected biocides. Soil Biol Biochem 26:41–47

Coyne R, Hiney M, O'Conner B, Cazabon D, Smith P (1994) Concentration and persistence of oxytetracycline in sediments under a marine salmon farm. Aquaculture 123:31–42

Dojmi di Delupis G, Macrì A, Civitareale C, Migliore L (1992) Antibiotics of zootechnical use: effects of acute high and low dose contamination on *Daphnia magna* Straus. Aquatic Toxicol 22:53–60

Donoho AL (1984) Biochemical studies on the fate of monensin in animals and in the environment. J Anim Sci 58:1528–1539

Froehner K, Backhaus T, Grimme LH (2000) Bioassays with *Vibrio fischeri* for the assessment of delayed toxicity. Chemosphere 40:821–828

Gavalchin J, Katz SE (1994) The persistence of fecal-borne antibiotics in soil. J AOAC Intern 77:481–485

Gilbertson TJ, Hornish RE, Jaglan PS, Koshy KT, Nappier JL, Stahl GL, Cazers AR, Napplier JM, Kubicek MF, Hoffman GA, Hamlow PJ (1990) Environmental fate of ceftiofur sodium, a cephalosporin antibiotic. Role of animal excreta in its decomposition. J Agric Food Chem 38:890–894

Gomez J, Mendez R, Lema JM (1996) The effect of antibiotics on nitrification processes. Appl Biochem Biotechnol 57/58:869–876

Halling-Sørensen B (2000) Algal toxicity of antibacterial agents used in intensive farming. Chemosphere 40:731–739

Hamscher G, Sczesny S, Abu-Qare A, Höper H, Nau H (2000) Stoffe mit pharmakologischer Wirkung einschließlich hormonell aktiver Substanzen in der Umwelt: Nachweis von Tetracyclinen in güllegedüngten Böden. Dtsch tierärztl Wschr 10:293–348

Hansen PK, Lunestad BT, Samuelsen OB (1992) Effects of oxytetracycline, oxolinic acid and flumequine on bacteria in an artificial marine fish farm sediment. Can J Microbiol 38:1307–1312

Hartmann A, Alder AC, Koller T, Widmer RM (1998) Identification of fluoroquinolone antibiotics as the main source of *umuC* genotoxicity in native hospital wastewater. Environ Toxicol Chem 17:377–382

Hartmann A, Golet EM, Gartiser S, Alder AC, Koller T, Widmer RM (1999) Primary DNA damage but not mutagenicity correlates with ciprofloxacin concentrations in German hospital wastewaters. Arch Environ Contam Toxicol 36:115–119

Hektoen H, Berge JA, Hormazabal V, Yndestad M (1995) Persistence of antibacterial agents in marine sediments. Aquaculutre 133:175–184

Hirsch R, Ternes T, Haberer K, Kratz KL (1999) Occurrence of antibiotics in the aquatic environment. Sci Total Environ 225:109–118

Holm JV, Rugge K, Bjerg PL, Christensen TH (1995) Occurrence and distribution of pharmaceutical organic compounds in the groundwater downgradient of a landfill. Envrion Sci Tech 29:1415–1420

Holten Lützhøft HC, Halling-Sørensen B, Jørgensen SE (1999) Algal toxicity of antibacterial agents applied in Danish fish farming. Arch Environ Contam Toxicol 36:1–6

Hossian AKM, Alexander M (1984) Enhancing soybean rhizosphere colonization by *Rhizobium japonicum*. Appl Environ Microbiol 48:468–472

Jacobsen P, Berglind L (1988) Persistence of oxytetracyline in sediment from fish farms. Aquaculture 70:365–370

Klaver AL, Matthews RA (1994) Effects of oxytetracycline on nitrification in a model aquatic system. Aquaculture 123:237–247

Koller G, Hungerbühler K, Fent K (2000) Data ranges in aquatic toxicity of chemicals. Consequences for environmental risk analysis. Environ Sci Pollut Res 7:135–143

Kümmerer K, Al-Ahmad A, Mersch-Sundermann V (2000) Biodegradability of some antibiotics, elimination of the genotoxicity and affection of wastewater bacteria in a simple test. Chemosphere 40:701–710

Lanzky PF, Halling-Sørensen B (1997) The toxic effect of the antibiotic metronidazol on aquatic organisms. Chemosphere 35:2553–2561

Lunestad BT (1992) Fate and effects of antibacterial agents in aquatic environments. Chemotherapy in Aquaculture: From theory to reality. Office Internat. des Epizooties, Paris, pp 152–161

Lunestad BT, Goksøyr J (1990) Reduction in the antibacterial effect of oxytetracycline in sea water by complex formation with magnesium and calcium. Diseases of Aquatic Organisms 9:67–72

Lunestad BT, Samuelsen OB, Fjelde S, Ervik A (1995) Photostability of eight antibacterial agents in seawater. Aquaculture 134:217–225

Macrì A, Stazi AV, Dojmi di Delupis G (1988) Acute toxicity of furazolidone on *Artemia salina, Daphnia magna*, and *Culex pipiens molestus* larvae. Ecotoxicology and Environmental Safety 16:90–94

Marengo JR, O'Brian RA, Velagaleti RR, Stamm JM (1997) Aerobic biodegradation of (^{14}C)-sarafloxacin hydrochloride in soil. Environ Toxicol Chem 16:462–471

Marking LL, Howe GE, Crowther JR (1988) Toxicity of erythromycin, oxytetracycline and tetracycline administered to lake trout in water baths, by injection, or by feeding. The Progressive Fish Culturist 50:197–201

Migliore L, Brambilla G, Grassitellis A, Dojmi di Delupis G (1993) Toxicity and bioaccumulation of sulphadimethoxine in *Artemia* (Crustacea, Anostraca). Int J Salt Lake Res 2:141–152

Migliore L, Lorenzi C, Civitareale C, Laudi O, Brambilla G (1995) La flumequina e gli ecosistemi marini: emissione con l'acquacoltura e tossicita su *Artemia salina* (L.). Atti S.I.T.E. 16

Migliore L, Civitareale C, Brambilla G, Dojmi di Delupis G (1997) Toxicity of several important agricultural antibiotics to *Artemia*. Wat Res 31:1801–1806

Nygaard K, Lunestad BT, Hektoen H, Berge JA, Hormazabal V (1992) Resistance to oxytetracycline, oxolinic acid and furazolidone in bacteria from marine sediments. Aquaculture 104:21–36

Oka H, Ikai Y, Kawamura N, Yamada M, Harada K, Ito S, Suzuki M (1989) Photodecomposition products of tetracycline in aqueous solution. J Agric Food Chem 37:226–231

Patten DK, Wolf DC, Kunkle WE, Douglass LW (1980) Effect of antibiotics in beef cattle faeces on nitrogen and carbon mineralization in soil and on plant growth and composition. J Environ Qual 9:167–172

Pearson M, Inglis V (1993) A sensitive microbioassay for the detection of antibacterial agents in the aquatic environment. J Fish Diseases 16:255–260

Plate P (1991) Bodenlose Folgen? Antibiotika in Gülle und Boden. Veto 27:15–17

Pouliquen H, Le Bris H, Pinault L (1992) Experimental study of the therapeutic application of oxytetracycline, its attenuation in sediment and sea water, and implication for farm culture of benthic organisms. Mar Ecol Progr Ser 89:93–98

Qiting J, Xiheng Z (1988) Combination process of anaerobic digestion and ozonization technology for treating wastewater from antibiotics production. Wat Treat 3:285–291

Rabølle M, Spliid NH (2000) Sorption and mobility of metronidazole, olaquindox, oxytetracycline and tylosin in soil. Chemosphere 40:715–722

Richardson ML, Bowron JM (1985) The fate of pharmaceutical chemicals in the environment. J Pharm Pharmacol 37:1–12

Samuelsen OB (1989) Degradation of oxytetracycline in seawater at two different temperatures and light intensities, and the persistence of oxytetracycline in the sediment from a fish farm. Aquaculture 83:7–16

Samuelsen OB, Solheim E, Lunestad BT (1991) Fate and microbiological effects of furazolidone in a marine aquaculture sediment. Sci Total Environ 108:275–283

Samuelsen OB, Torsvik V, Ervik A (1992) Long-range changes in oxytetracycline concentration and bacterial resistance towards oxytetracycline in fish farm sediment after medication. Sci Total Environ 114:25–36

Samuelsen OB, Lunestad BT, Fjelde S (1994) Stability of antibacterial agents in an artificial marine aquaculture sediment studied under laboratory conditions. Aquaculture 126:183–290

Stanislawska J (1979) Communities of organisms during treatment of sewage containing antibiotics. Pol Arch Hydrobiol 26:221–229

Ternes T (1998) Occurrence of drugs in German sewage treatment plants and rivers. Wat Res 32:3245–3260

Thomulka KW, McGee DJ (1993) Detection of biohazardous materials in water by measuring bioluminescence reduction with the marine organism *Vibrio harveyi*. Environ Sci Health A28(9):2153–2166

Tomlinson TG, Boon AG, Trotman CNA (1966) Inhibition of nitrification in the activated sludge process of sewage disposal. J Appl Bact 29:266–291

Watts CD, Crathorne M, Fielding M, Steel CP (1983): Identification of non-volatile organics in water using field desorption mass spectrometry and high performance liquid chromatography. In: Angeletti G, Bjørseth A (eds) Analysis of organic micropollutants in water. Reidel Publ. Corp., Dordrecht, pp 120–131

Weerasinghe CA, Towner D (1997) Aerobic biodegradation of virginiamycin in soil. Environ Toxicol Chem 16:1873–1876

Wiethan J, Henninger A, Kümmerer K (1999) Antibiotikaresistenz – Vorkommen und Übertragung in Abwasser, Oberflächenwasser und Trinkwasser. Teil 2. Resistenzausbildung und Verbreitung durch Antibiotikaeintrag in Abwasser und Kläranalgen. Untersuchung mittels Chemotaxonomie und Kläranlagensimulation. 2. Zwischenbericht BMBF Projekt

Wiethan J, Al-Ahmad A, Henninger A, Kümmerer K (2000) Simulation des Selektionsdrucks der Antibiotika Ciprofloxacin und Ceftazidim in Oberflächengewässern mittels klassischer Methoden. Vom Wasser 95:107–118

Wollenberger L, Halling-Sørensen B, Kusk KO (2000) Acute and chronic toxicity of veterinary antibiotics to *Daphnia magna*. Chemosphere 40:723–730

Antibiotics in the Environment: Zinc Bacitracin – Environmental Toxicity and Breakdown

T. Midtvedt

8.1
General Introduction

If one accepts the statement that any pharmaceutical or its breakdown product(s) may represent potential hazard(s) to the environment, it is implicit that antibiotics stay in the first row as candidates capable of influencing upon the environment. As mentioned in greater details in Chap. 18, many studies have been carried out in order to study the half-life of antibiotics in natural sediments as well as development of resistant microorganisms. The term "eco-shadow" has been introduced as a mode of describing alteration(s) in an ecosystem following exposure of the system to an antibiotic (or any other pharmaceutical). It has been shown that some groups of antibiotics, such as tetracyclines and especially the newer fluoroquinolones, can be present in the environment for weeks, months or even years after they have been given for prophylactic or therapeutic reasons.

Obviously, the importance of following a few safety-first principles listed in Chap. 18 (i.e. the drug should be rapidly broken down to inactive substances, and neither the drug nor any of the breakdown products should be concentrated in any part of the environment) is self-explaining. However, it is a sad fact that these important points are not included in official guidelines for registration of new pharmaceuticals, including antibiotics. Consequently, the pharmaceutical industry has paid little attention to the environmental part of half-life, etc., of drugs. Following our introduction of the term eco-shadow a few years ago, I have had many discussions with major pharmaceutical companies producing antibiotics with large or long-lasting eco-shadows; the fluoroquinolones and tetracyclines. It goes without saying that companies having compounds with smaller eco-shadows, such as penicillin G and V, had no difficulties in accepting this way of thinking. In the following I want to present some data reflecting what is known (and not known) about zinc bacitracin (ZB), a drug that for many years has been extensively used in animal husbandry as a growth promoting agent. Over the years, many tons of ZB have reached the environment. The therapeutic usage of ZB in human and veterinary medicine has always been negligible. ZB was mentioned in the Swann report 40 years ago (Swann 1969) and seems to fulfil most, if not all, of the principles listed by Swann for a proper use of antibiotics as growth promoting agents.

8.2
Zinc Bacitracin

8.2.1
Structure and Pharmacology

Bacitracin is a complex of polypetides produced by *Bacillus licheniformis* and was first described as early as in 1943 (for further details, see Walter and Heilmeyer 1975). Its main components are the dodecapeptides, bacitracin A, B1, B2 and B3. Zinc is added in order to stabilise these molecules. ZB has a very low acute oral toxicity. Mice tolerate daily doses of 3 000–5 000 mg kg^{-1} d^{-1} body weight for more than 30 days without any visible effects. High doses of ZB have also been given to rats, rabbits and dogs, all without any deaths or significant clinical symptoms (for further details, see Torsvik et al. 1990, that has 96 references).

In an extensive study of radiolabelled ZB, (labelled in the L-isoleucine moiety of the molecule) it was found that out of orally given ZB, 102% was recovered in rat faeces and 96% in piglet faeces while in chickens 95% of the dose was recovered in the combined faeces and urine (Al Pharma 1992). However, only a minor part of the recovered radiolabelled substands antibacterial activity (see below). When radiolabelled ZB was given orally to rats, chickens and piglets, it was found that urine from rats and piglets contained 3.2 and 3.6% respectively of the administered dose of labelled ZB – in the form of degradation products of ZB, mostly smaller peptides. Comparable values for bile were 0.5% and 0.03% respectively. However, no bacitracins or their near derivatives were detected in the bile or urine, nor was there any labelled free isoleucine. Taken together, these data strongly indicated that nearly all ZB given orally is excreted by faeces into the environment and neither ZB itself nor any of the breakdown products are concentrated in the animals receiving ZB.

8.2.2
ZB and Environmental Fate

From data presented in Al Pharma (1992), it can be mentioned that when ZB is added to chicken and piglet feed at the 100 ppm level, 5–10% of the native, active material is generally recovered from the excreta. The microbiologically active bacitracins are initially converted to analogous inactive bacitracins (by oxidation of the thiazoline ring) and desamido-bacitracins (by deamidation of the L-asparagine moiety) and further hydrolysed to smaller peptides and individual amino acids. When ZB is added at the level of 100 ppm to pig faeces, the half-life at 37 °C, 20 °C and 4 °C is less than 1 day, 2 days and less than 30 days, respectively. The kinetics of elimination in chicken excreta is stated to be similar. When faeces from pigs fed 100 ZB were mixed with clay, mould or sandy soil and stored at 4 °C and 37 °C, the recovery was close to detection level (0.1 mg kg^{-1}) after one day of storage, indicating a very rapid degradation in soil.

The effects of ZB on aquatic life has been studies in several set-ups. In concentrations up to 10 mg l^{-1} it does not inhibit the growth of a green algae, *Chlorella ellipsoidea*; LC$_{50}$ of ZB to *Daphnia magna* and *Salmo gairdneri* were 34 mg l^{-1} (48 hours) and 74 mg l^{-1} (96 hours), respectively. The concentrations mentioned are several logs above concentrations that can be expected to be found even with maximum environmental exposure of the drug.

It has been shown that isolates of *Rhizobium trifolii*, i.e. main nitrogen fixation microorganisms in soil, show high tolerance to ZB. However, whether and to what extent ZB may influence upon other parts of the flora present in soil has not been satisfactorily investigated. The mere fact that one gram of soil may contain a very high number of microbial species (Torsvik et al. 1990), makes it reasonable to assume, but difficult to prove that it really takes place. At any rate, the very rapid environmental breakdown of ZB indicates that its eco-shadow might have a short range. However, it goes without saying that this question should be studied in greater detail, and so should the question of alterations in tolerance to ZB in the soil ecosystem.

8.3
Conclusions

The eco-shadow concept was applied on available data concerning ZB, an antibiotic used nearly exclusively as a growth promoting agent. ZB is not absorbed in mammalian organisms but excreted into the environment where it is rapidly broken down. Neither the drug nor its main metabolites seems to be concentrated in any particular part of the environment. The drug seems to undergo a very rapid degradation. The rapid degradation makes it reasonable to assume ZB has a short or small eco-shadow. However, whether an environmental exposure gives rise to decreased sensitivity to the compound among members of soil ecology has not been studied in any detail.

References

Al Pharma (1992) Documentation for registration, FAD 70/524/EEC. Oslo, Norway
Swann MM (1969) Joint committee on the use of antibiotics in animal husbandry and veterinary medicine. Her Majesty's Stationary Office, London (Report 1969)
Torsvik V, Gogsoyr J, Dae FL (1990) High diversity in DNA in soil bacteria. Appl Environ Microbiol 56:782–787
Walter AM, Heilmeyer L (1975) Antibiotika-Fibel, 4. Aufl. Georg Thieme Verlag, Stuttgart

Pharmaceutical Residues in the Aquatic Environment and their Significance for Drinking Water Production

C. Zwiener · T. J. Gremm · F. H. Frimmel

9.1
Introduction

Pharmaceuticals belong to the environmentally relevant compounds. They are produced and administered for human and animal medical care. Due to the amount and types of applications pharmaceuticals can reach the environment, in particular the aquatic systems. Being produced and applied with the aim of causing a biological effect, their occurrence in the environment is of ecotoxicological interest. In particular this is of importance for antibiotics, but also for antineoplastics, hormones (compounds with endocrinic effects) and various compounds and metabolites that have already been detected in sewage plant effluents and surface waters in considerable concentrations (e.g. bezafibrate, clofibric acid, ibuprofen) (Stumpf et al. 1999; Hirsch et al. 1999). In particular, clofibric acid – a therapeutically active metabolite of clofibrate ethyl, etofibrate and ethofyllinclofibrate – shows a highly persistent behaviour in the aquatic environment and was already found in ground and drinking water in the city of Berlin (Heberer et al. 1998; Heberer and Stan 1996) as well as in the North Sea (Buser et al. 1998).

The occurrence of pharmaceuticals in the aquatic and the terrestrial environment can be linked to different sources such as emission from production sites, direct disposal of surplus drugs in households, excretion after application for human and animal medical care, therapeutic treatment of livestock on fields, and finally effluents of fish farms (Halling-Sørensen et al. 1998). Therefore, we have to consider both point sources such as production effluents and waste disposals as well as diffuse sources such as runoff from fields and anthropogenic effluents as possible routes of the pharmaceutical compounds to the environment.

The fate of pharmaceuticals can be followed beginning from the consumption of the active drug by a patient. After administration, the pharmaceuticals and their metabolites are excreted and reach the sewage system. In addition, surplus drugs in households are disposed mainly in the wastewater. Mass balances of the input and output of pharmaceuticals in sewage treatment plants reveal that during sewage treatment not all pharmaceuticals are totally removed (Ternes 1998). Consequently they are discharged into surface waters. This is of special importance, since surface water is a possible source for drinking water production. In drinking water treatment the pharmaceuticals can be removed by several technical processes such as flocculation, filtration, adsorption, or oxidation. In case of river water treatment, bank filtration is often used as the first treatment step. The compounds which are not removed by the drinking water treatment processes reach the consumer, which is shown to be the case for some pharmaceuticals in the city of Berlin (Heberer et al. 1998). However, it should be noticed that here an exceptional situation for the groundwater exposition – which can not be generalised for the rest of Germany – was found. Even though the resulting concentrations of pharmaceuticals in the aquatic system can be expected to be fairly low and the toxicity of the medical compounds are within the approved application limits, there has been no reliable information on the long-term effect on humans.

9.2
Pharmaceuticals in the Aquatic Environment

In the aquatic environment several specific pharmaceutical compounds have been detected in Germany. In Table 9.1 examples of pharmaceuticals for different medical applications like lipid regulators, antiphlogistics, beta blockers as well as antibiotics are shown.

Table 9.1. Estimated amounts of some selected pharmaceuticals applied in Germany and concentrations found in secondary effluents and surface waters (from Heberer and Stan 1998; Stumpf et al. 1996; Hirsch et al. 1999; Ternes 1998)

Agent	Applied mass (t yr^{-1})	Concentration in sewage water (µg l^{-1})	Concentration in surface water (µg l^{-1})
Lipid regulators			
Clofibric acid	15–21	0.46–1.56	0.005–0.30
Bezafibrate	38–57	0.25–4.56	0.005–0.38
Gemfibrozil	–	1.5[a]	0.51
Fenofibric acid	11–15	0.05–1.19	0.005–0.17
Antiphlogistics			
Ibuprofen	48–96	0.05–3.35	0.05–0.28
Diclofenac	48–72	0.005–1.59	0.005–0.49
Phenazone	–	0.41[a]	0.95[a]
Acetylsalic. acid	23–116	0.05–1.51	<0.05
Betablockers			
Bisoprolol	112	0.37[a]	2.9[a]
Betaxolol	16	0.19[a]	0.028[a]
Metoprolol	50	2.2[a]	2.2[a]
Propanolol	3	0.29[a]	0.59[a]
Antibiotics			
Clarithromycin	1.3–2.6	0.24[a]	0.26[a]
Erythromycin	3.9–19.8	6.00[a]	1.70[a]
Roxithromycin	3.1–6.2	1.00[a]	0.56[a]
Chloramphenicol	–	0.56[a]	0.06[a]
Sulfamethoxazole	16.6–76	2.00[a]	0.48[a]
Trimethoprim	3.3–15	0.66[a]	0.20[a]

[a] Maximum values.

Table 9.2. Concentrations of pharmaceuticals found in groundwater influenced by bank filtration and wastewater (from Heberer et al. 1997)

Pharmaceutical	Concentration range ($\mu g\,l^{-1}$)
Acetylsalic. acid	–
Ibuprofen	N.d.–0.2
Diclofenac	N.d.–0.3
Phenazon	<0.01–1.25
Clofibric acid	0.07–7.3
Fenofibric acid	N.d.–0.045

N.d. = not detected.

The substances are prescribed in high amounts up to 100 t yr^{-1} in Germany (Schwabe and Pfaffrath 1996) and found in the effluents of sewage treatment plants and surface waters in the $\mu g\,l^{-1}$ or ng l^{-1} range respectively. Most substances are known to have no acute toxicological or ecotoxicological effects – with the exception of antibiotics of course – but nevertheless they are important regarding their high amount of application and of their occurrence in the environment. Furthermore, long-term ecotoxicological effects can not be excluded totally up to now. Our studies focused in particular on the three substances: (1) clofibric acid, the active metabolite of a lipid regulator; (2) ibuprofen, an antiphlogistic; (3) diclofenac, an antirheumatic compound. Regarding these classes of compounds for example, maximum concentrations of 3.35 $\mu g\,l^{-1}$ were reached for ibuprofen, and of 4.56 $\mu g\,l^{-1}$ for bezafibrate in wastewater. In river water these substances were identified in much lower concentrations. Compared to sewage water a dilution of about a factor of ten was observed for the maximum concentrations of pharmaceuticals in river water (Table 9.1, Stumpf et al. 1996; Heberer and Stan 1998; Ternes 1998). As a consequence, sewage effluents may be regarded as the major source of pharmaceuticals in river water.

Compared to sewage water, the concentrations of pharmaceuticals in drinking water and the corresponding raw waters are normally very low. Data from 17 water samples collected from groundwater wells of a drinking water catchment area are shown in Table 9.2. The pharmaceuticals were found in the ng l^{-1} range in groundwater, which is influenced by infiltrated river water or channel water loaded with sewage effluents (Heberer et al. 1998).

The occurrence of pharmaceuticals in groundwater demonstrates that these substances are not being removed totally on their way through the underground or during river bank filtration. As a consequence, the knowledge of physical, biological, and chemical processes in the aquatic system such as adsorption, degradation, and hydrolysis is of great importance for a comprehensive risk assessment of pharmaceuticals in the environment. Only very limited information on these processes is available to date. This is especially true for the metabolites of the pharmaceutical compounds introduced into the environment.

9.3
Pharmaceuticals in Sewage Water Treatment

The biodegradability of pharmaceuticals characterises their persistence in the aquatic environment as well as in sewage treatment plants. Biodegradation tests can be performed following several test protocols such as the Closed Bottle test (OECD 301D) or the Zahn-Wellens test (OECD 302B). In general, the experiments are carried out with several hundred milligrams of a substance and can give answers to the question on biodegradability only for certain and very often unrealistic conditions. Therefore, conclusions from these experiments regarding the degradability of pharmaceuticals in a sewage treatment plant are limited. It is also important to note that the low $\mu g \, l^{-1}$ range of pharmaceuticals is accompanied by a high amount of easily digestible compounds in the sewage water. It is known that the kinetics and the extent of degradation of individual compounds are influenced by the simultaneous utilisation of mixed substrates. Furthermore, threshold concentrations for the utilisation of individual substances are reported in the order of $1-100 \, \mu g \, l^{-1}$ (Alexander 1994). Therefore, the degradability testing should be carried out ideally in a sewage plant or at least in a comparable test system. In this context, laboratory simulations of sewage treatment systems (STS) are of increasing interest. At the Engler-Bunte-Institut we have set up two test systems for testing the biodegradation: (1) a model STS, and (2) biofilm reactors. These two systems allow the degradation tests under "close to real life" conditions.

Degradation experiments for the pharmaceuticals ibuprofen, diclofenac and the metabolite clofibric acid were carried out in a pilot sewage plant. The pilot sewage plant was run in a three stage process with denitrification, activated sludge process and final settling (Fig. 9.1).

The total volume was about 25 l and the feed consisted of synthetic wastewater with a DOC concentration of about 60 mg l^{-1}, composed of peptone, meat extract, urea, and

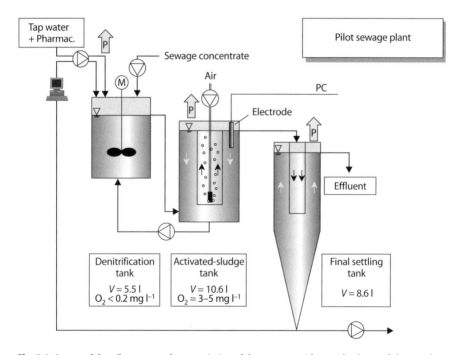

Fig. 9.1. Set-up of the pilot sewage plant consisting of three stages with a total volume of about 25 l

salts (DIN 1999; OECD 1992). The pharmaceuticals were dosed at a concentration of 10 μg l^{-1} each. To test the influences on pharmaceutical degradation, the operating parameters could be varied as well as the dosage of additional interfering compounds. From the investigated pharmaceuticals, only ibuprofen was eliminated significantly to about 60% of its initial concentration, whereas only about 5% of clofibric acid and of diclofenac were eliminated (Table 9.3, Zwiener 1999).

These results are comparable to those from a municipal sewage plant where ibuprofen was eliminated to a much greater extent than clofibric acid (Buser et al. 1999; Buser et al. 1998; Ternes 1998). The occurrence of clofibric acid in the North Sea reveals its persistence in the aquatic environment. However, despite the efficient elimination of 96–99.9% of ibuprofen in some wastewater treatment plants in Switzerland, the substance was detected in sewage effluents and surface waters (Buser et al. 1999). This may be attributed to different elimination efficiencies of sewage treatment plants, or to direct discharges of wastewater to rivers. Therefore, our further investigations will show the influence of operating parameters and the role of adaptation and threshold concentrations on the elimination efficiency.

An easy-to-use and a fast responding model system for biodegradation was realised with biofilm reactors (Fig. 9.2).

They consist of columns filled with pumice stones on which a biofilm was developed by feeding the columns with sewage water from a municipal sewage plant. The biofilm reactors were run under both oxic and anoxic conditions. The feed was synthetic sewage water with a DOC concentration of about 15 mg l^{-1} and 10 μg l^{-1} of each of the pharmaceuticals. The lower feed concentration for the biofilm reactors is used to control the biomass increase and therefore to prevent the columns from clogging. Under the applied operating conditions ibuprofen was eliminated in the range of 64–70% and diclofenac and clofibric acid in the range of 5–1% in the oxic biofilm reactor (Table 9.3). These results resemble those obtained for the pharmaceutical elimination in the pilot sewage plant. The average residence times of a volume element is about 8 h in the pilot sewage plant and about 1.5 h in the oxic biofilm reactor. However, the stratification of the biofilm in the flow direction of the feed due to the nutrient gradient in the column results in a much lower residence time based on bioactivity of about 0.5 h. A quite different elimination was found for the anoxic biofilm reactor (Table 9.3). Ibuprofen was eliminated only in the range of 17–21%. A different elimination mechanism based on the anoxic conditions may be the reason for these findings. The biofilm reactors proved to be attractive model systems for investigating the biological degradation of target compounds. They showed similar results, but had a

Table 9.3. Elimination of pharmaceuticals in a pilot sewage plant and biofilm reactors

Pharmaceutical	Elimination (%)		
	Pilot STP	Biofilm, oxic	Biofilm, anoxic
Clofibric acid	2–6	1–5	26–30
Ibuprofen	57–60	64–70	17–21
Diclofenac	1–6	1–5	34–38

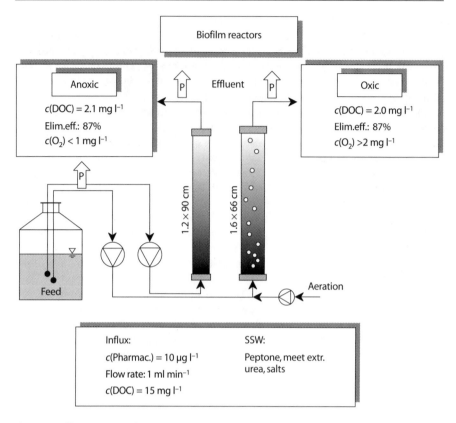

Fig. 9.2. Biofilm reactors and their principal operating conditions

faster response and a higher robustness compared to the pilot sewage plant. Further investigations should compare the microbial communities and its shift during operation of the biofilm reactors, the pilot sewage plant, and of sewage sludge from a municipal sewage treatment plant. No shift in microbial metabolic response was shown for laboratory-scale testing that applied continuous activated sludge and semicontinuous activated sludge units fed with wastewater or a synthetic wastewater over a period of 16 weeks (Kaiser et al. 1998).

9.4
Pharmaceuticals in Drinking Water Treatment

The occurrence of pharmaceuticals in surface waters has also an impact on drinking water production (Heberer and Stan 1996, 1998). Since surface waters contain considerable amounts of pharmaceuticals, the possibility of pharmaceutical reduction in several treatment steps of the drinking water production is of special interest. The treatment steps in question are the natural processes before raw water intake such as bank filtration or passage through the underground and the technical processes within a drinking water plant such as flocculation/filtration, slow sand filtration, ozonation, and activated carbon (AC) adsorption.

Only few data based on laboratory experiments are available on the behaviour of the pharmaceuticals carbamazepine, diclofenac, primidone, bezafibrate, and the metabolite clofibric acid in drinking water production. Flocculation doesn't seem to be suitable for reliable elimination of these pharmaceuticals. However, AC-adsorption resulted in a significant elimination. Ozonation was only effective for specific compounds like diclofenac (Ternes et al. 1999; Sacher et al. 1999). The limited ozone concentration in the aqueous phase and limited ozone contact time in drinking water treatment processes demand the application of more intensive oxidation methods like the so-called advanced oxidation processes (AOP). AOP are combined processes (e.g. UV/ozone, hydrogen peroxide/ozone) with the aim of OH-radical production as their common feature. OH-radicals are non-selective oxidants that react with many inorganic and organic water constituents with fast reaction kinetics.

We have carried out oxidation experiments with pharmaceuticals and ozone in a laboratory reactor (Fig. 9.3). The pharmaceuticals ibuprofen, diclofenac and the metabolite clofibric acid were spiked at a concentration of $2\ \mu g\ l^{-1}$ each. Ozonation with $1\ mg\ l^{-1}$ ozone in distilled water resulted only for diclofenac in an almost quantitative elimination of 96.8%. Ibuprofen and clofibric acid elimination was only 12% and 8%, respectively.

The application of AOP (hydrogen peroxide/ozone) improved the degradation efficiency of all investigated pharmaceuticals. Due to the radical scavenging capacity of tested river water, elevated oxidant concentrations were necessary to reach quantita-

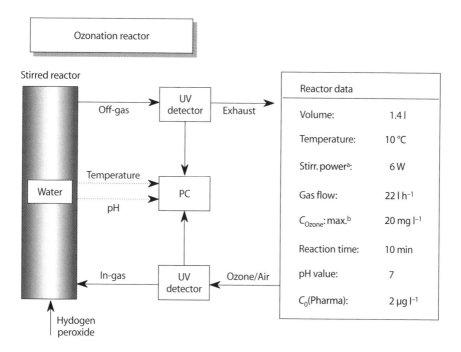

Fig. 9.3. Ozonation reactor and the reaction parameters ([a] applied electrical power; [b] in solution)

Table 9.4. Elimination of pharmaceuticals in a laboratory reactor by application of an AOP (ozone/hydrogen peroxide) at different concentrations of the oxidants in river water. (C_0(pharmaceutical) = 2 μg l^{-1}; reaction time = 10 min)

Pharmaceutical	Elimination in (%)		
	O_3/H_2O_2 1 mg l^{-1}/0.4 mg l^{-1}	O_3/H_2O_2 3.7 mg l^{-1}/1.4 mg l^{-1}	O_3/H_2O_2 5 mg l^{-1}/1.8 mg l^{-1}
Clofibric acid	21.8	92.7	97.9
Ibuprofen	29.2	94.0	99.4
Diclofenac	99.4	99.5	99.9

tive elimination of the pharmaceuticals (Table 9.4, Zwiener and Frimmel 2000). A sound assessment of the efficiency of the process and of its physiological relevance needs further information on the main degradation products and on the pathway of their formation.

It is beyond any question that drinking water has to be of special cleanness, and can not be the carrier for pharmaceuticals and health care substances. And it would not matter whether these substances were added on purpose or unwillingly as pollutants.

9.5
Future Research Needs

Pharmaceutical compounds are used in high amounts in human and veterinary medicine and reach the aquatic environment mostly via sewage treatment systems. The concentrations in the sewage systems can reach the μg l^{-1} range, whereas the concentrations of the pharmaceuticals in surface water, groundwater, and drinking water are generally very low (ng l^{-1} range). Despite the increasing research activities in this field, there is still a considerable need for future research. The most important research topics from our point of view are:

1. Development of analytical methods and verification of the results for pharmaceutical compounds and their metabolites in complex matrices, including extraction methods and clean-up procedures.
2. Investigation of the physical, chemical and biological processes in the aquatic system such as adsorption on particles, colloids and organic matter with the influences on transport in the aquatic system and aquifer; on transformation and biodegradation, including the formation of metabolites; and on the fate of the compounds in wastewater treatment.
3. Development and application of test systems that allow the investigation to be under "close to real life" conditions.
4. Investigation of the behaviour in drinking water treatment, especially determination of the elimination potential of the main treatment steps of drinking water production (ozonation, flocculation, adsorption, slow sand filtration)
5. Assessment of the toxicological relevance of the occurring concentrations ranges, including synergistic and antagonistic effects.

References

Alexander M (1994) Biodegradation and bioremediation. Academic Press, San Diego, California

Buser H-R, Müller MD, Theobald N (1998) Occurrence of the pharmaceutical drug clofibric acid and the herbicide mecoprop in various Swiss lakes and the North Sea. Environ Sci Technol 32:188–192

Buser H-R, Poiger T, Müller MD (1999) Occurrence and environmental behavior of the chiral pharmaceutical drug ibuprofen in surface waters and in waste water. Environ Sci Technol 33:2529–2535

DIN 38412 L24 (1999) Bestimmung der biologischen Abbaubarkeit unter Anwendung spezieller Analysenverfahren. Wiley-VCH, Weinheim, Beuth, Berlin (Deutsche Einheitsverfahren zur Wasser-, Abwasser- und Schlamm-Untersuchung, 44. Lieferung)

Halling-Sørensen B, Nielsen SN, Lanzky PF, Ingerslev, F, Holten Lützhøft HCH, Jørgensen SE (1998) Occurrence, fate and effects of pharmaceutical substances in the environment – a review. Chemosphere 36:357–393

Heberer T, Stan H-J (1996) Occurrence of polar organic contaminants in Berlin drinking water. Vom Wasser 86:19–31

Heberer T, Stan H-J (1998) Pharmaceutical residues in the aquatic system. Wasser und Boden 50:20–25 (Arzneimittelrückstände im aquatischen System)

Heberer T, Dünnbier U, Reilich C, Stan H-J (1997) Detection of drugs and drug metabolites in ground water samples of a drinking water treatment plant. Fresenius Environ Bull 6:438–443

Heberer T, Schmidt-Bäumler K, Stan H-J (1998) Occurrence and distribution of organic contaminants in aquatic systems in Berlin. Part I: Drug residues and other polar contaminants in Berlin surface and groundwater. Acta hydrochim hydrobiol 26:272–278

Hirsch R, Ternes T, Haberer K, Kratz K-L (1999) Occurrence of antibiotics in the aquatic environment. Sci Total Environ 225:109–118

Kaiser SK, Guckert JB, Gledhill DW (1998) Comparison of activated sludge microbial communities using biolog microplates. Wat Sci Technol 37:57–63

OECD (1992) Guidelines for testing of chemicals: 301 D, 302 B, 303 A. Organization for economic cooperation and development, Paris

Sacher F, Haist-Gulde B, Brauch H-J (1999) Untersuchungen zur Adsorbierbarkeit ausgewählter Arzneimittelstoffe und Metabolite an Aktivkohle. Jahrestagung der Fachgruppe Wasserchemie der Gesellschaft Deutscher Chemiker, Regensburg, 10.–12. Mai 1999

Schwabe U, Pfaffrath D (1996) Drug prescribing report '95 – Actual data, costs, trends, and comments. Gustav Fischer Verlag, Stuttgart (Arzneimittelverordnungsreport '95 – Aktuelle Daten, Kosten, Trends und Kommentare)

Stumpf M, Ternes TA, Haberer K, Seel P, Baumann W (1996) Determination of pharmaceutics in sewage plants and river water. Vom Wasser 86:291–303

Stumpf M, Ternes TA, Wilken R-D, Rodrigues SW, Baumann W (1999) Polar drug residues in sewage and natural waters in the state of Rio de Janeiro, Brazil. Sci Total Environ 225:135–141

Ternes TA (1998) Occurrence of drugs in German sewage treatment plants and rivers. Wat Res 32:3245–3260

Ternes TA, Meisenheimer M, Welsch H, Wilken R-D (1999) Verhalten von Pharmaka in der Trinkwasseraufbereitung. Jahrestagung der Fachgruppe Wasserchemie der Gesellschaft Deutscher Chemiker, Regensburg, 10.–12. Mai 1999

Zwiener C (1999) Beurteilung der biologischen Eliminierbarkeit von Arzneimittelrückständen in Wasser. Vortrag auf der Jahrestagung der Fachgruppe Wasserchemie der Gesellschaft Deutscher Chemiker, Regensburg, 10.–12. Mai 1999 (Assessment of the biological elimination of pharmaceutical residues in water)

Zwiener C, Frimmel FH (2000) Oxidative treatment of pharmaceuticals in water. Wat Res 34:1881–1885

Chapter 10

Pharmaceuticals as Environmental Contaminants: Modelling Distribution and Fate

A. Di Guardo · D. Calamari · E. Benfenati · B. Halling-Sørensen · E. Zuccato · R. Fanelli

10.1
Introduction

Concern is growing over the environmental consequences of the use of drugs for human and animal health. Long term treatments for several illnesses are a common mass practice in human health care (e.g. diuretics, beta blockers, antibiotics), a number of females are taking daily hormones to prevent unwanted pregnancies, modern life stress is handled very frequently through sedatives and tranquillizers, moreover there is in animal farming a general trend towards the intensification of production methods and production gains based on greater reliance on pharmaceuticals, feed additives, hormones and potent parasiticides (Halling-Sørensen et al. 1998).

The extent of the problem has not yet been fully evaluated, and the information for risk management is far from adequate. Human and environmental implications resulting from the massive use of human and animal drugs should be quickly evaluated. These days an increasing number of research groups are involved on this subject. Most of the approaches utilised in these studies follow the classical risk assessment procedures: calculating or assessing mass balances on consumptions and uses and monitoring the presence of the most common chemical substances in different environmental compartments in order to evaluate potential exposure (Calamari 1993). Other groups produce original experimental data on ecotoxicology and degradation.

The difficulties, however, are huge, the lack of data for environmental assessment is bigger than expected, and testing methods are not appropriate for these types of substances. Therefore, even if strategies for the evaluation are available, there is a need for adaptation, reconsideration and possibly new approaches.

In this chapter, a methodological attempt to evaluate the environmental distribution and fate of pharmaceuticals is presented, starting from their physicochemical properties and modelling through a stepwise procedure from a generic scenario towards a specific site situation. It comprises 4 stages: data evaluation, the use of generic models, the use of regional models and the use site-specific models (Fig. 10.1). The main requirements and a simple illustration will be presented.

10.2
Data Evaluation

This is the first stage in the process of understanding the fate of the chemical of interest. It involves the collection and critical assessment of structural formulas and physicochemical data such as molecular weight, vapour pressure, solubility in water, K_{ow}, and pK_a. These data are necessary to characterise the chemicals and select the type of

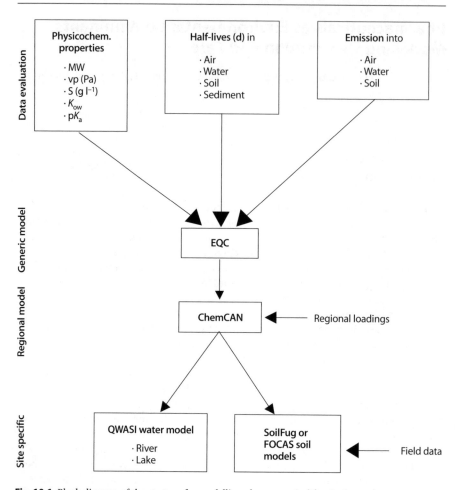

Fig. 10.1. Block diagram of the strategy for modelling pharmaceutical fate in the environment

model in order to run the simulations. (Mackay et al. 1996a). Chemicals can be classified as several "types", according to the scheme reported by Mackay et al. (1996a). The classification depends on the characteristics of the chemical and can be listed as follows:

- Type 1: Chemicals for which vapour pressure and water solubility are measurable and meaningful
- Type 2: Involatile chemicals
- Type 3: Insoluble chemicals
- Type 4: Chemicals that are both involatile and insoluble
- Type 5: Speciating chemicals (e.g. mercury)

According to the type of chemical the user can select the appropriate model "engine". For example, ionised chemicals cannot be modelled with a partitioning model based on equations that are used to estimate soil-water partitioning from K_{ow} to K_{oc} and K_d. Among the desired parameters, pK_a values are also important to understand whether the chemical will dissociate (and to what extent) at environmental pH values. Half-lives have to be collected whenever possible for the main 4 phases (air, water, soil, sediment). Wastewater treatment plant half-lives are also invaluable.

Among the data needed, discharges and emission patterns in a defined area or drainage basin are to be sought. The emissions can generally be into air, water and soil. For pharmaceuticals, the water compartment can be reached directly or at a later stage, from leaching or runoff of chemicals from the soil compartment. This may happen when sewage sludge, resulting from municipal sewage treatment plants, is applied to soil.

For pharmaceuticals it might be necessary to measure all such properties. Some physicochemical data are available for parent compounds, while very often the properties for the excreted metabolites are not known. It might then be necessary to measure such properties with the methods available. Some problems may arise for environmental half-lives.

Data at this stage will be critically evaluated and selected. Gaps could be filled by QSPR (quantitative structure-property relationships) methods whenever possible.

10.3
Generic Model

This stage is necessary to understand the main environmental pathways of the chemicals in a generic regional environment with predefined emission scenarios (in water only, in air only, in soil only). This stage will give important information on the mobility and overall persistence of a chemical in the different phases.

As stated from the authors (Mackay et al. 1996a,b,c) in the fate assessment, the focus is on understanding how the diverse properties of the chemical control its distribution among compartments, how it is transported and transformed, and its general persistence. Only the parent compound is treated. None of the metabolites or degradation products are treated, because they will require separate evaluations.

The scenario adopted is that of a generic environment at 25 °C, the common temperature for data acquisition. Because environmental conditions are evaluative, validation is not normally possible. Mackay et al. (1996b) have suggested an evaluative area of 10^5 km^2 with about 10% of the area being covered with water. The reasons to conduct an evaluative fate assessment are that it reveals general features of chemical behaviour and focuses efforts on obtaining information on the most important characteristics of the chemical, whether it is of no concern, or it is of definite concern.

Key information obtained in this stage includes the tendency for intermedia transport (e.g. evaporation), for bioconcentration and bioaccumulation, and the persistence of the substance, which is a function of reaction and advection rate.

It should be noticed that similar systems are nowadays utilised both in Europe and the USA (Cowan et al. 1995).

A detailed description of the equilibrium criterion model (EQC) is given in Mackay et al. (1996b), as well as the data requirements, the environmental scenario and the equation used to calculate partitioning, transport and transformation.

The physical chemical data and half-lives used in the simulation are given in Table 10.1.

Table 10.1. Physical chemical data and half-lives used in the simulation of cyclophosphamide, diazepam and ivermectin with the EQC model

Property	Chemical		
	Cyclophosphamide	Diazepam	Ivermectin
Molecular weight (g mol^{-1})	279.1	284	875
Melting point (°C)	49.5–53[a]	125–126[b]	155–157[c]
Vapour pressure (Pa)	1.00×10^{-6} [d]	5.00×10^{-5} [e]	1.00×10^{-6} [d]
Solubility in water (g m^{-3})	40 000[c]	41[f]	4[c]
Log K_{ow}	0.97[g]	2.99[h]	6.5[i]
Half-life in air (h)	200[j]	200[j]	200[j]
Half-life in water (h)	2 000[j]	2 000[j]	2 000[j]
Half-life in soil (h)	2 000[j]	2 000[j]	2 000[j]
Half-life in sediment (h)	20 000[j]	20 000[j]	20 000[j]

Note: Because of lack of property data, some values were assumed for comparison purposes.
[a] Parfitt (1999).
[b] Verschueren (1996).
[c] Budavari (1989).
[d] Assumed as low volatile.
[e] Assumed as slightly more volatile than cyclophosphamide and Ivermectin.
[f] Newton et al. (1981).
[g] Taken from Syracuse Research Corporation Database (http://esc-plaza.syrres.com).
[h] Hansch et al. (1995).
[i] Estimated with PALLAS 2.0 (CompuDrug Chemistry Ltd.,1994–95).
[j] Assumed half-lives.

As shown in the table, not all the data were available in the literature, therefore some assumptions were made for some of the physicochemical properties. The least frequently found data were vapour pressure together with half-lives in the main compartments. Considerable efforts should therefore be devoted to measurement and/or estimation of these properties for pharmaceuticals before reliable modelling exercises could be performed. The simulation shown later must therefore be considered as an attempt to show the probable behaviour in the environment of three pharmaceuticals.

Basically, Level I represents an environmental situation in which a fixed quantity of chemicals is introduced in a closed system under steady state and equilibrium conditions. The model calculates their partitioning among compartments. This gives an idea of the potential for distribution or more generally the "affinity" towards one or more environmental phases. The results of the Level I simulations for three chemicals (cyclophosphamide, diazepam and ivermectin) are shown in Fig. 10.2.

The six main compartments (air, water, soil, sediment, suspended sediment and fish) reach a different equilibrium for the selected chemicals: cyclophosphamide (Fig. 10.2a) will partition mainly into water (>99%), with negligible amounts in the other compartments, while diazepam (Fig. 10.2b) will concentrate almost equally in water and soil. The last chemical, ivermectin (Fig. 10.2c), reaches equilibrium with about 97% in soil. Level II shows the same percent distribution as in the Level I, but in this case the chemical is continuously discharged at a constant rate and achieves a steady state and equilibrium condition where input and output rates are equal. Degradation rates in

Fig. 10.2. Level I simulations for the selected pharmaceuticals; **a** cyclophosphamide; **b** diazepam; **c** ivermectin

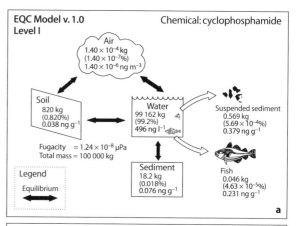

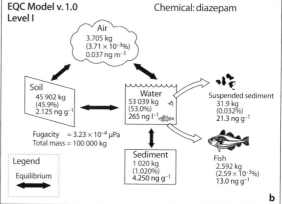

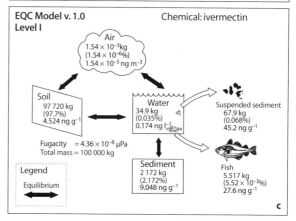

the compartments are calculated from half-life and advection by calculating the output rates through a fixed advection flow of air and water in the unit of world. Figure 10.3 reports the results for the Level II simulation of the chemicals chosen for the illustra-

Fig. 10.3. Level II simulations for the selected pharmaceuticals; **a** cyclophosphamide; **b** diazepam, **c** ivermectin

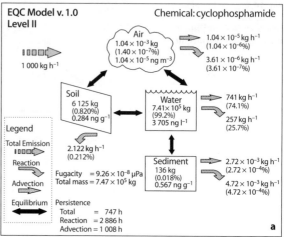

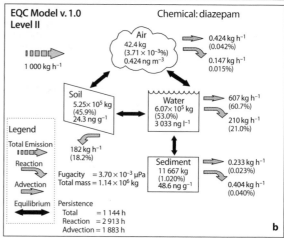

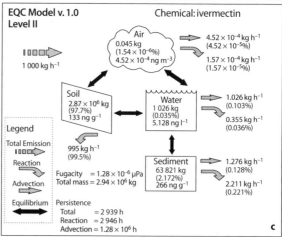

tion. The amounts at equilibrium are as in Level I, while the information obtained at this stage regards the most relevant phenomenon for the disappearance of the chemical from the environment. In fact, the most relevant disappearance mechanism for cyclophosphamide (Fig. 10.3a) is advection in water (74%, which is flow of water out of the environment), while for diazepam (Fig. 10.3b) three phenomena are relevant: advection and degradation in water (61% and 21% respectively) and degradation is soil (18%). For ivermectin (Fig. 10.3c), the only important disappearance phenomenon is degradation in soil, where most of the chemical is present.

Figures 10.4, 10.5 and 10.6 show Level III simulations for the selected chemicals. Since in Level III the user can select the media in which emission takes place, two scenarios were adopted for each chemical: the first is emission into water only (1 000 kg h^{-1}), while the second is into soil only (1 000 kg h^{-1}), to allow for direct discharge into the surface water compartment or the possible addition of the chemical as included into sewage sludge applied to soil. This last scenario was done to evaluate the extent of water contamination resulting from soil distribution of the investigated chemicals.

Level III simulations depict a steady-state application of chemicals in a typical non-equilibrium situation among compartments, due to the resistance of chemical transfer from one medium to another. Among the Levels outlined, Level III is the one more reflecting realistic conditions. Figure 10.4 shows Level III results for cyclophosphamide.

When the emission is into water (Fig. 10.4a), most of the chemical will be present there, and the most important disappearance phenomenon is advection in water. When initially applied to soil (Fig. 10.4b), about 68% of the chemical partitions in soil, while a certain amount will move towards the water compartment (about 650 kg h^{-1}) and then advect out of the water compartment. Practically no cyclophosphamide will move to the air phase.

The picture is slightly different for diazepam (Fig. 10.5). When discharged to water only (Fig. 10.5a), diazepam will concentrate in it, at steady state. The main removal mechanism is still advection in water. When discharged to soil (Fig. 10.5b), the situation changes dramatically: because of the resistance to transfer to other compartments, most of the chemical will stay in the soil environment, with moderate transfer to the water compartment. This clearly shows how different patterns of discharge can result in profoundly diverse distributions.

Ivermectin, when discharged to water (Fig. 10.6a), will substantially "escape" from it and reach the sediment compartment, in which the removal mechanisms are predominant: degradation (about 400 kg h^{-1}) and burial (230 kg h^{-1}). When discharged to soil (Fig. 10.6b), it will basically "stick" to it, degradation (1 000 kg h^{-1}) being the only removal mechanism.

The results of these sequences of Level I, II and III can show the general trend of the distribution behaviour in terms of percent distribution and most important removal phenomena.

10.4
Regional Model

Following the diagram depicted in Fig. 10.1 and the results outlined above, regional modelling represents the following stage in the strategy (Mackay et al. 1996a,c). The use of a regional model (for example the regional model ChemCAN) implies the collection of regional environmental data and the simulations in these regional scenarios.

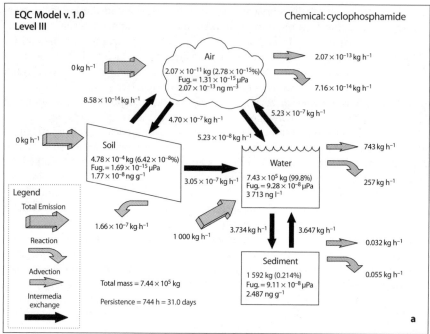

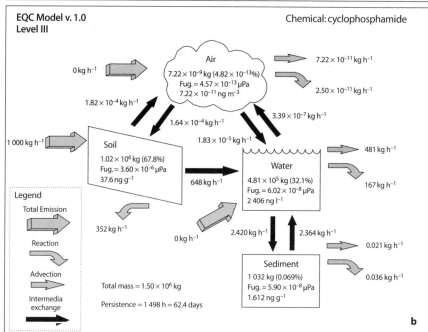

Fig. 10.4. Level III simulations for cyclophosphamide; **a** emission into water only; **b** emission into soil only

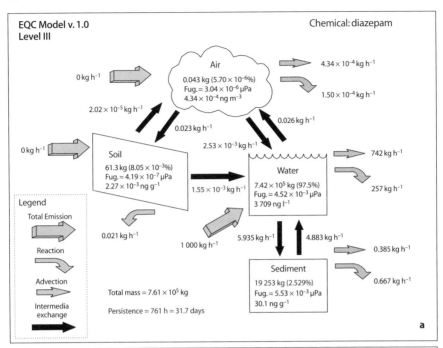

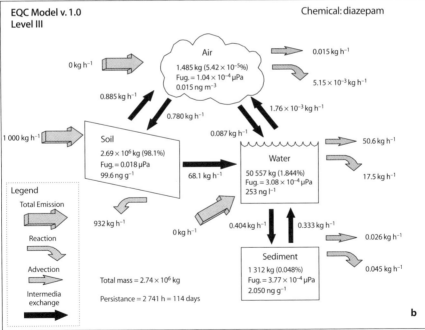

Fig. 10.5. Level III simulations for diazepam; **a** emission into water only; **b** emission into soil only

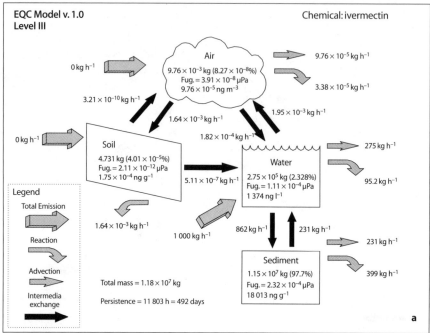

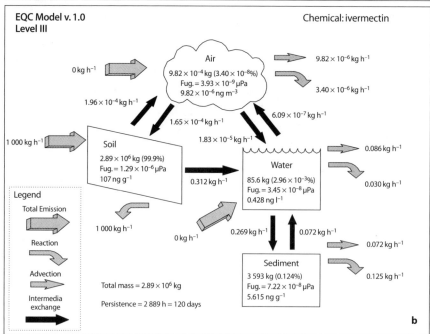

Fig. 10.6. Level III simulations for ivermectin; **a** emission into water only; **b** emission into soil only

The region in question could be, for example, Lombardy (Italy), for which approximate real use emission into the three main compartments can be employed. The results will be average estimates of concentrations in the different phases. The advantages of the use of a regional model are in the more realistic simulation of the area of interest, given the specific input data required (extent of soil and water compartments, depths, organic carbon composition of soil and sediment, average temperature etc.) and the pattern of distribution of the chemical in the environment, for example discharged to water or soil or both. A regional model gives realistic (order of magnitude) concentrations of the chemical in the main compartments. When better estimates of concentrations in a certain compartment are needed or when a regional evaluation shows that the major target for the distribution and fate of a chemical in the environment is a specific medium (e.g. soil or water), a site specific model can be employed, generally providing more accurate results.

10.5
Site Specific Models

When regional modelling exercises confirm that one medium (such as soil or water) is the environmental compartment that is relevant for the fate of a certain chemical, the use of a site specific model is required in order to predict its environmental concentrations with a satisfying level of accuracy. As an example we can cite the SoilFug (Di Guardo et al. 1994a) and FOCAS (Di Guardo et al. 2001) models, which can be used to evaluate chemical runoff from treated soil and the fate of amended- associated chemicals in soil respectively. Both models could theoretically be modified to be adapted to waste disposal sites or contaminated soils. The use of a such a local model requires that scenarios for simulations will comprise a detailed description of rain events, soil conditions etc.

Water compartment models, such as the QWASI models, can be used to calculate the fate, distribution and concentrations of chemicals in lakes and rivers (Mackay 1991). Again, these site specific models require a certain amount of additional environmental parameters in order to simulate the adopted scenario properly. In a number of cases the SoilFug model has been validated for research purposes (Di Guardo et al. 1994a,b; Barra et al. 1995) and in some cases utilised for risk assessment when analytical data were not available (Baldry et al. 1995; Calamari 1998).

10.6
Discussion and Conclusions

The general strategy outlined above can be utilised to assess the fate of pharmaceuticals in the environment. Some use-derived features may influence the fate of these compounds and in some cases disorient the assessor. For example, drugs emitted into water (through the sewer) will typically end up in sewage treatment plants, where they can be degraded to a larger extent and be transformed to metabolite products (with different chemical properties) or they can persist and largely reach the environment, still contained in water or in sewage sludge. An example of such a chemical is ibuprofen, which was measured in surface waters and wastewater treatment plant samples (Buser et al. 1999). When sludges are added to soil as amendments, they may release such chemicals into the soil environment, therefore reaching a different compartment from the one of entry. Some other chemicals may be persistent and not very mobile and therefore they can build up in a compartment such as soil and sediment. In these compartments they may exert effects on non target organisms and even return to human beings through the food chain.

A strategy for the understanding the fate and distribution of pharmaceuticals in the environment by using modelling approaches has been described.

Models can be invaluable tools to formerly describe and capture the mass balance of a chemical in the environment. It is suggested here that a strategy should start with a proper data collection, continue with generic scenario modelling to "grasp" the typical behaviour of a chemical in different discharge possibilities, proceed with a regional simulation that can provide information on the concentrations reached in the environment (given proper emissions), and eventually gain insight on the fate at a very detailed scale with a site specific modelling.

References

Baldry D, Calamari D, Yameogo L (1995) Environmental impact assessment of settlement and development in the Upper Leraba Basin: Burkina Faso, Cote d'Ivoire, and Mali. World Bank Technical Paper 302

Barra R, Vighi M, Di Guardo A (1995) Prediction of runoff of chloridazon and chlorpyrifos in an agricultural watershed in Chile. Chemosphere 30:485–500

Budavari S (ed) (1989) The Merck Index. An encyclopedia of chemicals, drugs and biologicals. Rahway, NJ, USA

Buser HR, Poiger T, Müller MD (1999) Occurrence and environmental behavior of the chiral pharmaceutical drug ibuprofen in surface waters and wastewater. Environ Sci Technol 33:2529–2535

Calamari D (ed) (1993) Chemical Exposure Predictions. Lewis Publishers Inc. Chelsea, MI, USA

Calamari D (1998) Initial environmental risk assessment of pesticides in the Batangas Bay Region, Philippines and the Xiamen Seas, China. GEF/UNDP/IMO and FAO. Manila, Philippines (Regional Programme for the Prevention and Management of East Asian Seas)

Cowan CE, Mackay D, Feijtel TCJ, Meent D van de, Di Guardo A, Davies J, Mackay N (1995) The multimedia fate model: a vital tool for predicting the fate of chemicals. SETAC Press, Pensacola, FL, USA

Di Guardo A, Calamari D, Zanin G, Consalter A, Mackay D (1994a) A fugacity model of pesticide runoff to surface water: development and validation. Chemosphere 28:511–531

Di Guardo A, Williams RJ, Matthiessen P, Brooke N, Calamari D (1994b) Simulation of pesticide runoff at rosemaund farm (UK) using the SoilFug model. Environ Sci Pollut Res 1:151–160

Di Guardo A, Mackay D, Cowan C (2001) Modelling the long-term fate of amended associated chemicals in soil with the FOCAS model. (in preparation)

Halling-Sørensen B, Nielsen SN, Lanzky PF, Ingerslev F, Holten Lützhøft HC, Jørgensen SE (1998) Occurrence, fate and effects of pharmaceutical substances in the environment – a review. Chemosphere 36:357–393

Hansch C, Leo A, Hoekman D (1995) Exploring QSAR. Hydrophobic, Electronic and Steric Constants. ACS Professional Reference Book, Washington DC

Mackay D (1991) Multimedia environmental models. The fugacity approach. Lewis Publishers Inc., Chelsea, MI, USA

Mackay D, Di Guardo A, Paterson S, Kicsi G, Cowan CE (1996a) Assessing the fate of new and existing chemicals: a five-stage process. Environ Toxicol Chem 15:1618–1626

Mackay D, Di Guardo A, Paterson S, Kicsi G, Cowan CE (1996b) Evaluating the environmental fate of a variety of types of chemicals using the EQC model. Environ Toxicol Chem 15:1627–1637

Mackay D, Di Guardo A, Paterson S, Kicsi G, Cowan CE, Kane DM (1996c) Assessment of chemical fate in the environment using evaluative, regional and local-scale models: illustrative application to chlorobenzene and linear alkylbenzene sulfonates. Environ Toxicol Chem 15:1638–1648

Newton DW, Driscoll DF, Goudreau JL, Ratanamaneichatara S (1981) Solubility characteristics of diazepam in aqueous and mixture solutions: theory and practice. Am J Hosp Pharm 38:179–182

Parfitt K (ed) (1999) Martindale. The complete drug reference, 32nd edn. Pharmaceutical Press, London

Verschueren K (1996) Handbook of environmental data on organic chemicals, 3rd edn. Van Nostrand Reinhold, New York

Part II
Risk Assessment

Chapter 11

Risk Assessment of Organic Xenobiotics in the Environment

P. Hartemann

11.1
Introduction

It seems appropriate to begin this paper with a brief presentation of some definitions that will clarify this discussion, taking into account the possible absence of background of some readers in risk assessment. These definitions will present the different steps necessary for performing risk assessment, the activity of collective expertise, and finally the role of risk managers which has to be perfectly differentiated from the assessment process.

Then the two classical approaches for risk assessment of organic xenobiotics in the environment will be presented: the global approach, the more general one trying to determine safe levels (threshold level), and the specific approach, appropriate for some very well defined situations for the evaluation of a probable effect for a given exposure. Examples of such approaches performed with pharmaceutical compounds released in the environment are very scarce, thus it is necessary to implement this way of research.

11.2
Definitions

What are "Risk" and "Hazard"?

Risk is defined as the probability that a substance or situation will produce harm under specified conditions. Risk is a combination of two factors:

a the probability that an adverse event will occur (such as a specific disease or type of injury),
b the consequences of the adverse event.

Risk encompasses impacts on public health and on the environment, and arises from exposure and hazard. Risk does not exist if exposure to a harmful substance or situation does not occur.

Hazard summarises the intrinsic stressor's characteristics (toxicity, physicochemical properties, degradability). Hazard is determined by whether a particular substance or situation has the potential to cause a harmful effect.

A *stressor* is any physical, chemical or biological entity that induces a change in the homeostasis of an environment. This term is broadly used for entities that cause primary effects and those primary effects that can cause secondary (i.e. indirect) effects. Stressors may be chemical (e.g. toxics or nutrients); physical (e.g. radiation, dams, fishing nets, or suspended sediments); or biological (e.g. exotic or genetically engineered organisms). While risk assessment is concerned with the characterisation of adverse responses, under some circumstances a stressor may be neutral or produce beneficial effects to certain ecological components.

What is "Exposure"?

Exposure is the contact or co-occurence of a stressor with a receptor (individual or population). Exposure applies to physical (e.g. radiations, heat, …) and biological (pathogens, …) stressors as well as to chemicals. Exposure is also applicable to higher levels of biological organisation, such as the exposure of a benthic community to dredging, or exposure of an owl population to habitat modification.

The receptor is the ecological component exposed to the stressor. This term may refer to tissues, organisms, populations, communities, and ecosystems.

Exposure characterisation consists of identifying contact between the stressor and one or several target species and quantifying the intensity of this contact (for a chemical stressor, this means a concentration in air, water, food, or even in an organ).

A *source* is an entity or action that releases to the environment or imposes on the environment a chemical, physical, or biological stressor or stressors. Sources may include a waste treatment plant, a former chemical or military installation, a pesticide application, a logging operation, introduction of exotic organisms, or a dredging project.

Some changes caused by stressors may be hazardous for human or animal health. Events that disrupt ecosystems, community, or population structure may, in fact, change resource and substrate availability. A physical environment may also be altered after the introduction of a stressor.

What is "Risk Assessment?"

Risk assessment is an activity performed by federal agencies for the past two or three decades, depending on the country. This activity is derived from further setting of threshold limit values for workers and acceptable daily intakes for dietary pesticide residues and food additives and application to different kinds of hazards for human health. According to different scenarios of exposure, and taking into account predictable effects, Federal agencies like the FDA and EPA in the US used some models to develop assessment strategies. According to the framework developed both by the US EPA and National Research Council, environmental risk assessment is composed of three main phases (Fig. 11.1):

a Problem formulation:
   Formal process for generating and evaluating preliminary hypotheses about ecological effects. Management goals are evaluated to establish objectives and a conceptual model. The plan for collecting and analysing data and characterising risk is determined.
b Risk analysis:
   Data collection and evaluation in terms of ecological exposure and the relationships between a stressor and ecological effects. This phase is composed of two principal activities: characterisation of exposure, characterisation of effects.
c Risk characterisation:
   Final phase in which analysis risk results are interpreted to estimate risk to individuals or populations identified.

Fig. 11.1. Framework proposed by US EPA for environmental risk assessment (Risk Assessment Forum US EPA 1996)

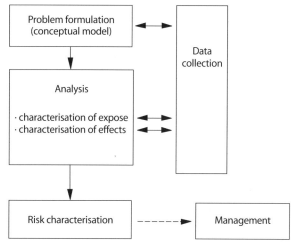

The first step of a risk assessment, the design of a conceptual model, includes three parts: *(a)* a contamination (diffusion) model, which summarises the main physico-chemical (environmental) changes due to the presence of the stressor (source), *(b)* an effect model, which describes the possible effects of the stressor on living organisms, and *(c)* an exposure model. Conceptual models must account for spatial and temporal boundaries. They should also be flexible enough to allow a set of working hypotheses.

Risk assessments are constrained by the availability of data, scientific understanding and financial resources. Because of these constraints, it is vitally important that risk managers and risk assessors discuss the nature of the assessment, including available resources; opportunities for increasing the resource base; and the output that will provide the best information for the required decision-making.

Part of the complexity of risk assessment is due to uncertainty. Part of the risk assessment process includes identifying various sources of uncertainty and then quantifying that uncertainty. The level of acceptable uncertainty dictates the nature of the risk assessment. For instance, the lower the level of acceptable uncertainty, the greater the scope and complexity needed in the risk assessment. Risk assessments completed in response to legal mandates may be challenged in court, and therefore require rigorous attention to acceptable levels of uncertainty to ensure that the assessment will be used for decision-making. Risk assessments should be iterative in nature and include explicitly defined steps. These steps may take the form of "tiers" that represent increasing levels of complexity and investment, with each tier designed to reduce uncertainty. The plan may include an explicit definition of iterative steps with a description of levels of investment and decision criteria for each tier.

What is "Ecological or Environmental Risk Assessment"?

Ecological risk assessment estimates risks that may result from events in the environment (air, water and soil) when xenobiotics are added to soil, and organisms living in and near the soil are exposed. This exposure may cause both physical and chemical changes to the fauna and flora living and near the soil.

What is "Risk Management"?

Risk management is the process of identifying, evaluating, selecting, and implementing policy actions to reduce risk. These actions must be scientifically-sound yet cost-effective, and they should be considered for social, cultural, ethical, political, and legal constraints. For instance, risk managers should consider the economic, social, cultural, ethical, legal, and political implications associated with implementing each option, as well as any worker health, community health, or ecological hazards the options may cause. Likewise, laws or procedures hinder risk managers from considering those implications and impacts.

During the traditional risk management process, decision-makers (typically government officials and other risk managers) gather information about a situation posing a risk to human health or an ecosystem's stability. Air pollution, water and soil pollution, workplace exposures, or the introduction of new pharmaceutical or consumer products are examples of situations that could pose risks to humans and ecosystems. Risk managers use this information they have gathered to consider the:

- nature and magnitude of risks,
- need for reducing or eliminating the risks,
- effectiveness and costs of options for reducing the risks.

Risk management has been defined in the US Presidential and Congressional Commission on Risk Assessment and Risk Management (Presidential/Congressional Commission on Risk Assessment and Risk Management 1997). This framework for environmental health risk management has six stages (Fig. 11.2):

Fig. 11.2. Framework proposed by US Presidential and Congressional Commission for risk management (Presidential/Congressional Commission on Risk Assessment and Risk Management 1997)

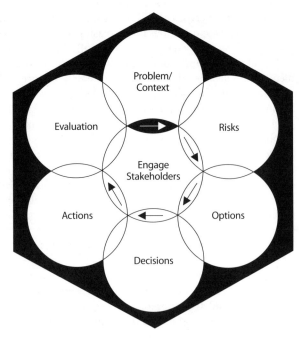

- define the problem and put it in context,
- analyse the risks associated with the problem in context,
- examine options for addressing the risks,
- make decisions about which options to implement,
- take actions to implement the decision,
- conduct an evaluation of the actions.

The Framework is conducted:

- in collaboration with stakeholders,
- using iterations if new information is developed that changes the need for or nature of risk management.

11.3
Global Approach

This approach identifies a target species, determines a species specific no observed effect level (NOEL), and then determines the corresponding level of contamination in environment.

11.3.1
Assessment Endpoints

Measurement endpoints are quantities such as LC_{50} values or diversity indices measured by toxicologists or field biologists. Some of these values may be generically defined (e.g. water-quality criteria) for use in standardised assessments; others are defined and measured on an assessment-specific basis.

Since endpoints may refer to characteristics of populations and ecosystems defined over fairly large spatial scales and long time periods, it may be impractical to directly measure changes in these characteristics as part of an assessment. In many cases (e.g. pesticide registration and new chemical review), an assessment must be made before any large-scale release can be allowed to occur. Thus, some form of extrapolation based on expert judgement, statistical methods, or simulation models is usually required to link the measurement endpoints to assessment endpoints. Assessment endpoints are generally connected to levels of biological organisation above the individual organism and measurement endpoints are frequently set at the level of individuals. Therefore, effects on individuals usually need to be aggregated or extrapolated to infer effects on population or ecosystem-level assessment endpoints.

Assessment endpoints are critical to problem formulation because they link the risk assessment to management concerns, and they are central to conceptual model development. They are "explicit expressions of the actual environmental value that is to be protected" according to the US EPA.

Three principal criteria are used when selecting assessment endpoint:

- ecological relevance,
- susceptibility to the known or potential stressors,
- represention of a form of management goals.

Ecologically relevant endpoints reflect important characteristics of the system and are functionally related to other endpoints. They may reflect information about the food base (e.g. primary production); habitat; regeneration of critical resources (e.g. decomposition or nutrient cycling); or the structure of the community and ecosystem. Ecological relevance becomes most important when there are potential cascading effects. This could result from the loss or reduction of one or more species or when human health is endangered through the food chain.

Susceptibility refers to how readily an ecological entity is affected. It is directly related to the mode of action of the stressors. Sensitivity may be related to the life stage of an organism such as juvenile animals, which are frequently more sensitive than adults. Species with long life cycles and low reproductive rates will be more vulnerable to extinction from increases in mortality than those with short life cycles and high reproductive rates. Measurement of sensitivity may include mortality or morbidity; reproductive effects from exposure to toxins; or behavioural abnormalities. *Exposure* (frequency, duration and intensity) is another determinant of susceptibility, since exposure may occur during sensitive life stages of the organism. Delayed and chronic effects as well as multiple-stressor exposures add complexity to evaluations of susceptibility, and conceptual models need to reflect these factors.

During the development of a conceptual model for ecological risk assessment, the following questions must be addressed:

- What ecological entities are affected?
- What is the nature of the effect(s)?
- What is the intensity of the effect(s)?
- Where appropriate, what is the time scale for recovery?
- What causal information links the stressor with any observed effects?
- How do changes in measures of effects relate to changes in assessment end points?
- What is the uncertainty associated with the analysis?

11.3.2
Determination of Exposures and Effects

The data used for exposure assessment may come from laboratory or fields studies, or may be produced as output from a model. Field surveys may be more representative of both exposures and effects, however, because conditions are not controlled; field data variability and uncertainty may be higher than are estimates generated from laboratory studies or theoretical models.

Several indices are used to evaluate effects:

- biomarkers
- toxicity bioassays
- mesocosms studies (or multiple species bioassays)
- field studies (population measurements, index of biotic integrity)

It is also possible to evaluate the toxicity of new chemicals using structure-activity relationships (SARs) (Auer et al. 1994) or with more advanced applications the quantitative structure-activity relationship (QSARs) (Lipnic 1995).

The determination and characterisation of *exposure* is based on measures of the stressor and its metabolites in environment, as well as the extent and pattern of contact or co-occurrence with the receptor. The primary objectives of exposure assessment are to characterise the source, type, magnitude, and duration of contact with the xenobiotic in terms of its spatial and temporal distribution stressors that come in contact with individuals and populations via pathways (for environmentally-transported processus) and routes (for biologically-transported processes). For xenobiotics in soil, pathway assessment includes evaluating chemical concentration in various media pathways. Analysis must also account for physicochemical properties such as solubility, vapour pressure, and hydrophobicity. Secondary stressors can be formed through biotic or abiotic transformation processes, and may be more or less toxic than the primary one. Therefore, it is necessary to measure concentrations of metabolites or degradation products as well as the chemical itself.

Exposure is a function of the a stressor concentration and behaviour. Exposure is estimated from the total potential dose, which is the amount available to an organism from all exposure pathways (e.g. ingestion, inhalation, absorption). *Uptake* is a term used when considering the amount of the stressor that is internally incorporated into an organism. Uptake is a function of the stressor (e.g. chemical structure and valence state); the medium (e.g. sorptive properties); the biological membrane (e.g. integrity, permeability); and the organism (e.g. age, sickness, active uptake) (Suter et al. 1994). Because of interactions among these four factors, uptake will vary on a case specific basis. Biomarkers and tissue residues can not only provide valuable evidence that exposure has occurred, but also they can help estimate internal dose.

The conceptual model of exposure must include both exposure scenarios and exposure pathways. The principal products of the conceptual model include

- a set of risk hypotheses that describe predicted relationships between stressor(s), exposure and assessment endpoint (target) response, along with the rationale for their selection.
- a diagram that illustrates the relationships presented in the risk hypotheses.

It is clear from this discussion that given the types of data available and the uncertainty associated with the assessment techniques for xenobiotics in the environment and in organisms, there will be high amounts of variability associated with any type of risk assessment. Variability can be described by using a distribution, for example, cumulative-distribution functions (CDFs) and probability-density functions (PDFs) as:

a   qualitative categories such as low, medium, or high,
b   single points estimates of exposure and effects (exposure concentration divided by an effects concentration),
c   stressor-response relationships,
d   variability in exposure and effects estimates,
e   process models,
f   empirical approaches including field data.

Another important aspect of the risk assessment process is determining which stressor-response relationship should be needed.

The stressor-response relationships used depends on the scope and nature of the risk assessment as defined in problem formulation. The choice of stressor response relationship is important because it is widely used a point estimate of on *effect* such as:

- median effects: expressed in terms of median effects concentration or lethality known as LC_{50} (in the diet or in water), LD_{50} (mg kg^{-1}), or in terms of median effects concentrations for growth (EC_{50} or ED_{50});
- no effect: expressed in terms of highest concentration for which effects are not statistically different from the controls (NOAEC: no observed adverse effect concentration) or lowest concentrations at which effects were statistically significant from the control (LOAEC: lowest observed adverse effect concentration). The range between the NOAEC and the LOAEC is sometimes called the maximum acceptable toxicant concentration (MATC).

The determination of the NOEC is based on "worst-case" conditions, that is, conditions minimising interactions, or interferences, and maximising exposure of target species. To make the assessment more realistic, these worst-case scenarios may be adapted by focusing on case-specific data.

11.3.3
Determination of Acceptable Level in Environment – Example of an Application: Determination of Safe Levels for PAHs in Urban Sewage Sludges

Polycyclic aromatic hydrocarbons (PAHs) are present in sewage sludges. Many of these are carcinogens, others are possibly carcinogenic, genotoxic, or insufficiently characterised. PAHs may occur in sewage sludges from direct discharge or road run-off. Many PAHs are hydrophobic, and therefore they are strongly sorbed onto solid particles in the different stages of the wastewater treatment plant process. Almost all urban sludges contain various levels of PAHs, but it is unclear whether PAHs in sludge is safe in terms of soil fertility, terrestrial ecosystem, or human health stability.

There are many PAHs, but this example will focus on those included in the Borneff's series: fluoranthene, benzo(b)- and benzo(k)fluoranthene, benzo(a)pyrene, benzo-(ghi)perylene, indeno-pyrene (Table 11.1). This example comes from a research project (Agence de l'Eau Rhin Meuse 1996), which was designed to determine safe levels for (organic) xenobiotics in sewage sludges. Funding was provided by the six French Water Agencies, and the work was done by a team including private consultants and 2 departments of the Ecole Polytechnique Fédérale de Lausanne.

11.3.3.1
Conceptual Model

The *dissemination* model includes six compartments (Fig. 11.3) including *soil* (microflora, -fauna), *plants, fauna, humans, groundwater,* and *surface water.* All compartments may be affected through various transfers by sludge components. Obviously, this representation is a simplification. For example, annual plants are decomposed by the soil microflora, but that process is not included in the model, and therefore planned decomposition via soil microflora may be underestimated.

Table 11.1. Borneff's series of PAH

Name	CAS number	Formula	LogK_{ow}
Fluoranthene	206-44-0	C_{16}-H_{10}	5.20
Benzo(b)fluoranthene	205-99-2	C_{20}-H_{12}	6.57
Benzo(k)fluoranthene	207-08-9	C_{20}-H_{12}	6.84
Benzo(a)pyrene	50-32-8	C_{20}-H_{12}	6.35
Benzo(ghi)perylene	191-24-2	C_{22}-H_{12}	6.90
Indeno-pyrene	193-39-5	C_{22}-H_{12}	7.66

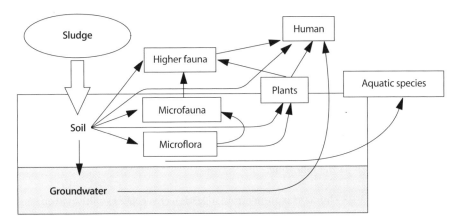

Fig. 11.3. Dissemination model of PAHs

For this particular risk assessment, each compartment was assigned a "quality ob-jective" (goal) (Table 11.2). Since safe levels must be relevant at a very large scale, these goals are rather broad and vague. In a site-specific assessment, they should be defined more accurately.

For each compartment, the assessment is based first on a "worst-case" approach. In a further step, the assessment can be refined on a more realistic basis, either for one of or all the compartments. The "quality objective" is first converted to an "assessment endpoint" (parameter(s) and associated value(s) that allow examination of the goal). Then a worst-case scenario is described; there is an assumption that all or most of the xenobiotic is bioavailable to the target species, and thus, this amount represents the assessment endpoint). The determination of a "PNEC" (probable no-effect concentra-tion of the xenobiotic in the considered compartment) is made using conservative hypotheses for xenobiotic transfer and degradation; using these conservative hypoth-eses it is then possible to calculate the corresponding concentration in the sludge.

The assessment endpoints for the different compartments are summarised in Table 11.3. When this risk assessment was performed, human health was of primary concern, and therefore, further discussion will focus on the human health compart-

Table 11.2. Quality objectives for the selected compartments

Compartment	Objectives
Soil	No long-term adverse effect on soil fertility should occur
Plants	No long-term adverse effect should occur
Fauna	No long-term adverse effect should occur, including bioconcentration and biomagnification
Human	No long-term adverse effect should occur, including bioconcentration and biomagnification
Groundwater	No impact (water should remain drinkable without additional treatment)
Surface water	No impact (water should remain drinkable without additional treatment, and there should be no impact on aquatic ecosystems)

ment. However, although the aspects of the results would be different, the procedure would be simpler for any of the compartments.

11.3.3.2
Human Health

According to the conceptual model, four pathways of exposure should be considered as presented in Fig. 11.4 (*dark lines*). The exposure pathways after sewage sludge has been applied include the following:

- Soil $\longrightarrow$ plant $\longrightarrow$ human: exposure from ingestion of vegetables cultivated on land treated with sludge.
- Soil $\longrightarrow$ plant $\longrightarrow$ animal $\longrightarrow$ human: exposure from ingestion of meat, animal products (from animals raised with plants cultivated on sludge-treated land).
- Soil $\longrightarrow$ animal $\longrightarrow$ human: exposure from ingestion of meat, animal products, from animals raised on sludge-treated pasture lands.
- Soil $\longrightarrow$ human: direct ingestion of soil (mainly a pathway for children).

Of these identified pathways, two were characterised as primary pathways and the other two secondary. Secondary pathways include those in which humans were exposed via livestock. These pathways were judged to be less important, because animals are able to metabolise PAHs in the liver, and therefore they have not been found to accumulate PAHs. Therefore, the (soil $\longrightarrow$ plant $\longrightarrow$ human) and the (soil $\longrightarrow$ man) pathways were used as the primary focus of the study.

For this study, the chosen end point for PAHs was carcinogenicity (gastric tumours). As in most risk assessments, there is a lack of relevant data about the lifetime risk dose for most PAHs. Of the xenobiotics in this study, benzo(a)pyrene was found to have the most reliable value for lifetime risk dose, which was reported as 20 ng kg^{-1} d^{-1}, and corresponds to a 10^{-6} additional risk. This value means there will be one additional case of cancer in 10^{-6} persons among those exposed over their lifetimes, assuming exposure from the two primary pathways mentioned above. Any lifetime risk dose found

Table 11.3. Assessment endpoints for the selected compartments

Compartment	Relevant species	Parameters or effects
Soil: a) Microflora	–	Respiration (14–90 days); nitrogen assimilation (non-symbiotic assimilation excluded); intra-cellular enzymatic activities; etc.
b) Microfauna	Earthworms; insects etc.	Survival, growth
Plants	Cultivated species; species used in standardised bioassays	Germination, growth, root-elongation, …
Fauna	Mammals (herbivorous), rodents...	Survival, growth
Human	–	Survival, metabolism, carcinogenicity
Groundwater	–	Maximum allowable levels for drinking water
Surface water	Algae, crustaceans, fish	Survival, growth, reproduction, or maximum allowable levels for drinking water

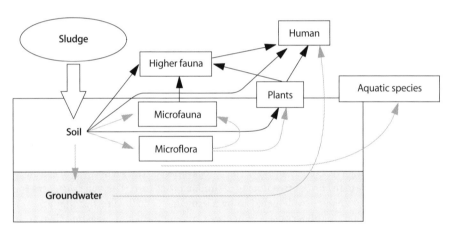

Fig. 11.4. Pathways of exposure of PAHs for human health risk assessment from field application of sewage sludge

above this value would be unacceptable. It is clear from the discussion above that there are very large safety margins incorporated into the calculation and estimation.

The next step in the risk assessment process includes making some assumptions about the individual exposed to the xenobiotic. With these assumptions, it is then possible to illustrate how risk assessors calculate lifetime risk dose (or limit values). The first assumption is that an average adult weighs 70 kg. The next assumption is the individual's diet, including: 20% of the daily ingested benzo(a)pyrene originates other from sources than diet; this diet equals 500 g (dry weight) of food per day, which includes, as usually considered, 65% vegetables. With these assumptions, it is possible to calculate the concentration of benzo(a)pyrene corresponding to the lifetime risk dose:

- Total daily intake (human) of benzo(a)pyrene:

$$0.02 \times 70 = 1.4 \ \mu g \, d^{-1} \tag{11.1}$$

- Total dietary daily intake of benzo(a)pyrene:

$$1.4 \times 0.8 = 1.1 \ \mu g \, d^{-1} \tag{11.2}$$

- Concentration of benzo(a)pyrene in vegetables:

$$\frac{1.1}{0.65 \times 0.5} = 3.38 \ \mu g \, d^{-1} \tag{11.3}$$

Using the value of vegetable concentration above, it is then possible to calculate a concentration in soil using a bioconcentration factor (BCF). The selection of a BCF depends on the focus of the assessment. In this case, since the protection of human health is the focus, the BCF should be conservatively high (within limits of reliability). For PAHs, the highest BCFs are 1.2 (fluoranthene) and 0.6 (other PAHs) representing bioconcentration in carrots from uptake in soil.
Concentration of benzo(a)pyrene in soil is

$$\frac{3.38 \ \mu g \, kg^{-1}}{0.6} = 6 \ \mu g \, kg^{-1} \tag{11.4}$$

This corresponds to a sludge concentration of 0.6 mg kg^{-1} considering a dilution factor of the sludge in the soil of 10^{-2}. The calcuations for the second exposure pathway (soil $\longrightarrow$ human) are derived using a similar procedure. The soil concentration of PAH for this pathway is calculated to be 2.5 mg kg^{-1}, which signifies that an individual may be more highly exposed to benzo(a)pyrene from soil ingestion than from diet. Also, for this risk assessment it is assumed that benzo(a)pyrene concentrations less than 0.4 mg kg^{-1} are "safe".
For a value of lifetime risk dose, 0.6 mg kg^{-1} in the sludge is considered by risk assessors as reliable, because the data used are considered to be reliable and because of safety factors, it is considered to be protective. At each step of the procedure the most restricting values were selected.
For the five other PAHs, it was necessary to derive the lifetime risk dose in the sludge by extrapolation, because no reliable values are available. The extrapolation is based on the comparison of the respective toxicities to that of benzo(a)-pyrene (Table 11.4)
Finally, adjustments can be made to the limiting values in order to take into account environmental factors. For instance, in this risk assessment it was found that PAHs strongly adsorb onto soil and sludge particles. Therefore, risk assessors decide to apply an adjustment factor, and the final values were doubled (thus, the limit value became 1.2 mg kg^{-1} for benzo(a)pyrene rather than 0.6 mg kg^{-1}).

Table 11.4. Limit values (worst-case) for 6 PAHs using human health pathways described in Fig. 11.4

Name	Ratio (respective toxicities)	BFC	Limit value (sludge, mg kg^{-1})
Fluoranthene	0.06	1.2	2.0
Benzo(b)fluoranthene	0.14	0.6	0.4
Benzo(k)fluoranthene	0.10	0.6	0.6
Benzo(a)pyrene	1.00	0.6	0.6
Benzo(ghi)perylene	0.03	0.6	2.0
Indeno-pyrene	0.23	0.6	0.3

This procedure appears to be rather arbitrary. However, risk assessors are confined because they are required to evaluate regional or national safety levels. It is unrealistic to place limiting values on every case, since adequate data does not exist. Many risk assessments are now being conducted with distributions of values (for diet, toxicity, etc.), but this type of study requires very large sets of data, many of which are still unavailable. Furthermore, these approaches are very complex, mathematically. Although most scientists agree that this approach is more scientifically valid than calculations of point toxicities, it is not clear that estimates for many individuals wouldn't be similar using the two different methods. Given the goal of risk assessors, which is to provide a practical tool to discriminate between safe and unsafe sludges, the procedure followed here appears to be adequate.

11.4
Specific Approach

For this example, instead of trying to determine safe levels (threshold level), the aim of this section will be to evaluate a probable effect for a given exposure. This second approach is based on the same concepts as the first example, but used in a different way. As in the previous section, this approach will consist of four main parts including: *(a)* identification of target species, *(b)* description of the stressor's effects on these species, *(c)* description of the stressor's fate, *(d)* exposure characterisation. This type of procedure will be more convenient for existing situations (brownfields, landfills), and will allow the setting of priorities or the comparison of remediation scenarios. Nevertheless, procedures such as these are rather complex and expansive, because the analysis needed is case by case based. In some cases, the analysis could be limited to hazard assessment, without characterisation of exposure.

Hazard assessment includes three terms: source description, fate assessment, and effects assessment. The first one implies analytical techniques (GC/MS, or /ECD etc.). The fate of the contaminants associated with the matrix under study (soil, sludge or waste) may be assessed through lixiviation and degradation protocols. Effects are measured with toxicity bioassays. There is a need for improving both fate assessment methods and ecotoxicity bioassays because of a lack of standardised protocols, and sometimes even a lack of relevant methods.

Another consideration of the risk assessment process is the method used for aggregating the results. Many studies have shown various mathematical methods for manipulating risk evaluation data. However, the (ecological and health) relevance of these models should be addressed more thoroughly before mathematical solutions are considered to be as important or reliable as other risk management techniques. These methods of analysis should probably be considered as tools for qualitative priority setting rather than quantitative safe level setting. This corresponds well with a need for classification, as mentioned above. However, this type of approach might be helpful for actual problems with contaminated sites, toxic wastes, or sludges.

The example of paper mill effluents on the quality of the Nancy drinking water is presented here as a case study for illustrating the principles discussed above. This part of the study might be interpreted as a preliminary risk assessment. When the results showed sufficient agreement between all parts, risk assessors decided to conclude the study to maintain controls and vigilance and to limit the expenses after this preliminary approach.

The previous environmental impact study predicted only limited effects of the effluents of a new paper mill on the quality of the Moselle River. This was because of wastewater treatment and elimination of previously-discharged DOC in the river from different factories and communities. But this first environmental impact assessment did not take into account the use of the river for drinking water for the French city Nancy (350 000 inhabitants) located approximately 70 km downstream. One possible effect that was not considered was chlorination by-product formation through the substitution of biologically-degradable carbon by less biodegradable carbon sources.

In this study the identification of target species was straightforward. Humans were assumed to be affected by drinking water containing halogenated compounds such as trihalomethanes (THMs) or chlorophenols. The descriptions of effects for these compounds were taken from extensive literature surveys. The literature showed two main concerns from these compounds in drinking water, including carcinogenesis and mutagenesis.

Source Description

The new paper mill is situated near the town of Golbey, which lies on the Moselle River. An investigation program was initiated in 1991 during construction of the mill. For this paper mill the industrial process does not include conventional bleaching with chlorine or chlorine dioxide, which produces high quantities of halogenated compounds, but instead the mill uses a new bleaching process with ozone, that decreases pollution.

The first phase of production included only one machine with a capacity of 850 t d^{-1}. Three other machines were planned after the first one was operational. The wastewater treatment plant included primary and secondary biological stages. There was a final clarification objective of 90 to 95% BOD, COD and SM elimination. Thus, the plant did not rejected halogenated compounds. The plant did reject, however, "hard" organic carbon compounds resistant to biological degradation that entered the flow of the Moselle River. The strong temporal variability in water flow (4 to 128 m^3 s^{-1}, mean value 35 m^3 s^{-1}) implies that the paper mill effluent concentrations are highly variable in terms of the conditions investigated. These conditions were selected to reflect minimal dilution and negligible degradation of organic matter in the river. Before operations, the river water quality was in the Category A2 of the European regulations (Communauté Européenne 1975) containing (mean values): 0.45 mg l^{-1} NH$_4$; 9.5 mg l^{-1} suspended matter; 4 mg l^{-1} DOC (ranging from 2–17 mg l^{-1}); and 0.4 mg l^{-1} total organic carbon (TOC). This amount of organic matter allowed a potential of trihalomethane formation (pTHM) of 60 µg l^{-1}.

Fate Assessment

The possible impact of the Golbey mill effluents on the Nancy drinking water is a combined effect of several factors:

- the amount and composition of the effluent,
- the dilution, retention and transformation of organic matter in the Moselle River,
- the interaction between raw water quality and treatment processes at the waterworks of Nancy.

For the experimental study, effluents from a Scandinavian paper mill with similar expected production of the proposed Golbey mill were used. The chemical parameters sampled in the Moselle River did not indicate retention or transformation products within 70 km downstream. Thus, only dilution was taken into account. The study was designed to estimate the combined effect of a high effluent concentration and an organic matter background concentration. This refers to a situation with minimum river water flow and typical discharge from the paper mill. The dilution factors were determined in such a way that the TOC values of the river water samples increased with 1, 4 and 10 mg l^{-1} respectively. These samples were used for chemical analysis (TOC; AOX; EOX; POX; THMs; pTHMs, chlorophenols and gas-phase chromatography, and mass spectrometry GC/MS). Mutagenicity testing (Ames test) was performed before, during, and after laboratory production of drinking water.

The waterworks in Nancy is located approximately 10 km from the raw water intake of the Moselle River. As a first treatment, water is pre-chlorinated to the breakpoint and transported to the waterworks through two aqueducts with a residence time of about 4 hours. At the waterworks, the treatment includes alum coagulation and sedimentation, sand filtration, ozonation, CAG filtration, and postchlorination. Thus pilot plants at laboratory scale were used for simulation of treatment. These preliminary results confirmed that laboratory contaminant concentrations in reproduced drinking water corresponded to actual drinking water samples measures at the treatment plant.

TOC reduction was approximately 50%. The increase of the AOX value was most pronounced for samples with high concentration of paper mill effluents. When the compound concentrations were measured with a GC, the values were considerably larger, along with higher chlorine doses. When the raw water was more charged, it was sometime necessary to use as much as 9 mg l^{-1} of chlorine for prechlorination at the waterworks. The combined impact of simultaneous increase in chlorine dose and concentration of organic matter is significant, especially for AOX, THMs and 2,4,6-trichlorophenol concentrations.

In conclusion, the results of the chlorination by-products study showed that under normal flow conditions in the Moselle River, effluents from the Golbey mill will have a very small impact. A low dilution factor resulted in elevated concentrations of AOX and certain specific organohalogens such as chloroform (until 120 μg l^{-1}), which had a maximal concentration of 120 μg l^{-1}.

Effects Assessment

Since the formation of chloroform during water chlorination was discovered in the mid 1970s, the potential health effects of chlorination by-products has achieved considerable attention.

The three major areas of study have included:

1. epidemiological studies of cancer rates in relation to exposure to chlorinated drinking water,
2. whole animal bioassays of the genotoxicity of specific compounds identified in chlorinated drinking water,
3. short-term bioassays of mutagenic activity of complex mixtures of chlorination by-products.

Among the compounds found during this study, only chloroform and 2,4,6-trichlorophenol have been quantitatively assessed (in 1991) for possible human carcinogenicity. A 10^{-6} life time cancer risk was estimated for a concentration of 20 μg l^{-1} for both chloroform and 2,4,6-trichlorophenol, and at this point most countries have defined a maximum admissible chloroform concentration between 10 μg l^{-1} and 100 μg l^{-1}.

Chloroform concentrations of 50 μg l^{-1} have sometimes occurred in the Nancy drinking water. The formation of 2,4,6-trichlorophenol was very limited and at this concentration. The only possible effect is the methylation to 2,4,6-trichloroanisol in the distribution system, which changes the taste of the water. Thus, it was decided to limit the TOC concentration in the water after clarification, corresponding to a level of 6–7 mg l^{-1} in the raw water. Legal standards were taken for the limitation of discharge from paper mills at this level of concentration.

A tertiary physicochemical process was added to the treatment at the wastewater plant, effluent in the Moselle River was monitored for concentrations of TOC, and a new clarification and filtration plant was installed adjacent to the raw water intake, decreasing the need for prechlorination and allowing transportation of clear water to the waterworks located 12 km away.

These changes were adopted to limit chloroform concentration to 30 μg l^{-1} at any point of the distribution networks.

11.5
Conclusion: Application to Pharmaceuticals

Risk assessment is a useful analytic process that provides valuable contributions to risk management, public health, and environmental policy decisions. Risk assessment was developed because politicians, regulators, and the public require scientists to go beyond scientific observations of relationships between exposures to chemicals and pollutants and their effects on people, the environment, or test systems. Risk assessors as scientists must rely on scientific inferences and assumptions to evaluate and estimate risk. When judgements regarding a chemical's toxicity to humans are unresolved, however, sophisticated and complex risk assessments cannot substitute for basic ignorance about the chemical's toxicity to humans.

Ecological risk assessment is even less understood than human health risk assessment. Furthermore, a significant amount of research is needed to validate and improve the risk assessment process itself; the quantification and prediction of the biological effects (aquatic and terrestrial toxicology); and to better understand the behaviour of toxic chemicals in the environment (chemistry, fate, and modelling). Therefore, risk assessment of pharmaceuticals in the environment is only in the infancy stage, and there are only a few examples throughout Europe. Their toxicity for humans are well-known; this is fatally different for their impact on environment.

Of course the situation is very difficult in the field of ecological risk assessment, because at present there is a very limited data base for comparative biochemistry and physiology of most non-mammalian organisms of ecotoxicological concern. Predicting ecosystem effects from environmental residues means accounting for biotic and abiotic processes as well as transport and transformation of the pharmaceuticals. As an example, we have absolutely no information about the degradation of antibiotics and disinfectants in wastewaters and their potential impact on the development of resistant microorganisms. There is some information about the possible transfer of plasmidic resistance between bacteria during biological treatment processes. But data on the influence of selective pressure through the presence of residues are very scarce. There are also some reports on the effect of molecules acting as endocrine disrupters on fish or other organisms in polluted waters, but no real knowledge of the phenomenon. Thus, a new field is now open, and it seems necessary to produce new concepts for pharmaceuticals taking into account their fate in the environment and ecological risk assessment.

References

Agence de l'Eau Rhin Meuse (1996) Détermination de valeurs seuil pour les micropolluants organiques dans les boues d'épuration. AERM (ed), Metz (vol I: Méthodologie, vol II: APS)

Auer CM, Zeeman M, Nabholz JV, Clements RG (1994) SAR. The US regulatory perspective. SAR QSAR Environ Res 2:21–38

Communauté Européenne (1975) Directive concernant la qualité requise des eaux superficielles destinées à la production d'eau alimentaire dans les états membres. J.O. CEE L 194/26 à L 194/31 du 25.07.1975

Lipnic RL (1995) Structure activity relationships. In: Rand GM, Retrocelli SR (eds) Fundamentals of aquatic toxicology. Taylor & Francis, London, pp 609–655

Presidential/Congressional Commission on Risk Assessment and Risk Management (1997) Framework for environmental health risk management. Final Report

Risk Assessment Forum US EPA (1996) Proposed guidelines for ecological risk assessment. US EPA, Washington DC (US EPA/630/R-95/002B)

Suter GW, Gillet JW, Norton SB (1994) Issue paper on characterization of exposure. In: Risk Assessment Forum US EPA (ed) Ecological risk assessment issue paper. US EPA, Washington DC (US EPA/630/R-94/009)

Chapter 12

Ecotoxicological Evaluation of Pharmaceuticals

J. Römbke · T. Knacker · H. Teichmann

12.1
Introduction

From an ecotoxicological point of view, pharmaceuticals were not considered to be a problem until the early 1990s (Wolf 1995). In Europe, Hekstra (1991) from the Netherlands was the first author who identified the need of data on the fate and effects of pharmaceuticals, especially veterinary pharmaceuticals, in the environment. Some isolated reports, published as early as in the late 1960s or early 1970s were related to hormones in the aquatic environment, and their potential effects on human beings (e.g. Sonneborn 1978). The measured and/or estimated concentrations of these medicinal products were believed to be harmless, since the exposure concentrations of the hormones were far below the concentration levels prescribed for medical treatment. In the meantime and based on improved knowledge, the risk caused by pharmaceuticals was re-evaluated in general. (e.g. Römbke et al. 1996). This time, also potential ecotoxicological effects were discussed, since quite a few pharmaceuticals were detected in different environmental compartments (e.g. Ternes et al. 1998; Daughton and Ternes 1999). Therefore, governmental authorities on the national (e.g. Germany) as well as on the international level (e.g. the European Union) began to discuss whether and how pharmaceuticals should be dealt with from an ecotoxicological point of view. For the pharmaceutical industry, it would be advantageous if an environmentally relevant registration procedure for pharmaceuticals were eventually accepted and would follow the same procedures world-wide (Schnick 1992).

In this paper, first the current legal status in Germany, the European Union and the United States with regard to the environmental aspect of the registration procedure for new medicinal products is briefly outlined. In all these countries it is common sense that environmental risk assessments (ERA) for pharmaceuticals should follow the same general rules that have been established for other chemicals. In the third section, these rules and their application to some human and veterinary medicinal products are shown. The following section outlines a test strategy and a specific ERA proposed for medicinal products. Afterwards, this proposal is compared with ERA procedures currently used in the EU and the USA. Finally, in the last section, our conclusions and recommendations concerning the environmental risk assessment for medicinal products are summarised.

12.2
Legal Situation

In all industrialised countries, human and veterinary medicinal products have to be registered before they can be placed onto the market. Furthermore, the relevant regulations refer more or less to the need of assessing potential environmental risks for medicinal products, which will be briefly outlined for some countries in the following sections.

12.2.1
Germany

Until 1998, environmental aspects were only indirectly mentioned in the Act on Pharmaceuticals (Arzneimittelgesetz (AMG); Pabel 1995). In § 11.16a of the AMG it was stated that "if necessary, special precautions have to be considered for the waste treatment of (human) non-used drugs." Based on § 23.3a of the AMG which refers to safety aspects of the use of veterinary medicinal products, only some basic environmental fate data of these drugs have been investigated in Germany (Kroker 1994). Methodological details and results of these studies have not been published. Medicinal products for pet animals like mice, parrots or aquarium fish have been exempted from many data requirements within the registration process (Grove 1990). Since 1995, ecotoxicological data are required for the registration of veterinary drugs (Gärtner 1998a). The 8th amendment of the AMG (1998) in accordance with relevant Directives of the European Union (EU 1997) provides guidance how to proceed with veterinary medicinal products, if environmental effects have been determined. The growing concern with regard to environmental aspects of medicinal products is expressed by the participation of the Federal Environmental Agency (Umweltbundesamt) in the registration procedure since 1998. Requirements to assess the environmental risks of human medicinal products are still under discussion.

12.2.2
European Union

Since January 1, 1995, innovative drugs as well as certain medicinal products manufactured by biotechnological methods are registered by the new European Medicines Evaluation Agency (EMEA) located in London, UK. For all other types of drugs, the rule has been established that the registration of medicinal products by one national competent authority should be approved by all other national competent authorities within the EU. In the case of an objection by one member country, EMEA is asked to settle the case by arbitration. EMEA consists of two committees, one of which (CPMP: Committee for Pharmaceutical Medicinal Products) is responsible for human and the other for veterinary (CVMP: Committee for Veterinary Medicinal Products) medicinal products. Additionally, the committees develop guidelines for the registration of medicinal products which are regularly published (e.g. "Notices for Applicants"; Irwin 1995). All regulations for drugs within the EU are based on the Directive 65/65/EEC, extended and amended by Directive 75/318/EEC and 93/39/EEC, respectively. In the latter, § 4.6 states that each application for the registration of a medicinal products must provide information on whether the product may cause a risk to the environment (see also Gärtner 1998b).

In the years 1994/95, several EU working groups discussed various test requirements as a prerequisite for the ecotoxicological risk assessment of human medicinal products. At first it was thought to use the same procedure as described for industrial chemicals in Directive 67/548/EEC, including its 7th amendment (Directive 92/32/EEC) and the related Technical Guidance Documents (TGD 1996) as a starting point. In these documents and guidance papers, the required environmental data as well as the environmental risk assessment procedures for existing and new chemicals are laid down. Some of the early draft documents on environmental data requirements for medicinal products were very far reaching and beyond practicability. Later the discussion focused on the value for predicted environmental concentration (PEC), which should be used as a trigger value. Estimated PECs higher than the trigger value would then initiate further investigations, in particular, on environmental effects of the drug. Estimated PECs lower than the trigger value would lead to the conclusion that the drug is of no concern for the environment. In an earlier version of the draft documents, $0.001 \; \mu g \, l^{-1}$, later $0.01 \; \mu g \, l^{-1}$ was chosen as the trigger value for the aquatic medium, while $10 \; \mu g \, kg^{-1}$ was determined to be the trigger value for drugs in soil. However, the various draft documents on human medicinal products have not been finalised.

The requirements for the registration of veterinary medicinal products within the EU were harmonised by Directive 81/852/EEC, amended by Directive 92/18/EEC. In contrast to the Directive 93/39/EEC for human medicinal products, this document for the very first time contained data requirements for "ecotoxicity" (§ 3.5). Based on these directives, the EMEA/CVMP published a detailed "Note for Guidance" (EU 1997) for the registration of all veterinary medicinal products that do not contain genetically modified organisms. Since January 1998, an environmental assessment based on the EMEA note is necessary for the registration of veterinary drugs in Europe (see http://www.eudra.org for actual examples). A similar paper was prepared by FEDESA (European Federation of Animal Health) two years earlier (FEDESA 1993). Finally, the "Veterinary Medicine Directorate" of the UK proposed an ERA especially for drugs in aquaculture, which very closely resembles the one proposed by the EU for pesticides and existing chemicals (VMD 1996).

12.2.3
United States of America

Until 1995 human and veterinary medicinal products were registered by the Food and Drug Administration (FDA) in the USA according to the requirements of the "Federal Food, Drug and Cosmetic Act (FFDCA)" until 1995 (Eirkson et al. 1987; Velagaleti 1995). Part of the registration process was an "Environmental Assessment (EA)," which resulted either in an "Environmental Impact Statement (EIS)" or, more often, in a "Finding of No Significant Impact on the Environment (FONSI)." According to Bloom and Matheson (1993), "A FONSI does not necessarily mean that no environmental effects are anticipated, but rather that under the conditions of use, the product under assessment is not predicted to cause significant effects in the environment." Furthermore, other regulations like "The Endangered Species Act" can influence the registration of a drug, like in the case of the anticancer product taxol, which is extracted from the bark of the tree *Taxus brevifolia*, an endangered species (Mandava 1995). The data requirements for the EA are based on rather general rules, which in some cases can lead to specific tests, i.e. runoff studies for ivermectin (Bloom and Matheson 1993). The view of the pharmaceutical industry can be summarised by the following statement: "The currently used system has worked well in ensuring that there has been *no* significant damage to the environment due to the use of animal health products. However, the system has not worked well in providing the needed products in timely manner" (Mangels 1995).

In November 1995, the FDA published a new "Guidance for Industry" for the registration of human medicinal products as part of the deregulation politics of the US government (current version: FDA 1998). According to this document, hardly any EA for drugs is required. This change has taken place, because almost all EAs have ended with a FONSI-statement in the past (Van Leemput 1998). A comparable guidance for veterinary medicinal products is under way.

12.2.4
International Harmonisation

Currently the registration procedure for human and veterinary medicinal products is about to be harmonised within the European Union, Japan and the United States. The Veterinary International Co-operation on Harmonisation (VICH) is responsible for the harmonisation process of veterinary drugs. In 1996 the VICH Steering Committee authorised the formation of a working group to develop harmonised guidelines for conducting the environmental risk assessment (here called environmental impact assessment, EIA) for veterinary medicinal products. The mandate of this VICH Ecotoxicity/Environmental Impact Assessment Working Group is to elaborate tripartite guidelines on the design of studies and the evaluation of the environmental impact of veterinary drugs. It was suggested to follow a tiered approach based on the general principles of risk analysis. Categories of products to be covered by different tiers of these guidelines should be specified. Existing or draft guidelines in the USA, the EU and Japan should be taken into account. The working group consists of six members from each of the three regions, one expert from industry and one expert from competent authorities).

In October 1999 the draft for the Phase I EIA guideline was on Step 5 of the VICH procedure. The final guideline will be submitted at Step 7. It has to be expected that the VICH guidelines will be adopted by the European Commission and will replace the existing EMEA guideline. In principle, the existing draft for the Phase I EIA guideline follows the EMEA guideline, nevertheless, there are some relevant changes. For instance, the trigger value for predicted environmental concentration in soil for conducting the Phase II assessment has been increased (from 10 μg kg^{-1} to 100 μg kg^{-1}) and the trigger value for the compartment groundwater has been eliminated (EU 1998). The latest draft version of the guideline can be found on the internet (http:// www.eudra.org/ vetdocs/vet/VICH.htm).

12.3
Environmental Risk Assessment

12.3.1
General ERA Principles

Since it was not intended to reinvent the wheel for medicinal products, general principles of the environmental risk assessment (ERA) scheme that are widely accepted in the industrialised countries are used as a starting point (see also OECD 1989 and Chap. 11). Basically, an ERA consists of the following steps (Fig. 12.1):

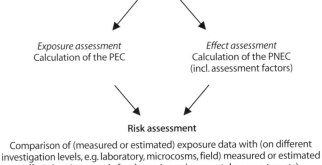

Hazard identification

Evaluation, which environmental compartments (e.g. surface water, soil) are likely to be affected, based on the properties of the compound and the use pattern

Exposure assessment
Calculation of the PEC

Effect assessment
Calculation of the PNEC
(incl. assessment factors)

Risk assessment

Comparison of (measured or estimated) exposure data with (on different investigation levels, e.g. laboratory, microcosms, field) measured or estimated effect data (separately for the main environmental compartments)

Risk characterisation
Assessment of the probability that an environmental risk is likely to occur by calculating the PEC/PNEC ratio (< or >1)

Risk management

Measures in order to avoid or to minimise an environmental risk as part of the registration or re-registration decision

Fig. 12.1. General principles of an environmental risk assessment (ERA) process (modified according to various authors)

1. Hazard identification
2. Exposure (predicted exposure concentration) and effect (predicted no-effect concentration) analysis
3. Risk characterisation (PEC/PNEC ratio)
4. Risk management

According to Barnthouse (1992), ERA is "simply a systematic means of developing a scientific basis for regulatory decision making." It has been developed in the USA for the notification of chemicals (Fava et al. 1987), but it is also used by the American FDA for the registration of medicinal products. The European Union started off using ERAs for the registration of pesticides. Later ERAs were also required for the notification of new and existing chemicals and for the registration of biocides. The whole ERA is an iterative process, i.e. in a tiered approach; in particular, exposure and effect analysis can be repeated twice with increasing complexity. Probably the example of an ERA best suited for medicinal products is the process currently used in the European Union for existing and new chemicals (TGD 1996). There assessment classes are defined to categorise the outcome of the ERA:

- PEC/PNEC > 1: Improvement of exposure and effect analysis necessary
  (EU-Class 1)
- PEC/PNEC < 1: No indication of environmental risk potential (EU-Class 2)
- PEC/PNEC > 1: Risk management necessary (EU-Class 3)

12.3.2
ERAs for Selected Medicinal Products

In the following section, ERAs for several human and veterinary medicinal products are presented according to Römbke et al. (1996); more recent publications have also been taken into consideration. The examples have been chosen in a way that the above given assessment classes are represented. The first step (hazard identification) is not given in detail, since all chemicals listed here have already been measured in the environment or are likely to occur in the environment due to their high production volume.

12.3.2.1
Risk Assessment for Acetylsalicylic Acid

- Exposure analysis: Measured concentration in surface water: $0.34\ \mu g\,l^{-1}$
  $\longrightarrow PEC = 0.34\ \mu g\,l^{-1}$
- Effect analysis: Acute laboratory test with *Daphnia magna*: $LC_{50} \approx 167.5\ mg\,l^{-1}$
  Assessment factor according to EU (TGD 1996): 1 000
  $\longrightarrow PNEC = 167.5\ \mu g\,l^{-1}$
- Risk characterisation: PEC/PNEC ratio: 0.002 (EU Class 2)
- Comment: There is no indication of a risk for the environment. The same result would be found when using the assessment factor used for pesticides (= 100). However, due to the high production volume, monitoring samples in surface waters should be taken from time to time. Additionally, the performance of environmentally relevant long-term tests is recommended.

Low PEC/PNEC ratios (EU-Class 2) have also been found for the psychiatric drug diazepam, the broncholyticum theophylline and the antibiotic erythromycin (Römbke et al. 1996).

12.3.2.2
Risk Assessment for Salicylic Acid (Metabolite of Acetylsalicylic acid)

- Exposure analysis: Measured concentration in surface water: $0.01-28.8\ \mu g\,l^{-1}$
  Measured concentration in urban STP effluent water (biologically treated): $<1\ \mu g\,l^{-1}$
  $\longrightarrow PEC\ 1.0\ \mu g\,l^{-1}$
- Effect analysis: Acute laboratory test with *Enchytraeus albidus*: $LC_{50} = 16\ mg\,l^{-1}$ (not valid)

Acute laboratory test with *Daphnia magna*: $EC_{50} = 180$ mg l^{-1}
Chronic laboratory tests with *Daphnia magna*:
NOEC = 10 mg l^{-1}
Assessment factor according to EU (TGD 1996): 50
$\longrightarrow$ PNEC = 200 µg l^{-1}

- Risk characterisation: PEC/PNEC ratio: 0.005 (EU-Class 2)
- Comment: Based on rather old studies (1968–1977) in which non-stand-ardised methods were used, the PEC/PNEC wasdetermined as being 1.8 by Römbke et al. (1996). Afterwards, Kalbfus and Kopf (1998) recalculated the PEC/PNEC ratio after perform-ing monitoring studies and several (acute and chronic) labo-ratory tests as being 0.01. According to TGD (1996), the assess-ment factor is even lower than considered by these authors (50 instead of 100), so this compound can surely be put in EU-Class 2. However, the authors recommend that due to the specific mode of action, a chronic cell growth inhibition test should be conducted (e.g. with *Pseudomonas putida*; ISO 1995).

12.3.2.3
Clofibric acid/Clofibrate

- Exposure analysis: Measured concentrations in surface water: 0.001–1.75 µg l^{-1}
$\longrightarrow$ PEC = 1.75 µg l^{-1}
- Effect analysis: Acute laboratory tests with two species: $EC_{50} = 12$–28.2 mg l^{-1}
Assessment factor according to EU (TGD 1996): 1 000
$\longrightarrow$ PNEC = 12 µg l^{-1}
Chronic laboratory tests with two species:
NOEC = 0.01–5.4 mg l^{-1}
Assessment factor according to EU (TGD 1996): 50
$\longrightarrow$ PNEC = 0.2 µg l^{-1}
- Risk characterisation: PEC/PNEC ratio: 8.75 (EU-Class 3)
- Comment: Compared to the fairly large data basis for the exposure analy-sis, the effect analysis should be improved. In a recent publi-cation, Kalbfus and Kopf (1998) calculated a PEC/PNEC ratio of 5, using their own exposure measurements and acute and chronic effect data derived from 5 different species and also an assessment factor of 50. Again, an indication of risk would still be there if the assessment factor would be based on the pesticide guidelines (e.g. 10). It should be kept in mind that this risk assessment was performed with effect data obtained from studies in which clofibrate was applied while the expo-sure data were measured for clofibric acid. This might be ac-ceptable, because the transformation of the ester to the acid occurs in water as well as in organisms.

12.3.2.4
Risk Assessment for Ethinyloestradiol

- Exposure analysis: Measured concentration in surface water: 0.062 mg l^{-1}
  $\longrightarrow$ PEC = 0.062 mg l^{-1}
- Effect analysis: NOEC from two chronic tests (Algae, *Daphnia*): 10–54 mg l^{-1}
  Assessment factor according to EU (TGD 1996): 100
  $\longrightarrow$ PNEC = 0.1 mg l^{-1}
- Risk characterisation: PEC/PNEC ratio: 0.62 (EU-Class 2)
- Comment: No indication of environmental risk potential. However, en-
  docrine effects (e.g. an increase of the vitellogenin concentra-
  tion) on fish, especially trout, were found in non-standardised
  laboratory studies at approx. 1 ng l^{-1} (Purdom et al. 1994).

12.3.2.5
Risk Assessment for Ivermectin (Antiparasiticum)

Probably the best investigated veterinary drug is the antiparasitic ivermectin, due to its very high acute toxicity to many invertebrates (Campbell 1989). An ERA has been performed as early as 1986 (US Federal Register, vol. 51, no. 145). Since then, many stud-ies (but only few according to standardised guidelines) have confirmed that exposure and effects are likely to happen in the environment (Römbke et al. 1996). Labels are already in use to avoid damage for the aquatic compartment.

- Exposure analysis: Measured concentration in cow dung: 0.4–9 mg kg^{-1}
  $\longrightarrow$ PEC = 9.0 mg kg^{-1}
- Effect analysis: LC_{50} from an acute tests (earthworm): 15.8–315 mg kg^{-1}
  Assessment factor according to EU (TGD 1996): 1000
  $\longrightarrow$ PNEC = 0.016 mg kg^{-1}
- Risk characterisation: PEC/PNEC ratio: 562 (EU-Class 1)
- Comment: When reassessing the environmental concentration of ivermectin concentrations (maximum 1.70 mg kg^{-1}; see Montforts,
  this volume) and assuming that the low effect concentration
  for earthworms (15.8 mg kg^{-1}) might not be valid, i.e. (Barth,
  pers. comm.) the PEC/PNEC ratio would still behigher than 1.
  Hence a data refinement seems to be necessary. For the fauna
  of the specific sub-compartment dung, a risk has been identified. However, the ERA performed for the compartment soil, in
  general, leads to the conclusion that there is no risk for the environment (Bloom and Matheson 1993). The results of some field
  studies confirm the risk, whereas in other investigations no effects
  on the meadow ecosystem were found (e.g. Barth et al. 1994; Herd
  et al. 1993; Strong 1993). These seemingly contradictory results are
  probably caused by the application of different, usually not standardised methods. Furthermore, the example of ivermectin shows
  that ERAs should be conducted for defined environmental compartments and with standardised and validated methods.

12.3.2.6
Further Experiences

The experience gained in the German Federal Environmental Agency when performing ERAs for three veterinary medicinal products following the EMEA note for Guidance (EU 1997) were not satisfying. These examples cover various exposure scenarios (e.g. internal or external application), animal species (e.g. dogs or pigs and drug classes (e.g. antibiotics or antiparasitics)). Further testing was not necessary for an injectable drug but for an antibiotic (PEC in soil > 10 µg kg^{-1}), whereas for an antiparasitic drug, risk management measures had to be taken into consideration (Gottmanns-Wittig 1998). However, looking at the quantity and quality of the data provided by industry, in the above mentioned cases it was not be possible to complete an ERA in a scientifically satisfactory way, due to the lack of information or non-validity of data (Kolossa 1998). Obviously, the Note for Guidance needs further improvement (cf. the following two sections).

For 64 selected human drugs, Webb (1998) assessed the environmental risk for the aquatic compartment in the UK. Based on short-term effect data and worst-case assumptions for assessing the environmental concentrations (no metabolism, no removal in wastewater plants, no dilution in surface water), only 7 compounds showed a PEC/PNEC ratio higher than 1. When taking into account a dilution factor of 10, the number of drugs was reduced to one (paracetamol) with a PEC/PNEC ratio higher than 1. Paracetamol, however, can be metabolised and has not been found in field monitoring programs so far (Ternes 1998). However, the author identified data gaps for single compounds (e.g. concerning the fate and effects of metabolites or chronic ecotoxicity tests in general) which should be filled for a final assessment.

When treating medicinal products like "normal" industrial chemicals, i.e. when ignoring that drugs are specially designed to achieve defined biological effects, the following conclusions can be drawn with regard to ERAs:

- few valid data, especially very few exposure and effect data for one and the same compound were found in the literature;
- based on established short-term toxicity data, most medicinal products seem to cause no risk for the environment;
- there is an urgent requirement to adjust the ERA to the specific environmental compartments of concern and to investigate organisms and endpoints that are related to the biological activity of the medicinal product.

12.4
Proposal for an ERA Procedure for Medicinal Products

Human and veterinary medicinal products should be treated separately as well as the main environmental compartments of concern (cf. Cowan et al. 1995). In the case of many veterinary medicinal products (e.g. antibiotics in aquaculture or antiparasitics in agriculture), the proposed ERA procedure is similar to the ERA of pesticides due to their direct input into the environment, whereas drugs for pets and human medicinal products are more handled like existing and new chemicals. In the following, the four steps of an ERA modified for medicinal products are briefly described.

12.4.1
Hazard Identification

In this first step, it is investigated whether an ERA is necessary at all, and, if yes, in what direction the following steps of an ERA should be performed. The most important issues that should be addressed are:

- *Is contamination of the environment likely to occur at all?* If not, an ERA should not be performed. An example for such a case is the use of radioactive tracers for cancer treatment in hospitals. This group of substances is controlled by other regulations to avoid any release into the environment. Another example is the naturally occurring minerals, enzymes and organic compounds that might be used in small amounts for human health purposes.
- *Do the inherent properties of an active ingredient indicate environmental risks?* For example, high logP_{ow} values (>3) indicate that a chemical is liable to accumulate in biota. Data on inherent properties (e.g. water solubility or vapour pressure) as required for the so-called "base-set" when notifying new chemicals according to Directive EEC/67/548 should be compulsory for any ERA.
- *Which exposure pathways should be considered?* In general, drugs or their metabolites can reach the environment directly or indirectly via the "target" organism attended medically. The most important exposure pathway for human medicinal products is the entry in surface water after passage of a sewage treatment plant. Veterinary medicinal products applied in agriculture might be either released directly or indirectly as a diffuse source via dung or liquid manure on pasture, arable land and in surface water (e.g. with runoff after heavy rainfall). Those veterinary medicinal products used in aquaculture are released directly into limnic or marine compartments. In industrialised countries, releases during production are unlikely to occur, whereas in other regions such releases might happen more often due to the lack of appropriate regulations (Bisaya and Patil 1993). Further, it should be examined whether the medicinal product of concern is released to the environment due to other uses, for example, when acetylsalicylic acid (Aspirin®) is occurring in surface waters as a metabolite of naphthalene oil (Richardson and Bowron 1985).
- *Which environmental compartments (surface water, marine water, sediment, or soil) are likely to be at risk?* In the case of human medicinal products and veterinary drugs used in aquaculture, the most likely are surface waters and sediments in which the drugs are emitted directly or indirectly after passing a wastewater treatment plant. In the case of the other veterinary drugs, the most likely is the terrestrial compartment in which the residues are released via excretion in dung or via spreading of manure. A risk to the compartment air/atmosphere seems be very unlikely.

12.4.2
Exposure Analysis

Ecotoxicological fate and effect studies should be performed according to standardised and accepted international guidelines (e.g. published by the OECD). However, for many relevant test parameters, only national guidelines or test proposals described in the scientific literature are available; e.g. for the determination of the degradation of veterinary drugs in manure (Spaepen et al. 1997). In any case, expert knowledge is necessary not only for the assessment of test results but also for the selection of the best suited test methods (Chapman and Scott 1992; Aldridge 1995). Additionally, a suitable specific analytical method must be available. Since the active ingredient and the main metabolites of a new drug have to be analysed in various organic substrates like blood or tissue anyway, it should normally be no problem to adapt these methods to environmental compartments like water or soil.

In the following section, for the limnic compartment a tiered scheme for an exposure assessment of human medicinal products is presented. Exposure assessments for other environmental compartments could follow the same principal rules, but so far are less elaborated. At the beginning and on a regional scale, the predicted environmental concentration (PEC) of a human medicinal product in surface water should be related to the number of inhabitants in a given area, the amount of water used by the population of this area and the average number of prescriptions. Based on the estimated concentration determined in this step, a tiered scheme can be applied:

- *Level 1*: Evaluation of the PEC after passage of a sewage treatment plant
  In existing formulae, the degradation in the wastewater treatment plant is considered to be zero to simulate the "worst-case" situation. A more realistic approach might be to incorporate the results of appropriate biodegradation studies into the assessment of the PEC.
- *Level 2*: Improvement of the exposure assessment
  The PEC assessment can be improved by performing water/sediment simulation tests with environmentally relevant concentrations. Additionally, at this level the regional PEC should be specified by applying more realistic exposure scenarios; e.g. for drugs that are only used in a small part of the region or at restricted time periods (e.g. certain antiparasitics that are used only in summer).
- *Level 3*: Residue analyses in sewage treatment outflow and in surface water
  Based on the experiences and results gained at the first two levels, samples should be collected from the environmental compartments of concern and analysed. By measuring the concentration of the medicinal product in the environment, the data with the highest relevance for an ERA can be achieved. However, Level 3 data can only be requested for a product that is expected to have been released into the environment; i.e. if the product is re-registered or if further data are requested to be provided after a preliminary registration has been granted.

12.4.3
Effect Analysis

As stated earlier, effect studies should also be performed according to internationally standardised guidelines. Due to the usually low concentrations and long exposure periods of medicinal products, long-term studies and the determination of bioaccumulation should be preferred compared to short-term studies normally performed at the first level ("base set") of effect analysis for other chemicals (e.g. Wenzel and Schäfers 1998). Results obtained from effect studies are transferred into PNEC (= predicted no-effect concentration) values by applying assessment factors. Assessment factors have been introduced to take into account methodological uncertainties of the tests as well as the uncertainties when extrapolating laboratory data to field situations. The better the environmentally relevant data, the smaller the assessment factors become. According to the TGD (1996) the assessment factor is 1 000, if only acute data are available; if three NOEC-tests with species from different trophic groups are performed, the factor is 10 (TGD 1996). As mentioned already, other guidelines (e.g. for pesticides or veterinary medicinal products) use different assessment factors, but usually the final result would not be different.

It is important to keep in mind that medicinal products are designed to exhibit rather specific biological effects. For most of these specific effects, for example, endocrine or neurotoxic effects, test methods are not yet developed or are still in the standardisation/validation process. In particular, it doesn't seem to be justified to measure effects in cell cultures or use other in vitro techniques, when effects can be expected to occur at higher biological organisation levels (e.g. organisms, populations). In this paper, specific criteria (trigger values) for the performance of tests at Level 1 are presented, using the aquatic compartment as an example (Table 12.1). These trigger values are not applicable for medicinal products with known mutagenic effect potential.

It is proposed to select so-called "priority medicinal products" representing various indication and effect categories, which should undergo a specifically designed testing program. This program could be implemented jointly by industry and governmental agencies.

The determination of the PNEC in surface water also follows a tiered scheme. Due to the reasons given above, e.g. the specific effect mechanism of medicinal products, new tests need to be developed and incorporated into up-dated versions of the following approach for the effect analysis:

- *Level 1*: At least two long-term studies, e.g. Algae Growth Inhibition (OECD 201 1993) and *Daphnia* Reproduction (OECD 202 1993), should be performed. An assessment factor of 100 is recommended for Level 1. In the case of a persistent drug that might adsorb to the sediment (e.g. in aquaculture), a sediment dwelling organism like *Chironomus riparius* should also be tested (Streloke and Köpp 1995; currently discussed as an OECD draft guideline).
- *Level 2*: Additional long-term tests, e.g. Fish Early-Life-Stage (OECD 210 1993) should be performed. The assessment factor could then be 10. Studies related to specific effect mechanisms (e.g. endocrine and/or mutagenic effects) are also included at Level 2.

Table 12.1. Criteria (trigger values) for the performance of standardised effect tests at Level 1

Evaluated exposure-effect-concentration ($\mu g\ l^{-1}$)	Ready biodegradation	Low potential for bio-accumulation ($\log P_{ow} < 3$)	Tests
PEC < 0.001	Not relevant for decision	Not relevant for decision	No
$0.001 \leq$ PEC < 0.01	Yes	Yes	No
$0.001 \leq$ PEC < 0.01	No	No	Yes
PEC > 0.01	Not relevant for decision	Not relevant for decision	Yes

Further, the bioconcentration of the drug in fish (BCF_{Fish}) should be evaluated, if the $logP_{ow} \geq 3$ and the PEC < 0.01 mg l^{-1}. The BCF_{Fish} should be measured, if the $logP_{ow} \geq 3$ and the PEC $\geq$ 0.01 mg l^{-1}. Based on bioaccumulation data, the potential of secondary poisoning should be considered.

- *Level 3*: Taking into consideration that an ERA is not aimed to evaluate the risk to a single species or populations but to ecosystems, studies in micro- or mesocosms might be appropriate at this level. Further, at Level 3 biomonitoring studies might be required. As stated earlier, these data can either be requested for a product that is expected to be present in the environment and that is about to be re-registered or for a product that has been registered preliminarily under the condition of providing highly relevant ecological effect data. Biomonitoring of effects of a single medicinal product is extremely difficult, taking into account the vast amount of interactions with other chemicals and/or stress factors, the thousands of potentially affected species and the varying environmental conditions

12.4.4
Risk Characterisation

This step entirely follows the rules established by the EU for the ERA of existing and new chemicals (TGD 1996): the PEC/PNEC ratio is calculated. Depending on the result, the medicinal product is classified in one out of three classes.

- PEC/PNEC < 1: No indication of environmental risk potential (EU-Class 2)
- PEC/PNEC > 1: Refinement of exposure and effect analysis (EU-Class 1)

PEC/PNEC ratio after data refinement:

- PEC/PNEC < 1: No indication of environmental risk potential (EU-Class 2)
- PEC/PNEC > 1: Risk management necessary (EU-Class 3)

There is general consensus that in cases where a refinement of data is necessary, preferably a PEC-refinement should be performed before gathering improved effect data.

12.4.5
Risk Management

Recommendations for risk management measures, which might include socio-economic aspects, are not given in this paper. However, some thoughts are indicated, which might need further considerations:

- In a class of drugs that exhibit the same medicinal properties, the use of those with a minimum ecotoxicological risk potential should be preferred.
- Releases into the environment might be reduced by modifying the formulation or by recommending special treatments of non-used amounts.
- In aquaculture the application of veterinary drugs directly into surface waters could either be adjusted to the minimum of the required amount or banned for a limited period of time or, if found necessary, be eliminated from the market.

12.5
Comparison of Various ERA Proposals

In addition to the above-described ERA concept, other ERAs for medicinal products have been recommended. In particular, the concepts of the US Food and Drug Administration (FDA 1998) and the EU Committee for Veterinary Medicinal Products (EU 1997) are important examples. All of these concepts are based on the same principles, e.g. by proposing a comparison of exposure and effect data and by recommending a tiered test system approach.

The concept of the FDA, however, reveals also some considerable differences compared to the ERA presented in this paper. For example, values that trigger the process of an ERA (Expected Introduction Concentration, EIC) have been set by the FDA to 1 μg l^{-1} for human drugs in the outflow of wastewater treatment plants and to 0.1 μg l^{-1} in surface water (Velagaleti 1998). Drugs exhibiting EICs below these trigger values do not require a detailed ERA. To expect an environmental concentration of 1 μg l^{-1}, the sales of a drug has to be in the range of 40–50 t yr^{-1}, which is only rarely the case in the USA. The introduction of EIC trigger values has considerably reduced the regulatory burden on the pharmaceutical industry in the USA. However, it is well-known, for example for endocrine disrupters, that concentrations below 1 μg l^{-1} can be biologically active. For veterinary medicinal products, the trigger value has been set to 10 μg l^{-1} by the FDA.

Further, if an ERA needs to be performed, the FDA requires mainly standardised short- and long-term ecotoxicological tests. However, extraordinary circumstances such as environmental effects other than toxicity and/or lasting effects on ecological dynamics can be taken into consideration. Unfortunately, it is not exactly described when and how these further testing efforts should be performed. These decisions depend on laboratory test results divided by an assessment factor or on substance properties like a tendency for bioaccumulation (Daughton and Ternes 1999). In any case, it is difficult to imagine how specific effects can be assessed if hardly any ecotoxicological data for non-target species are required.

In Europe, the ERA for veterinary medicinal products published in the Note for Guidance (EMEA/CVMP/055/096; EU 1997) has been required since 1998. According to Lepper (1998), the two phases of the EMEA/CVMP note can be briefly described as follows: In Phase I the potential of exposure of the product, its ingredients or relevant metabolites to the environment is assessed by applying trigger values for concentrations in manure, dung, soil and groundwater. Products exceeding any trigger value have to be examined in the rather complex Phase II (many different studies can be required). The Phase II consists of Part A, in which the fate of the substance in relevant environmental compartments (including bioaccumulation) and, for the first time, its effects on organisms (e.g. earthworms) is studied. On the effect side, the testing procedure starts with short-term studies. However, if high persistence (DT$_{90}$ > 1 yr) and low adsorption (K_{oc} < 500) have been determined, even microcosm or field studies can be requested (Aldridge 1995). Based on an UK proposal (VMD 1996) medicinal products for fish are treated according to a specific testing regime, because of their direct release into the aquatic environment. If in Part A of Phase II no hazard has been found *or* an appropriate risk management strategy is proposed by the applicant, no further testing is necessary. Otherwise, in Part B, refined tests for the environmental compartment likely to be affected have to be performed, which to a large extent are subject to expert judgement. In contrast to other ERA proposals published so far, the EMEA/CVMP note mentions the need of risk management measures – but the guidance on measures is rather general. Van Leemput (1998) recommends that an "appropriate labelling should be accepted as a genuine risk management tool."

The EMEA/CVMP note has been criticised by scientists as well as governmental authorities (Lepper 1998): In addition, industry has proposed a modified testing strategy for veterinary drugs intending to reduce the numbers of medicinal products to be assessed (FEDESA 1993), since according to Montforts (Chap. 14), "all veterinary antibiotics intended for herd treatment will enter a Phase II assessment for the soil compartment (because the PEC_{soil} are higher than the trigger)." An ERA encompassing Phase I and II certainly demands considerable efforts with regard to time and costs.

In his comments on the EMEA/CVMP note, Lepper (1997) has expressed that especially Phase II "offers potential for an improvement and optimisation with respect to the environmental relevance of the recommended tests and the testing efforts." The same author has proposed to include effect data, possibly based on QSAR estimations, in Phase I, which might allow to avoid assessments for drugs in Phase II. In addition, a shift from various single-species tests to simple microcosm tests is recommended, since results from such studies are usually more reliable, show a better reflection of environmental conditions and are more cost-effective, especially if several metabolites have to be considered simultaneously. These comments are in agreement with the opinion of the authors of this paper and should be incorporated into the ERA procedures.

Further aspects of the EMEA/CVMP note should also be discussed:

- The assessment of the aquatic compartment for veterinary medicinal products released to the terrestrial compartment should not be explicitly excluded from an ERA, since these drugs can reach surface waters via wastewater or runoff (Kolossa 1998).
- It is not feasible that in Phase I of the note no-effect tests are required at all. Even in Phase II Part A, (mainly acute) effect tests have to be performed only if certain trigger values have been exaggerated (100 µg kg^{-1} in manure, 10 µg kg^{-1} in fresh dung, 10 µg kg^{-1} in soil and 0.1 µg l^{-1} in groundwater). However, effects can occur at lower concentrations than those defined for the trigger values. For example, the antiparasitic drug ivermectin induces aberrations in wings of a dung fly at the concentration of 0.5 µg kg^{-1} (Strong and James 1993; see also Montforts, this volume).
- Also, the exclusion of veterinary drugs for pets from ERAs is not justified, since adverse effects can be caused by any product released into the environment. An example issue is the antiparasitic veterinary drug bromocyclen that is closely related to some well-known plant protection products like dieldrin. This plant protection product has not been re-registered due to its high persistence and bioaccumulation potential. Bromocyclen, however, for which an ERA was not performed, was found at high concentrations in fish caught for human consumption. After proving that these findings were caused by the use of bromocyclen as a pet drug, the drug was voluntarily withdrawn from the market (Seel 1998).
- Montforts et al. (1998) summarise their analysis of this approach as follows: "At the moment the triggers that lead to further extensive testing are either useless, or at least inconsistent with each other. The current proposals for effect assessment are too diverse."

Due to this criticism, an improvement of the existing EMEA note for veterinary medicinal products is necessary. The lessons learned from this process should be implemented in any notes for the assessment of human medicinal products.

12.6
Discussion and Recommendations

There are only few data available on the exposure and effects of medicinal products in the environment. Nevertheless, these data indicate that some of these biologically highly active chemicals pose a potential risk to the environment (Römbke et al. 1996). There is a common understanding that a harmonised ERA should be applied to human and veterinary medicinal products, based on the following considerations:

- The ERA should be based on existing guidelines, including assessment factors (e.g. as developed by the EU for the notification of New and Existing Chemicals (TGD 1996)) and the precautionary principle.
- A tiered test strategy should be used in order to use resources efficiently including the possibility of using multi-species test systems (Lepper 1997).
- The performance of an ERA is not necessary, if exposure is unlikely.
- Effect and exposure (especially biodegradation) tests should start on Level 1 of the tiered test strategy. In general, NOECs or comparable endpoints should be used for effect assessments (e.g. in place of the acute fish test a fish embryo test; Wenzel and Schäfers 1998). Persistence, bioaccumulation and toxicity are the main assessment endpoints.
- The scenarios used to calculate the PEC values have to be harmonised, since even small changes can have considerable implications on the outcome of the calculation, and therefore for the risk assessment (Lepper 1997; Spaepen et al. 1997; Chap. 14).
- New test systems have to be developed for the detection of specific (e.g. endocrine) or indirect (e.g. resistance development of bacteria) effects.
- Not only parent compounds, but also "relevant" metabolites have to be considered.
- Risk management measures in addition to simple labelling should be developed (Gärtner 1998a,b).
- Finally, the international harmonisation of the use of ERAs for medicinal products is supported.

There is also an overall agreement that more and better, i.e. valid data are necessary; not only for new substances but also for those existing drugs which have never been assessed up to now (Kümmerer 1998). One possibility to improve the ecotoxicological risk assessment of these existing drugs would be the definition of "priority substances," which are typical for individual classes of medicinal products like cytostatics, antibiotics or sedatives and/or belong to certain subgroups with a common mode of action. Such "priority substances" could be tested intensively in order to identify those groups or classes of drugs that could cause an environmental risk. Such an approach has been successfully applied when investigating the environmental risk of existing chemicals in the European Union (e.g. Greim et al. 1993). However, avoiding the introduction of persistent chemicals into the environment would be better than all of the aforementioned activities (Vack 1996; Kümmerer 1998).

Despite the fact that the amount of data is very limited, it is clear that an environmental risk assessment is necessary for the registration of human and veterinary medicinal products. However, it should be kept in mind, especially when talking about risk management measures, that the use of medicinal products is necessary for the health of human beings and domestic animals. This statement is certainly not true for each individual drug or formulation, considering that the number of (human) medicinal products available on the German market is approximately 8 000 (BPI 1995). According to the German pharmaceutical industry, just 2 000 of these drugs cover 93% of the business of pharmacy prescriptions (FCI 1989). Newer data are more or less in the same order of magnitude.

References

Aldridge CA (1995) Environmental risk assessment for veterinary medicines in the EU, Phase II. In: Wolf PU (ed) Environmental risk assessment for pharmaceuticals and veterinary medicines. RCC Group, Basel, pp 67–79

AMG (Arzneimittelgesetz) (1998) Gesetz über den Verkehr mit Arzneimitteln (8. Novellierung vom 11.Dezember 1998). Bundesgesetzblatt I 1998, S 3586

Barnthouse LW (1992) The role of models in ecological risk assessment: A 1990's perspective. Environ Toxicol Chem 11:1751–1760

Barth D, Heinze-Mutz EM, Langerholff W, Roncalli RA, Schlüter D, (1994) Colonisation and degradation of dung pats after subcutaneous treatment of cattle with ivermectin or levamisole. Appl Parasitol 35:277–293

Bisaya SC, Patil DM (1993) Determination of salicylic acid and phenol (ppm level) in effluent from an aspirin plant. Res Industry 38:170–172

Bloom RA, Matheson JC (1993) Environmental assessment of avermectins by the US Food and Drug Administration. Vet Parasitol 48:281–294

BPI (Bundesverband der Pharmazeutischen Industrie) (1995) Rote Liste. Arzneimittelverzeichnis des BPI und VFA. ECV Editio Cantor, Aulendorf

Campbell WC (1989) Ivermectin and Abamectin. Springer Verlag, New York

Chapman MJ, Scott PW (1992) The role of the experts in the EC's medicines licensing procedures. In: Michel C, Alderman DJ (eds) Chemotherapy in aquaculture: From theory to reality. Office Internat. des Epizooties, Paris, pp 130–140

Cowan CE, Versteeg DJ, Larson RJ, Kloepper-Sams PJ (1995) Integrated approach for environmental assessment of new and existing substances. Regul Toxicol Pharmacol 21:3–31

Daughton CG, Ternes T (1999) Pharmaceuticals and personal care products in the environment. Agents of subtle changes? Environ Health Perspect 107:907–938

Eirkson C, Harrass MC, Osborne CM, Sayre PG, Zeeman M (1987) Environmental assessment technical assistance handbook. Food and Drug Administration. NTIS, Springfield, VA (PB 87-175345)

EU (European Union) (1997) Note for guidance: environmental risk assessment for veterinary medicinal products other than GMO-containing and immunological products. EMEA, London (EMEA/CVMP/055/96)

EU (European Union) (1998) Guideline on environmental impact assessment (EIAS) for veterinary medicianl products – Phase I. VICH Topic GL6 (Ecotoxicity Phase I). EMEA, London (EMEA/CVMP/592/98)

Fava JA, Adams WJ, Larson RJ, Dickson GW, Dickson KL, Bishop WE (1987) Research priorities in environmental risk assessment. SETAC Workshop Report, Breckenridge, Colorado

FCI (Fonds der Chemischen Industrie) (1989) Folienserie Arzneimittel. Fonds der Chemischen Industrie, Frankfurt

FDA (Food and Drug Administration) (1998) Guidance for industry: environmental assessment of human drug applications. CDER/CBER CMC 6 (rev. 1)

FEDESA (European Federation of Animal Health) (1993) Implementation of EC Directive 92/18/EEC. Guidelines for assessing environmental effects of veterinary medicinal products. Explanatory Memorandum. Brussels, Belgium

Gärtner S (1998a) Arzneimittel in der Umwelt: Umweltschutz im Arzneimittelrecht. UWSF-Z Umweltchem Ökotox 10:154–156

Gärtner S (1998b) Rechtliche Regelungen zu den Umweltauswirkungen von Arzneimitteln. In: Touissant B (ed) Arzneimittel in Gewässern? Hesssiche Landesanstalt für Umwelt, Wiesbaden, pp 59–64

Gottmanns-Wittig H (1998) The assessment process upon application to EMEA/CVMP/055/96. In: Lepper P (ed) Environmental risk assessment for veterinary medicinal products. Fraunhofer Institute for Environmental Chemistry and Ecotoxicology, Schmallenberg, pp 25–36

Greim H, Ahlers J, Bias R, Broecker B, Gamer AO, Gelbke H-P, Haltrich WG, Klimisch H-J, Mangelsdorf I, Schön N, Stropp G, Vogel R, Welter G, Bayer E (1993) Priority setting for the evaluation of existing chemicals. The approach of the German Advisory Committee on Existing Chemicals on Environmental relevance (BUA). Chemosphere 26:1653–1666

Grove H-H (1990) Arzneimittelrechtliche Voraussetzungen für die Behandlung von Zierfischen und anderen "Heimtieren". Tierärztliche Praxis 18:85–89

Hekstra GP (1991) Towards ecologically sustainable use of chemicals: the Netherlands policy approach. In: Ravera O (ed) Terrestrial and Aquatic Ecosystems. Perturbation and Recovery. Ellis Horwood Ltd., Chichester, pp 501–516

Herd R, Strong L, Wardhaugh K (eds) (1993) Environmental impact of avermectin usage in livestock. Vet Parasitol 48:1–340

Irwin V (1995) EU regulatory requirements affecting environmental risk assessments for human and veterinary medicinal products. In: Wolf PU (ed) Environmental risk assessment for pharmaceuticals and veterinary medicines. RCC Group, Basel, pp 48–57

ISO (International Standard Organisation for Standardisation) (1995) Water quality – *Pseudomonas putida* growth inhibition test. ISO 10712

Kalbfus W, Kopf W (1998) Erste Ansätze zur ökologischen Bewertung von Pharmaka in Oberflächengewässern. Münch Beitr Abwasser-, Fischerei- Flussbiol 51:628–652

Kolossa M (1998) Ökotoxikologische Bewertung umweltrelevanter Chemikalien. In: Touissant B (ed) Arzneimittel in Gewässern? Hessische Landesanstalt für Umwelt, Wiesbaden, pp 75–82

Kroker R (1994) Sicherung der Arzneimittelqualität für Tiergesundheit und Verbraucherschutz. Deut tierärztl Wochenschr 101:278–280

Kümmerer K (1998) Vorkommen von Arzneimitteln in der Umwelt – was ist zu tun? In: Touissant B (ed) Arzneimittel in Gewässern? Hesssiche Landesanstalt für Umwelt, Wiesbaden, pp 97–104

Leemput L Van (1998) Consequences for industry from restrictive application of EMEA/CVMP/055/96. In: Lepper P (ed) Environmental risk assessment for veterinary medicinal products. Fraunhofer Institute for Environmental Chemistry and Ecotoxicology, Schmallenberg, pp 37–44

Lepper P (1997) Prüfung der Umweltverträglichkeit von Tierarzneimitteln – Potential zur realitätsnäheren Gestaltung der Prüfung bei gleichzeitiger Verringerung des Testaufwands. IUCT (Institut Umweltchemie und Ökotoxikologie), Schmallenberg (Jahresbericht 1997, pp 65–68)

Lepper P (1998) Environmental risk assessment for veterinary medicinal products. Fraunhofer Institute for Environmental Chemistry and Ecotoxicology, Schmallenberg

Mandava NB (1995) Environmental risk assessment for human medicines by the FDA. In: Wolf PU (ed) Environmental risk assessment for pharmaceuticals and veterinary medicines. RCC Group, Basel, pp 93–114

Mangels GD (1995) Environmental risk assessment for veterinary medicines by the FDA. In: Wolf PU (ed) Environmental risk assessment for pharmaceuticals and veterinary medicines. RCC Group, Basel, pp 115–132

Montforts MHMM, Kalf DF, Vlaardingen PLA Van, Linders JBHJ (1998) The exposure assessment for veterinary medicinal products. SETAC Europe 8th Annual Meeting, Bordeaux (Abstract No. 4H/P006, p 300)

OECD (Organisation for Economic Development) (1989) Report of the OECD workshop on ecological effects assessment. OECD, Paris (Environment Monographs 26)

OECD (Organisation for Economic Development) (1993) Guidelines for testing of chemicals. OECD, Paris

Pabel H-J (ed) (1995) Arzneimittelgesetz mit Änderungsgesetzen und einer Kurzdarstellung. Deut Apotheker Verlag, Stuttgart

Purdom CE, Hardiman PA, Bye VJ, Eno NC, Tyler CR, Sumpter JP (1994) Estrogenic effects of effluents from sewage treatment works. Chem Ecol 8:275–285

Richardson ML, Bowron JM (1985) The fate of pharmaceutical chemicals in the aquatic environment. J Pharm Pharmacol 37:1–12

Römbke J, Knacker T, Stahlschmidt-Allner P (1996) Studie über Umweltprobleme im Zusammenhang mit Arzneimitteln. UBA-Texte (Berlin) 60/96:361

Schnick RA (1992) An overview of the regulatory aspects of chemotherapy in aquaculture. In: Michel C, Alderman DJ (eds) Chemotherapy in aquaculture: From theory to reality. Office Internat. des Epizooties, Paris, pp 71–79

Seel P (1998) Arzneimittel in Gewässern – Neue Umweltchemikalien. In: Touissant B (ed) Arzneimittel in Gewässern? Hesssiche Landesanstalt für Umwelt, Wiesbaden, pp 1–9

Sonneborn M (1978) Zum Vorkommen von Steroiden mit biologisch wirksamer Östrogenaktivität im Wasserkreislauf. In: Aurand K (ed) Organische Verunreinigungen in der Umwelt. E. Schmidt-Verlag, Berlin, pp 205–207

Spaepen KRI, Leemput LJJ Van, Wislocki PG, Verschueren C (1997) A uniform procedure to estimate the Predicted Environmental Concentration (PEC) of the residues of veterinary medicines in soil. Environ Toxicol Chem 16:1977–1982

Streloke M, Köpp H (1995) Long-term toxicity test with *Chironomus riparius*: development and validation of a new test system. Mittl Biol Bundesanst Land- und Forstwirtsch 315:1–96

Strong L (1993) Overview: the impact of avermectins on pastureland ecology. Vet Parasitol 48:3–17

Strong L, James S (1993) Some effects of ivermectin on the yellow dung fly *Scatophaga stercoraria*. Vet Parasitol 48:181–191

Ternes TA (1998) Occurrence of drugs German sewage treatment plants and rivers. Water Res 32:3245–3260

Ternes TA, Stumpf M, Schuppert B, Haberer K (1998) Determination of acidic drugs and antiseptics in sewage and river water. Vom Wasser 90:295–309

TGD (1996) Technical Guidance Documents in support of The Commission Directive 93/67/EEC on risk assessment for new notified substances and The Commission Regulation (EC) 1488/94 on risk assessment for existing substances. European Union, Brussels

Vack A (1996) Östrogene Wirkung von Xenobiotika. Forschungsstand und Konsequenzen für die Bewertung der Umweltrelevanz von Chemikalien. UWSF-Z Umweltchem Ökotox 8:222–226

Velagaleti RR (1995) Technical and schedule impacts of environmental assessments on the drug development process. Drug Inform J 29:171–179

Velagaleti RR (1998) Risk assessment of human and animal health drugs in the environment – A chemical fate and effects approach. In: Little CE et al. (eds) Environmental toxicology and risk assessment. ASTM, Philadelphia (ASTM STP 1333)

VMD (Veterinary Medicines Directorate) (1996) Ecotoxicology testing of medicines intended for use in fish farming: Note for guidance. VMD, Addlestone

Webb S (1998) An objective analysis of the environmental and indirect human health risks associated with pharmaceuticals. Presentation at the SETAC 19th Annual Meeting, Charlotte, USA

Wenzel A, Schäfers C (1998) Possibilities and limitations of standardised ecotoxicological tests – use of other ecologically relevant endpoints? In: Lepper P (ed) Environmental risk assessment for veterinary medicinal products. Fraunhofer Institute for Environmental Chemistry and Ecotoxicology, Schmallenberg, pp 153–160

Wolf PU (1995) Environmental risk assessment for pharmaceuticals and veterinary medicines. RCC Group, Basel, 132 pp

Worst-Case Estimations of Predicted Environmental Soil Concentrations (PEC) of Selected Veterinary Antibiotics and Residues Used in Danish Agriculture

B. Halling-Sørensen · J. Jensen · J. Tjørnelund · M. H. M. M. Montforts

13.1
Introduction

Antibiotics are used as drugs to kill or reduce the growth of bacteria both in the treatment of humans and animals. Despite a relatively high usage of some antibiotics, very little information on the environmental release of this group of substances is available (Halling-Sørensen et al. 1998, 1999). Antibiotics for humans are mostly given therapeutically, whereas for animals, veterinary antibiotics are also used as a precaution in feed additives.

If antibiotics are used as a precaution in husbandry, they are often named antimicrobial growth promoters. Since January 1, 2000, the use of antimicrobial growth promoters is abandoned in Denmark and therefore not assessed in this paper. Similarly they are named medical feed additives or medicated feed if used therapeutically. Antibiotics are primarily used in husbandry for pigs, calves and poultry, but also horses, sheep, fish and cows are treated therapeutically.

Most antibiotics are water-soluble (e.g. tetracyclines, sulfonamides and β-lactam antibiotics) and excreted with urine as parent compounds (e.g. tetracyclines and β-lactam antibiotics) or metabolites (e.g. sulfonamides and macrolides). Tylosin and tiamulin, on the other hand, are less water-soluble ($\log K_{ow} = 1.83$ and 5.93, respectively) and excreted with faeces. Table 13.1 shows, for the investigated compounds, excretion fractions excreted with urine and faeces, respectively after a different mode of dosage. *(i)* stands for administrated as injections, *(wpo)* for peroral administration with water and *(fad)* for feed administered drug. Table 13.2 shows $\log K_{ow}$ values for the selected drugs. Results are either cited references from the literature or calculated with the estimation program ACD logP (ACD 1995).

Compared to, e.g. industrial chemicals, the exposure routes of veterinary antibiotics to the environment are relatively easy to identify and related to specific scenarios. The release (route and quantity) of the drug determines the extent of the assessment and the scenario to be used. For veterinary antibiotic dosage, route of application (e.g. injection or oral as medical feed additive or antimicrobial growth promoter), type of target animals, excretion rates, route of entry into the environment, and agricultural practise determine the level of release. Figure 13.1 shows the two main exposure routes of veterinary drugs; *(a)* excretion of drugs via faeces and urine from grazing animals or *(b)* amendment of arable soil with manure or slurry containing drugs used for stabled animals. In the field, urine and faeces are dispersed separately, whereas in stables urine and faeces are collected, mixed and compiled before entering the environment. On the one hand, the use of manure or slurry as fertilisers on arable land may involve a risk for the environment, as residues of antibiotics are deposited on ar-

Table 13.1. Pharmacokinetic values and doses used of the selected antibiotics (information from Veterinærmedicinsk Produktkatalog 1999). Excretion data are for both parent compound and metabolites

Antibiotic	Daily Dosage Pigs	Excretion Urine	Faeces	Daily Dosage Cattle	Excretion Urine	Faeces
Sulfonamides						
Sulfadiazine	(i): 200 mg per 15 kg bw (fad): 30 mg per kg bw, 3–5 days	0.90	–	(i): 200 mg per 15 kg bw (fad): 30 mg per kg bw, 3–5 days (only calves)	0.90	–
Sulfatroxazole	(i): 200 mg per 15 kg bw	0.90	–	(i): 200 mg per 15 kg bw	0.90	–
Sulfadoxine	(i): 200 mg per 15 kg bw	0.90	–	(i): 200 mg per 15 kg bw	0.90	–
Sulfapyrazole	(i): 50–70 mg per kg bw.	0.90	–	(i): 50–70 mg per kg bw	0.90	–
Tetracyclines						
Tetracycline	–	–	–	–	–	–
Chlortetracycline	(fad): 40 mg per kg bw, 5–7days	0.65	–	–	0.65	–
Oxytetracycline	(i): 5–10 mg per kg bw (wpo): 25 mg per kg bw, 3–5 days	0.65	–	(i): 5–10 mg per kg bw (wpo): 25 mg per kg bw, 3–5 days (only calves)		
β-lactam antibiotics						
Benzylpenicillin (penicillin G)	(i): 10–20 mg per kg bw 10^6 IE = 0.6 g	0.90	–	(i): 10–20 mg per kg bw 10^6 IE = 0.6 g	0.90	–
Amoxicillin	(i): 15–30 mg per kg bw (fad): 10–20 mg per kg bw, 3–5 days	0.90	–	(i): 15–30 mg per kg bw	0.90	–
Ampicillin	(i): 15–30 mg per kg bw	0.90	–	(i): 15–30 mg per kg bw	0.90	–
Penethamate	–	–	–	-	–	–
Quinolones						
Enrofloxacin	(i): 2.5–5 mg per kg bw, 3–10 days (fad): 5–10 mg per kg bw, 5–10 days	0.35	–	(i): 2.5–5 mg per kg bw, 3–10 days	0.35	–
Macrolides						
Tylosin	(i): 5–10 mg per kg bw (fad): 4 mg per kg bw, 21 days (wp): 5–10 per kg bw, 3–6 days	1.0	–	(i): 5–10 mg per kg bw	1.0	–
Spiramycine	(wpo)	–	–	(i): 5–10 mg per kg bw (wpo): 20 mg per kg bw		
Aminoglycosides						
Dihydrostrepto–mycin	(i): 10–20 mg per kg bw	0.95	0.05	(i): 10–20 mg per kg bw	0.95	0.05
Neomycin	(wpo): 70–100 mg per kg bw, 3 days (fad): 10–20 mg per kg bw, 3–5 days			(wpo): 20–40 mg per kg bw, 3 days (fad): 10–20 mg per kg bw, 3–5 days		

Table 13.1. *Continued*

Antibiotic	Daily Dosage Pigs	Excretion Urine	Faeces	Daily Dosage Cattle	Excretion Urine	Faeces
Miscellaneous						
Spectinomycin	(i): 10–20 mg per kg bw, 3–5 days (fad): 5 mg per kg bw, 7 days (wpo): 10 mg per kg bw, 5 days	1.0	–	–	1.0	–
Tiamulin	(i): 10–20 mg per kg bw, 3–4 days (fad): 10–20 mg per kg bw, 14–21 days (wpo): 8 mg per kg bw, 5 days					
Trimethoprim	(i): 40 mg per 15 kg bw	0.65	–	(i): 40 mg per 15 kg bw	0.65	–
Florfenicol				(i): 20 mg per kg bw, repeated after 2 days		
Lincomycin	(i): 5–10 mg per kg bw, 3–5 days (fad): 5 mg per kg bw, 7 days (wpo): 10 mg per kg bw, 5 days	0.2	0.75		0.2	0.75

(i): Dose administrated by injection; *(wpo):* peroral administration with water; and *(fad):* feed administrated drug.

able land or pastures as a constituent of manure or slurry. On the other hand, the use of these products is desirable for recycling nutrients and hence an important part of the concept of a self-sustainable agriculture.

Very little is known concerning the fate ((micro)biological and chemical degradation) of antibiotics during storage of manure prior to spreading (Halling-Sørensen et al. 1999). The uncertainty in the PEC of antibiotics due to soil amendment with manure and slurry is therefore likely to be larger than in the calculations related to environmental release of antibiotics from grazing animals. This scenario is only based on pharmacokinetic parameters predicting the time-related exposure via urine and faeces. Several model approaches have been developed (Spaepen et al. 1997; Jørgensen et al. 1998; Montforts 1997 and Montforts et al. 1999).

The aim of this paper is to estimate and compare the environmental release of selected antibiotics to the soil compartment via the two aforementioned exposure routes. Groups of antibiotics that were investigated are: sulfonamides (sulfadiazine, sulfatroxazole, sulfadoxine, sulfapyrazole), tetracyclines (chlortetracycline, oxytetracycline), β-lactam antibiotics (benzylpenicillin, amoxicillin, ampicillin) quinolones (enrofloxacin), macrolides (tylosin, spiramycin (I, II and III)), aminoglycosides (dihydrostreptomycin, neomycin (A, B and E)), spectinomycin, penethamat, tiamulin, trimethoprim, florfenicol, lincomycin.

Table 13.2. Logarithm to the octanol/water partition coefficient $\log K_{ow}$

Antibiotic	$\log K_{ow}$	References
Sulfonamides		
Sulfadiazine	0.12 ±0.26	ACD (1995)
	−0.08 (pH 4.0 to 8.0, ion-corrected)	Agren et al. (1971)
Sulfatroxazol	−	
Sulfadoxine	0.34 ±0.43	ACD (1995)
Sulfapyrazol	1.98 ±0.50	ACD (1995)
Tetracyclines		
Tetracycline	−1.19 ±0.71	ACD (1995)
	−1.47 (measured at pH 6.9)	Hansch and Leo (1979)
Chlortetracycline	−0.04 ±0.72	ACD (1995)
Oxytetracycline	−1.22 ±0.75	ACD (1995)
β-lactam antibiotics		
Benzylpenicillin	1.67 ±0.20	ACD (1995)
	1.70	Tsuji et al. (1977)
Amoxicillin	0.61 ±0.38	ACD (1995)
Ampicillin	1.35 ±0.38	ACD (1995)
Cloxacillin	2.53 ±0.39	ACD (1995)
	2.43	Tsuji et al. (1977)
Penethamate	2.41 ±0.86	ACD (1995)
Quinolones		
Enrofloxacin	2.53 ±0.75	ACD (1995)
Macrolides		
Tylosin	2.50±0.84	ACD (1995)
Spiramycin (I, II and III)	(2.49–3.56) ±0.82	ACD (1995)
Aminoglycosides		
Dihydrostreptomycin	−3.57 ±1.01	ACD (1995)
Gentamicin D	−2.98 ±0.65	ACD (1995)
C1	−2.39 ±0.65	
C1A	−2.98 ±0.65	
C2	−2.63 ±0.65	
Neomycin A	−3.15 ±0.57	ACD (1995)
B	−4.73 ±0.83	
E	−4.34 ±0.84	
Miscellaneous		
Spectinomycin	0.83 ±0.72	ACD (1995)
Tiamulin	5.93 ±0.62	ACD (1995)
Trimethoprim	0.79 ±0.38	ACD (1995)
	0.91	Hansch and Leo (1979)
Florfenicol	0.37 ±0.64	ACD (1995)
Lincomycin	0.52 ±0.68	ACD (1995)

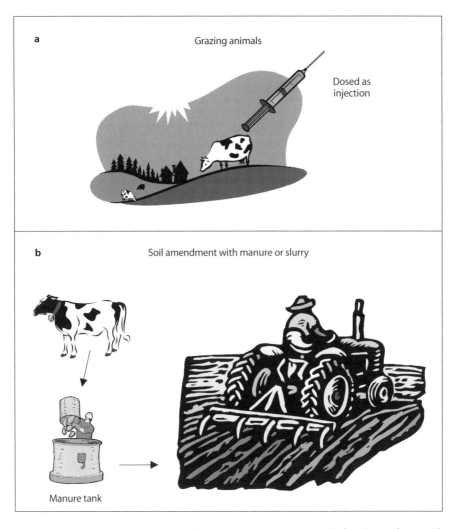

Fig. 13.1. Exposure routes to the terrestrial environment; **a** grazing animals; **b** soil amendment with manure or slurry

Estimations are made for pigs and cattle receiving different routes of applications of the drug. The selected antibiotic dosages are in accordance with recommendations in the Veterinærmedicinsk Produktkatalog (1999) and follow normal treatment patterns in Denmark. Experts checked doses. Doses and necessary duration of treatment are shown in Table 13.1. The management, storage and spreading of manure are in accordance with Danish regulations. These are to a very large extent based on EU ordinances. Predicted environmental soil concentration (PEC$_{soil}$) is estimated on a short-term scale, i.e. directly after the antibiotic enters the soil compartment. This is partly due to a limited knowledge of antibiotic degradation in soil and partly because the initial concentration represents a worst-case situation. Very little is known about the ability of ecosystems to recover after short term acute effects (e.g. Bender et al. 1984).

13.2
Models

The model descriptions for the two emissions and distribution routes, used to esti- mate the predicted soil concentrations (PEC_{soil}), are given below and were originally suggested by Montforts 1997. Model I presents the scenario of environmental release from grazing animals and Model II the scenarios of soil amendment with manure containing drugs from housed animals.

13.2.1
Grazing Animals on Arable Land

This is a model description for estimating the concentration of antibiotic in soil (PEC_{soil}) due to excretion of urine and faeces from grazing animals and subsequent leaching of antibiotics from dung.

Grazing animals urinate several times daily. The urine will penetrate into the top- soil following the normal routes of water flow. Antibiotics or residues of antibiotics might, depending of the physicochemical properties of the compound, leach from the dung into the soil. The water fraction and associated substances is assumed to be trans- ferred from the dung to the soil (e.g. at a rain event) and unevenly distributed in the first 3–5 cm of the topsoil.

The water flow from the dung to the soil will significantly decrease in cases of high temperature, due to evaporation. A pharmacokinetic model can be coupled to the model proposed in Montforts et al. 1999 and will be able to estimate the time-related excretion of drugs and drug residues from the animal. But if plasma half-life ($t_{1/2}$) is short, e.g. less than 12 hours, as in the case of most antibiotics, the majority of the dose is excreted during the first day of treatment.

The total amount of drug or drug residue excreted is:

$$Q_{drug\,excreted} = Q_{drug\,excreted,\,urine} + Q_{drug\,excreted,\,dung} \tag{13.1}$$

where Q is the quantity (mg) of drug or drug residue excreted with the urine or faeces.

$$Q_{drug\,excreted,\,urine} = D_{daily\,dose}\,m_{animal}\,F_{excreted,\,urine}\,T_{days\,of\,treatment} \tag{13.2}$$

where D is the daily dose of drug (mg (kg animal)$^{-1}$ day^{-1}), m_{animal} is the body weight of the animal (kg), $F_{excreted,\,urine}$ is the fraction (%) of the doses that is excreted with urine. T is the number of treatment days.

$$Q_{drug\,excreted,\,dung} = D_{daily\,dose}\,m_{animal}\,F_{excreted,\,dung}\,F_{leached,\,dung}\,T_{days\,of\,treatment} \tag{13.3}$$

where

$$F_{\text{leached, dung}} = \cfrac{F_{\text{water, dung}}}{F_{\text{water, dung}} + F_{\text{solid, dung}} \cfrac{F_{\text{oc, dung}} \, 0.41 \, K_{\text{ow}}}{1\,000} RHO_{\text{dung}}} \tag{13.4}$$

$F_{\text{water, dung}}$ and $F_{\text{solid, dung}}$ are the fraction of water ($m^3\,m^{-3}$) and solid ($m^3\,m^{-3}$) in the dung, respectively. $F_{\text{oc, dung}}$ is the fraction of organic carbon in dung. K_{ow} is the partitioning coefficient of the drug or drug residue between 1-octanol and water and RHO_{dung} the density of dung solids ($kg\,m^{-3}$).

$$PEC_{\text{soil}} \, (mg\,kg^{-1}) = (Q_{\text{drug excreted, urine}} + Q_{\text{drug leached, dung}}) \frac{N_{\text{animals on field}}}{RHO_{\text{soil}} \, F_{\text{spreading}} \, 10\,000 \, H_{\text{depth}}} \tag{13.5}$$

where RHO_{soil} is the soil density ($kg\,dwt\,m^{-3}$), $N_{\text{animals on field}}$ is the animal density (No hectare^{-1}). The conversion factor from hectares to m^2 is 10 000, $F_{\text{spreading}}$ is the fraction of the field area receiving drug or drug residue, and H_{depth} (m) is the depth of the soil in which the drug is (homogeneously) distributed.

13.2.2
Soil Amended with Manure from Stabled Animals

This is a model description for estimation of the concentration of drugs in the soil after spreading of manure or slurry.

The concentration of drug and drug residues in manure and slurry is given by the excreted amount of antibiotic, Q_{excreted}, the amount of produced manure and slurry, $Q_{\text{manure and slurry}}$, and the degradation of the antibiotics (T_{days}) in the interval between spreading. For the model calculations, it is assumed that the excretion of drug and drug residues into manure and slurry takes place within one day.

$$Q_{\text{drug excreted}} = D_{\text{daily dose}} \, T_{\text{days}} \, F_{\text{excreted}} \, m_{\text{animals}} \tag{13.6}$$

$$C_{\text{manure or slurry}} = \frac{Q_{\text{drug excreted}}}{Q_{\text{manure or slurry}}} \tag{13.7}$$

$$k_{\text{manure or slurry}} = \frac{\ln 2}{DT_{50, \text{manure or slurry}}} \tag{13.8}$$

The concentration in the soil (PEC_{soil}) depends on the following factors: the concentration of drug and drug residue in manure and slurry at the time of spreading, the regulation of manure spreading (i.e. nitrogen or phosphorus emission limits), mixing depth with soil and soil density.

$$PEC_{soil} = \frac{C_{N,\,total}\,Q_N}{RHO_{soil}\,10\,000\,H_{depth}} \qquad (13.9)$$

where

$$C_{N,\,total} = \sum_{Time,i=0}^{Time,i=i} \frac{Q_{excreted}}{T_{storage}P_N}\,e^{-k_{slurry\,or\,manure}\,T_{time,i}} \qquad (13.10)$$

$T_{storage}$ is the total storage time in the manure tank, which is typically between 6 months and 1 year. $T_{time,\,i}$ is the storage time of the drug from each individual treatment until spreading. If the compound is used at "i" occasions, during storage of manure it is necessary to calculate individual $C_{N,\,i}$ and sum up all treatment to $C_{N,\,total}$. P_N is the amount of manure (as kg N) produced during a day, multiplied with the storage period it gives the total amount of nitrogen produced.

Q_N (Eq. 13.9) is area based load of manure (kg N hectare^{-1}). In the calculations we have used the Danish regulations for nitrogen application on arable land.

13.2.3
Modelled Scenarios

The two presented models (Model I and II) are used to estimate worst-case soils concentrations (PEC_{soil}) for three different scenarios A, B, and C. Common aspects of all scenarios are that they are all based on short-term worst-case situations, i.e. the initial concentration shortly after the antibiotics entering the soil. In these short term scenarios, degradation in the soil is not considered. The different scenarios A, B, and C are described below:

Scenario A: Model I (field animals) is used to simulate the predicted soil concentration of antibiotics in fields with cattle and pigs. The scenario considers 10 beef cattle per hectare, each with a weight of 330 kg, or 15 fattening pigs per hectare, each with a weight of 100 kg. All estimations were based on a single injection of antibiotic (Veterinærmedicinsk Produktkatalog 1999) to all animals on a field area of 1 hectare. A considerable fraction of the total dose will be excreted within one day after treatment, with urine and/or faeces, depending on the pharmacokinetic of the substance and the method of application. Excretion fractions in both urine and faeces can be found in Table 13.1 for each substance. The excretion half-life for most veterinary antibiotics is less than 12 hours for both pigs and cattle. Therefore, it is anticipated that a substantial amount of the injected dose (F_{urine} and F_{dung} listed in Table 13.1) will be excreted during the day of treatment. Table 13.3 shows the model input parameters used in Scenario A.

Model II (stabled animals) is used to estimate the predicted soil concentration, PEC_{soil} after soil amendment with manure or slurry containing antibiotics. The antibiotics may be given as an injection (Scenario B) or orally as feed administered drugs (Scenario C).

Table 13.3. Parameters used in the three scenarios

Parameter		Value	Reference
Scenario A			
Number of fattening pigs (No per ha)	$N_{\text{animals field}}$	15	Pers. comm. Danish EPA
Number of beef cattle (No per ha)	$N_{\text{animals field}}$	10	Pers. comm. Danish EPA
Animal weight (fattening pig) (kg)	m_{animal}	100	Pers. comm. Danish EPA
Animal weight (beef cattle) (kg)	m_{animal}	330	Pers. comm. Danish EPA
Amount of urine (beef cattle), ($I\ d^{-1}$)		10	
Soil density (kg dwt m^3)	D_{soil}	1 500	
Dung density (kg dwt m^3)	D_{dung}	1 675	Montforts (1997)
Depth of field (m)	H_{depth}	0.05	
Conversion factor ($m^2\ ha^{-1}$)		10 000	
Fraction of field receiving urine and faeces	$F_{\text{spreading}}$	0.01 or 0.001	
Fraction of water in dung, fattening pig ($m^3\ m^{-3}$)	$F_{\text{water, dung}}$	0.88	Montforts (1997)
Fraction of water in dung, beef cattle ($m^3\ m^{-3}$)	$F_{\text{water, dung}}$	0.88	Montforts (1997)
Fraction of solid in dung, fattening pig ($m^3\ m^{-3}$)	$F_{\text{solid, dung}}$	0.12	Montforts (1997)
Fraction of solid in dung, beef cattle ($m^3\ m^{-3}$)	$F_{\text{solid, dung}}$	0.12	Montforts (1997)
Weight fraction of organic carbon in dung	$F_{\text{oc, dung}}$	0.44 correct	Montforts (1997)
Number of excretion events, fattening pigs (d^{-1})		10	
Number of excretion events, beef cattle (d^{-1})		10	Marsh and Campling (1970)
Scenario B and C			
Animal weight (fattening pig), (kg)	m_{animal}	100	Spaepen et al. (1997)
Animal weight (beef cattle), (kg)	m_{animal}	330	Spaepen et al. (1997)
Animal weight (piglets), (kg)	m_{animal}	20	Spaepen et al. (1997)
Nitrogen immision standard for pig manure on arable land (kg N $ha^{-1}\ yr^{-1}$)	$Q_{N, \text{pigs}}$	170	Pers. Comm. Danish EPA
Nitrogen immision standard for pig manure on arable land (kg N $ha^{-1}\ yr^{-1}$)	$Q_{N, \text{cattle}}$	210	Pers. Comm. Danish EPA
Daily production of manure (fattening pigs), (kg N d^{-1} $animal^{-1}$)	$P_{N, \text{pigs}}$	0.0263	Spaepen et al. (1997)
Daily production of manure (beef cattle), (kg N d^{-1} $animal^{-1}$)	$P_{N, \text{cattle}}$	0.0299	Spaepen et al. (1997)
Total storage time of manure (d)	T_{storage}	180	
Time from medication,i, to spreading of manure (d)	$T_{\text{time, } i}$	Variable	
Degradation of antibiotic in manure or slurry, (k slurry or manure)	$k_{\text{slurry or manure}}$	Variable	

Manure is often stored for 6 months or more before spreading. During storage, the degradation (abiotic and/or biotic) of the drug at 10 °C (average measured temperature in a Danish manure tank (Halling-Sørensen, unpublished results), may be described by a first order kinetic degradation rate. In the literature, information on degradation rates is very often only available in a different matrix and at a different temperature than 10 °C. Calculations presume that no nitrogen is stripped from the manure tank during storage. The applied 1st order kinetic degradation data in manure are preliminary experimental results obtained in our research group at 10 °C (Halling-Sørensen, unpublished). In Table 13.4 they were converted to half-lives ($t_{1/2}$, days).

All cattle or pigs in the husbandry are treated equally. No "dilution" with unmedicated manure was assumed. Manure is spread in accordance with the Danish regulations, i.e. 170 kg N ha^{-1} yr^{-1} and 210 kg N ha^{-1} yr^{-1} for pig and cattle manure, respectively, and ploughed down in the top 10 cm of soil.

Scenario B: Antibiotics are dosed as injection. Fattening pigs of a weight of 100 kg and beef cattle of 330 kg are all treated 1 to 3 times (at the 1st day, 60th day, 180th day of manure storage period) during the 6 months manure storage period.

Scenario C: Antibiotics are dosed orally as feed administered drugs. Fattening pigs of a weight of 100 kg and beef cattle of 330 kg are all treated 1 to 3 times, i.e. on the 1st day, 60th day, 180th day of the manure storage period of 6 months. The only difference between Scenario B and C is the dosage form. Table 13.3 shows the model input parameters both for fattening pigs, piglets and beef cattle, used in Scenario B and C.

13.3
Results and Discussion

Worst-case environmental soil concentration of veterinary substances and residues was estimated for two different exposure routes; excretion with urine and dung from field animals and as a consequence of soil amendment with manure containing residues of excreted antibiotics from animals in stables. Calculations were performed for three different scenarios, for both fattening pigs and beef cattle, as they are the primary consumers of veterinary antibiotics. Scenario A (field going animals): fattening pigs was included in this scenario because production of pigs in the field has increased recently and properly will become even more common in the coming years. Scenario B

Table 13.4. Degradation rate constants (degradation in manure) at 10 °C (pH = 8) used in Scenario B, and C. Data are from unpublished primary experiments obtained in our laboratory (Halling-Sørensen et al., unpublished)

Compound group	Half-lives $t_{1/2}$ (days)
Sulfonamides	30
Tetracyclines	100
β-lactams	5
Quinolones	100
Macrolides	21
Aminoglycosides	30
Default	100 (worst case)

and C: soil amendment of manure containing antibiotics dosed as an injection (B), as medicated feed (C), respectively.

13.3.1
Scenario A

Soil concentrations of antibiotics in the top 5 cm are estimated just after the antibiotics enter the soil compartment. In the absence of soil disturbance (e.g. tilling), as in Scenario A, it is assumed that the substances within a short term distribute over the first 5 cm of the topsoil.

The estimations assume that no degradation will take place in the soil compartment during the time needed for the complete dosage to be excreted. Two different estimations were attempted. First an uneven excretion of the urine and leaching from the dung to 10% of the field surface area was attempted. Table 13.5 shows the estimated soil concentrations. The PEC for sulfonamides, β-lactam antibiotics, macrolides and aminoglycosides was estimated to fall within the range of 25–1100 µg kg^{-1} soil and 75–2800 µg kg^{-1} soil for fattening pigs and beef cattle, respectively.

A second and even more conservative calculation was made by dividing the total amount of excreted drug by 10 (field pigs and cattle defecate or urinate approximately 10 times daily, Marhs and Campling 1970). This assessment gave the content of drug dispersed on 1 m^2 of field surface and in a depth of 5 cm per defecation or urination. Thus it spread on 0.1% of the total field area. The results from the second estimation resulted in PEC values two orders of magnitude higher than the first estimation. They seem unreasonable and are therefore neglected until they can be validated with field measurements. Note that in this scenario one should look at one treatment day only, so $T_{\text{treatment}}$ equals 1.

Highest soil concentrations, found with both methods, resulted for water-soluble antibiotics, whereas PEC for the more lipophilic antibiotics ($\log K_{\text{ow}} > 2.5$) excreted partly or totally via faeces (e.g. enrofloxacin, tylosin and tiamulin), was lower. This is primarily caused by the dosage, and has no relation to the hydrophobicity of the compounds. Residues and metabolites from these antibiotics will partly leach to the soil but mostly remain in the excreted dung due to adsorption to organic carbon. The majority (75 to 90%) of sulfonamides, β-lactam antibiotics, macrolides and aminoglyosides is excreted via urine.

More fattening pigs than beef cattle are permitted per hectare of arable land. However, due to higher animal weight and hence higher absolute doses, excretion from field going beef cattle results in higher soil concentrations. Excretion fraction and metabolisation are practically equal for fattening pigs and beef cattle for the selected compounds. If the excretion rate for a drug (expressed as $t_{1/2}$) is longer than half a day, it is necessary to include a pharmacokinetic model to Model I (Scenario A) to estimate the time related peak excretions of drug, Q_{urine} and Q_{faeces}. However, all investigated antibiotics have relatively short excretion half-lives (see Table 13.1), and are consequently nearly fully excreted within the same day as injected. Therefore, it was not necessary to include a pharmacokinetic model in the calculations presented in this paper. Fattening pigs and beef cattle defecate and urinate, as indicated above, about 10 times a day. The following "back on the envelope" calculation can therefore be performed: a single injection of antibiotic to a fattening pig of 100 kg of body weight may

Table 13.5. Estimated PEC soil concentrations taken the degradation rates from Table 13.4 into account

Antibiotic	Scenario A (Field scenario) Dosage as injection PEC soil µg kg^{-1}		Scenario B Dosage as injection 1 to 3 treatments PEC soil µg kg^{-1}		Scenario C Dosage as feed administrated drug (medicated drug) 1 to 3 treatment PEC soil µg kg^{-1}	
	Fattening Pigs	Beef Cattle	Fattening Pigs	Beef Cattle	Fattening Pigs	Beef Cattle
Sulfonamides						
Sulfadiazine	240	528	0.4–27.4	1.2–79.5	4.7–308	13.5–895
Sulfatroxazole	240	528	0.4–27.4	1.2–79.5	–	–
Sulfadoxine	240	528	0.4–27.4	1.2–79.5	–	–
Sulfapyrazole	1080	2772	2.2–144	6.3–418	–	–
Tetracyclines						
Chlortetracycline	–	–	–	–	155–921	–
Oxytetracycline	98	286	4–23.7	11.6–69	–	–
β-lactam antibiotics						
Ampicillin	540	360	10^{-8}–5.7	10^{-8}–55.3	–	–
Penethamate	–	–	0.4–29	–	–	–
Quinolones						
Enrofloxacin	26	770	10.8–63.9	31.2–186	21.5–128	–
Macrolides						
Tylosin	115	338	0.06–21.6	0.2–62.8	0.5–182	–
Spiramycin (I,II and III)	–	–	–	0.2–62.8	–	–
Aminoglycosides						
Dihydrostreptomycin	300	880	0.7–45.7	2.0–133	–	–
Neomycin (A,B and E)	–	–	–	–	3.1–205	9.0–597
Miscellaneous						
Spectinomycin	300	–	34.5–228	–	1.2–80	–
Tiamulin	0.0076	–	2.8–183	–	14.5–959	–
Trimethoprim	35	76	0.03–4	0.17–11.5	–	–
Florfenicol	–	–	–	4–265	–	–
Lincomycin	129	–	–	–	1.2–75.9	–

"–": Not calculated as the antibiotic due to pharmacological causes is not applied in the scenario.

be as high as 1 g of active antibiotic. If this amount is equally divided into 10 defecations or urinations. each will contain about 100 mg of active compound depending on excretion fractions and pharmacokinetics of the drug. It is therefore likely that high local soil concentrations can occur after treatment of field going animals.

13.3.2
Scenario B and C

As indicated previously, residues of veterinary antibiotics can also enter the environment when manure from treated animals in stables is used to fertilise soil. Based on the Danish limit for applying manure on arable land, and knowledge of the level of drug residues in manure, the PEC of drug residues was calculated for the soil compartment. In the EU regulations, good agriculture practise insures that land is not over fertilised with respect to nitrogen or phosphorus. These nitrogen and phosphorus limits thus directly determine the maximum allowed load of manure and thus the worst-case concentrations of residues of veterinary antibiotics. For pig holdings, the current Danish criterion is a maximum of 170 kg N ha^{-1} yr^{-1}. For cattle, the corresponding amount is 210 kg N ha^{-1} yr^{-1}. Estimations show (Table 13.5) that predicted soil concentrations (PEC$_{soil}$) depend on the dosage form. Scenarios were therefore based on different dosage forms to both fattening pigs and beef cattle treated up to three treatments (1st day, 60th day and 180th day) during a 180-day manure storage period. All animals in the husbandry were treated equally. Results showed that for the same antibiotic, higher PEC$_{soil}$ values were estimated when the drug was used as a medicated feed than as an injection simply due to application of higher doses. The tetracycline used on fattening pigs is an example of this. Depending in the number of treatments, PEC values were found in the range of 4 and 23.7 µg kg^{-1} soil when injected, and between 155 and 921 µg kg^{-1} soil when used as medicated feed. The variations are due to different prescribed doses and duration of treatment. The same overall tendency, i.e. an approximately 10 times higher concentration in soil, as a result of application of medicated feed, was observed for sulfonamides (sulfadiazine), tetracyclines (chlortetracycline), macrolides (tylosin) and tiamulin.

As for Scenario A, predicted soil concentrations were also higher here by a factor of three when amended with cattle manure in lieu of pig manure due to higher total dose for cattle and higher limits for nitrogen application for cattle manure.

As long as the storage time is long compared with the excretion rate, the excretion rates and routes are unimportant for animals in stables. The manure tank is utilised as a buffer tank where a primary degradation or mineralisation of the compounds may take place. Before spreading, manure is homogenised so that urine and faeces are mixed and distributed evenly on the soil. Physicochemical parameters, such as the lipophilicity, are therefore not as important factors for animals in stables (Scenario B, and C), as they are for field animals (Scenario A).

Degradation kinetic constants used in Scenario B, and C, for the different antibiotics were primary results from laboratory experiments performed in our lab (unpublished). Table 13.4 gives an overview of the used values. Manure is normally conserved under methanogenic conditions and at a temperature of 10 °C (unpublished result). For some of the antibiotics, it was completely impossible to provide degradation constants (spectinomycin, penethamat, tiamulin, trimethoprim, florfenicol and lincomycin). In these cases, a default half-life ($t_{1/2}$) of 100 days was selected. The uncertainty in the half-life estimations, imply that the soil concentrations have been underestimated for some of the antibiotics.

In Scenario B and C, three treatments, given on the 1st, 60th and 180th day of the manure storage period, were anticipated in the PEC calculations. Treatments made the

1st and 60th day were almost degraded during the 180-day storage period. The last treatment was hence more or less solely responsible for the relatively high estimated soil concentration, as soil concentrations based on only the first two treatments were estimated to less than 20 µg kg^{-1} soil. These computations show the importance of a long storage time relative to the disappearance time of the drugs in manure, as the most important aspect in Scenario B and C is to relate the length of the residence time in the storage tank to the disappearance time of the drug. According to Cowan et al. (1995), more than 90% of a substance should disappear between two subsequent introductions into the environment to avoid an increase in PEC. A residence time of manure long enough to ensure a 90% transformation could also be suggested as desirable.

13.4
Conclusion

This paper presents equations to calculate PEC$_{soil}$ of veterinary antibiotics and residues for two different exposure routes. Grazing animals excrete directly on grassland via urine and faeces or as part of soil amendment of manure. The first exposure route is based on the use pattern of the drug, drug excretion rate, fraction and routes, the lipophilicity of the drug, the number of daily animal defecations and animal husbandry practises. The latter is based on the use pattern of the drug (dose and dosage), on physiological parameters of the target animals, on existing regulations on manuring practises, on animal husbandry practises, and on the kinetics in the animal, in stored manure or in soil. Only few antibiotics remain partly in the dung. Antibiotics are primarily water-soluble and will leach to the ground and surface waters. Degradation studies determining better kinetics under different redox conditions are urgently needed. Already existing substances should be examined, because some of the realistic scenarios using realistic degradation kinetics indicate that PEC$_{soil}$ will exceed 10 µg kg^{-1} soils. Generally higher soil concentrations were found due to excretion from grazing animals than from drug residues coming from manure immersion.

Acknowledgements

This investigation was funded by a grant from the Danish Centre for Sustainable Land Use and Management of Contaminants, Carbon and Nitrogen under the Danish Strategic Environmental Research Programme, Part 2, 1997–2000.

References

ACD (1995) Advanced Chemical Development Log P software. Advanced Chemical Development, Toronto, Canada

Agren A, Elofsson R, Nielson SO (1971) Complex formation between macromolecules and drugs. VI. Correlation of binding parameters for the binding of sulfa drugs to human serum albumin (HSA) with partition coefficients. Acta Pharm Suec 8(5):475–484

Bender EA, Case TJ, Gilpin ME (1984) Perturbation experiments in community ecology: theory and practice. Ecology 65:1–13

Cowan EC, Versteeg DJ, Larson RJ, Kloepper-Sams PJ (1995) Integrated approach for environmental assessment of new and existing substances. Regul Toxicol Pharmacol 21:3–31

EU (European Union) (1996) Note for guidance: environmental risk assessment for veterinary medical products other than GMO-containing and immunological products. EMEA, London (EMEA/CVMP/055/96)

Halling-Sørensen B, Nielsen SN, Lansky PF, Ingerslev F, Holten Lützhøft HC, Jørgensen SE (1998) Occurrence, fate and effects of pharmaceutical substances in the environment – a review. Chemosphere 36(2):357–393

Halling-Sørensen B, Jensen J, Nielsen SN (1999) Environmental assessment of veterinary medicinal product in Denmark. Miljø og Energi Ministeriet (Miljøstyrelsesrapport)

Hansch C, Leo AJ (1979) Substitution constants for correlation analysis in chemistry and biology. Wiley, New York

Jørgensen SE, Holten Lützhøft H-C, Halling-Sørensen B (1998) Development of a model for environmental risk assessment of growth promoters. Ecological Modelling 107:63–72

Marsh R, Campling RC (1970) Fouling of pastures by dung. Herbage Abst 4:123–130

Montforts MH (1997) The environmental risk assessment for veterinary medicinal products. Part 1. Other than immunological or GMO-containing products. RIVM, Bilthoven, the Netherlands (RIVM Report 613310 001)

Montforts MH, Kalf DF, Vlaardingen PL van, Linders JB (1999) The exposure assessment for veterinary medicinal products. Sci Total Environ 225(1–2):119–133

Spaepen KRI, Leemput JJ van, Wislocki PG, Verschueren C (1997) A uniform procedure to estimate the prediction of the residues of veterinary medicines in soil. Environ Toxicol Chem 16(9):1977–1982

Tsuji A, Kubo O, Miyamoto E, Yamana T (1977) Physicochemical properties of beta-lactam antibiotics: oil-water distribution. J Pharm Sci 66(12):1675–1679

Veterinærmedicinsk Produktkatalog (1999) Veterinærmedicinsk Industriforening, Strødamsvej 50H, Copenhagen (ISSN 1395-7430, in Danish)

Chapter 14

Regulatory and Methodological Aspects Concerning the Risk Assessment for Medicinal Products; Need for Research

M. H. M. M. Montforts

14.1
Introduction

The EU has issued Directive 81/852/EEC (EU 1981) in which is stated that with a request for registration of a veterinary medicinal product, information is to be provided to enable an assessment of the safety for the environment. In 1997 the Committee for Veterinary Medicinal Products (CVMP) issued a Note for Guidance on the environmental risk assessment (EMEA 1997a) outlining procedures, trigger values and backgrounds to the proposed risk assessment methodology, in order to harmonise the assessment procedure in Europe. The proposed methodology is based on the hazard quotient approach, that is widely used in the environmental risk assessment frameworks of new and existing substances and of plant protection products and biocides (ECB 1996a; EU 1997a,b).

Methodologies to assess the environmental risk for human pharmaceuticals are currently being developed (draft guideline III/5504/94 of DGIII of the European Commission) and are harmonised with the approach developed by the United States Food and Drug Administration (EMEA 1997b).

This paper will shortly discuss the structure of the environmental assessment, and will elaborate on the exposure assessment with exposure models adapted to the Dutch agricultural situation for veterinary products as well as on the available information on the occurrence of human pharmaceuticals in surface water.

14.1.1
Risk Management

The environmental assessment is part of a risk management process consisting of two distinct phases: a risk assessment phase and a risk management phase (Van Leeuwen and Hermens 1995). Here only risk assessment will be considered.

Directive 81/852/EEC is the direct result of the hazard identification, the first step in risk assessment. The second step is the exposure assessment. Exposure assessment can either be done by measuring exposure concentrations or by predicting them with models. The latter involves determining the emissions, pathways and rates of movement of a substance and its transformation in order to obtain concentrations to which environmental compartments may be exposed (yielding PEC-values: predicted environmental concentrations). Underestimation of the exposure in a compartment is avoided by making worst-case assumptions. Worst-case assumptions can be modified to realistic worst-case assumptions, once reliable information is available.

What does the environmental risk assessment for veterinary medicinal products based on the CVMP Guidance document (EMEA 1997a) look like? Directive 92/18/EEC describes the ERA process as composed of two phases. The first phase (Phase I) shall assess the potential of exposure of the environment and is thus limited to product identification and exposure assessment. Several exemptions for further testing are given, such as trigger values for PECs: 100 µg kg^{-1} in slurry, 10 µg kg^{-1} in soil, 0.1 µg l^{-1} in groundwater, 10 µg kg^{-1} in dung; or trigger values for half-lives: DT$_{50,\ slurry}$ = 30 days. These values are the result of the negotiations in the EMEA working group between all interested parties and have no scientific basis. Their primary function is to serve as management tools. When exemptions do not apply and trigger values are exceeded, one enters Phase II.

Phase II includes effect assessment and risk characterisation, and here the notifier is facing considerable testing efforts. The possibility that the assessment may end at the exposure assessment is an 'escape route' that is welcomed by the pharmaceutical industry; as this could make the difference between an economically profitable product and a dead end. To the regulatory authorities, this escape route increases the demand for a thorough exposure assessment. Although in the effect assessment the uncertainties are relatively well-known, one has to realise that certainly the exposure assessment has a relatively high level of uncertainty. Models are drawn up based on literature studies and aiming at realistic worst-case situations. Validations hardly ever have been performed up to now.

One should also be aware that some parameters used in exposure and distribution assessment are directly used in the risk characterisation process. The substance properties of sorption capacity (K_{oc}) and transformation rate in soil and slurry (DT$_{50}$) are used as triggers in the risk characterisation process, because they are indicators of the outcomes of distribution routes and processes. This implies that attention should be paid to the reliability and usefulness of the studies investigating these parameters (Mensink et al. 1995).

Livestock breeding and rearing is an important industry in the Netherlands (Table 14.1). Considering the above and the diversity of target animals listed in Table 14.1, it is worthwhile to put a major effort into elaborating the exposure assessment. To illustrate the consequences, some exposure models based on the Dutch agricultural practice are given (Sect. 14.2). The proposed methodology for human drugs

Table 14.1. An overview of animal husbandry in the Netherlands (CBS 1996)

Category	Number of animal places (×1 000)	Number of farms
Dairy cows	1 675	36 000
Cattle	4 550	54 400
Pigs	14 400	21 250
Horses/ponies	107	20 000
Sheep	1 625	21 000
Broilers	44 000	1 200
Laying hens	39 500	2 700

is not elaborated in this paper. Sect. 14.3 will discuss the available data on occurrence in surface water. The results of these models are discussed in Sect. 14.4.

14.2
Exposure Assessment of Veterinary Products

One example is performed with data for oxytetracycline hydrochloride (oxytetracycline HCl) (CAS 2058-46-0), oxytetracycline (CAS 79-57-2) and chlortetracycline (CAS 57-62-5), used for sows and turkeys in rearing. The data are drawn from dossiers provided for the registration of oxytetracycline products in the Netherlands. Currently new data are available in the public literature that contradict some values used in this example (Rabølle and Spliid 2000).

Oxytetracycline HCl is dosed with 40 mg $(kg\,bw)^{-1}$ for 5 days. It was found that wethers (castrate sheep) excrete at least 21% of the oral dosage oxytetracycline and that young bulls excrete 17–75% of an oral dosage chlortetracycline as the parent compound (Roij and De Vries 1980). The $F_{excreted}$ used here is 0.75. Chlortetracycline is found to degrade in cattle manure with a DT_{50} of 1 week at 37 °C, increasing to a $DT_{50} > 20$ days when decreasing the temperature to 28 °C. Using the Arrhenius-Equation to recalculate the DT_{50} from 37 °C to 20 °C, the DT_{50} (20 °C) amounts to 30 days. From the data presented by Soulides et al. (1962), an average DT_{50} in soil of 4 days (25 °C) can be derived, and recalculated to a DT_{50} (20 °C) of 6 days. The estimated $logK_{ow}$ for oxytetracycline is –0.58 (calculated with the method according to Rekker 1977), which is compatible with the finding of Soulides et al. (1962) that oxytetracycline desorbs in moistened soils. However, oxytetracycline probably binds to clay minerals (Soulides et al. 1962). Based on the $logK_{ow}$ of –0.58 and the relationship $K_{oc} = 1.26\,K_{ow}^{0.81}$ (Linders and Jager 1997), the calculated K_{oc} is 0.427 l kg^{-1}. Although this QSAR is not validated for this type of compound, the order of magnitude of the K_{oc} is considered worst-case for the compound.

A realistic worst-case exposure assessment can be performed if the daily agricultural practice is taken into account. A calculation model for the concentration in soil is presented by Montforts et al. (1999), comparing the Dutch models with the approach presented by Spaepen et al. (1997). Some results are given in Table 14.2.

The results in Table 14.2 show that exposure concentrations differ by a factor of forty, depending on the model and the substance properties. The availability of a $DT_{50,\,soil}$ can lower the $PIEC_{soil}$ for grassland substantially.

The Dutch models give higher estimations for animals with long life cycles compared to the basic year-averaged model, whereas for animals with short life cycles

Table 14.2. Results of PEC_{soil} calculations for (oxy)tetracycline ($\mu g\,kg^{-1}$ dwt) in grassland for different distribution scenarios

$DT_{50,\,slurry}$	$DT_{50,\,soil}$	Sow ($\mu g\,kg^{-1}$ dwt)		Turkey in rearing 0–6 weeks ($\mu g\,kg^{-1}$ dwt)	
		Spaepen	Montforts	Spaepen	Montforts
None	None	315	400	1 550	1 710
30	6	4	180	980	280

(young turkeys, broilers) estimations can be lower, depending on the substance properties. These calculations show also that the choice of the trigger values ($DT_{50, slurry} = 30$ days, $PIEC_{soil} = 10$ µg kg^{-1}), as made by the EMEA, are not harmonised. For example: with a DT_{50} of <30 days further assessment is not necessary, but $PIEC_{soil}$ may still be >10 µg kg^{-1}.

This exposure route is also of interest to disinfectants (biocides) used for the cleaning of stables. Examples are trichlorfon, methomyl and diflubenzuron. Degradation of trichlorfon is highly pH-dependent: at pH 9 practically no residues will reach the soil; at pH 7 considerable amounts of parent compound and metabolites (including dichlorvos) will reach the soil, and possibly the groundwater. Registration of these products may therefore depend on the model parameters used (pH, redox potential, temperature in slurry basin) that determine the predicted environmental concentrations.

Evidently, many antibiotics intended for mass-treatment will enter a Phase II assessment for the soil compartment (because the PEC_{soil} are higher than the trigger) and for the groundwater compartment (because the K_{oc} will probably be <500 l kg^{-1}), unless the $DT_{50, slurry}$ is <30 days. This underlines the importance of a valid soil-slurry scenario, and the availability of validated tests to determine the $DT_{50, slurry}$.

14.2.1
Leaching to Groundwater

The concentration in groundwater depends on the concentration in the soil and the capacity of the substance to adsorb to the organic material in the soil. In Phase I the EU-approach (ECB 1996b, Chap. 2.3.8.6, p. 312) is used, where the concentration in the groundwater is set equal to the concentration in the porewater. Default settings of the module for groundwater are presented in Table 14.3.

Model for calculation of the concentration in groundwater:

$$PIEC_{gw} = PIEC_{porewater}$$

$$PIEC_{porewater} = \frac{PIEC_{soil}RHO_{soil}}{K_{soil-water}1000}$$

$$K_{soil-water} = Fair_{soil}K_{air-water} + Fwater_{soil} + Fsolid_{soil}\frac{Kp_{soil}}{1000}RHO_{solid}$$

$$Kp_{soil} = Foc_{soil}K_{oc}$$

$$K_{air-water} = \frac{VP\ MOLW}{SOL\ R\ TEMP}$$

with input:
- $PIEC_{soil}$ highest concentration in the soil (mg kg^{-1} soil)
- RHO_{soil} fresh bulk density of soil (kg m^{-3})
- RHO_{solid} density of soil solids (kg m^{-3})
- $Fair_{soil}$ fraction air in soil (m^3 m^{-3})
- $Fwater_{soil}$ fraction water in soil (m^3 m^{-3})
- $Fsolid_{soil}$ fraction solids in soil (m^3 m^{-3})
- Foc_{soil} fraction organic carbon in soil (w/dw) (kg kg^{-1})
- K_{oc} partition coefficient organic carbon-water (dm^3 kg^{-1})
- VP vapour pressure (Pa)
- $MOLW$ molar mass (g mol^{-1})
- SOL water solubility (mg l^{-1})
- $TEMP$ temperature at air-water interface (K)
- R gas constant (Pa m^3 mol^{-1} K^{-1})

intermediate results:
- $K_{soil\text{-}water}$ partition coefficient solids and water in soil (v/v) (m^3 m^{-3})
- Kp_{soil} partition coefficient solids and water in soil (v/w) (dm^3 kg^{-1})
- $K_{air\text{-}water}$ partition coefficient air and water in soil (m^3 m^{-3})
- $PIEC_{porewater}$ predicted initial concentration in porewater (mg l^{-1})

output:
- $PIEC_{gw}$ predicted initial concentration in groundwater (mg l^{-1})

Using the calculated concentrations in grassland and this model, the following concentrations in groundwater are calculated (Table 14.4).

Clearly the trigger of 0.1 μg l^{-1} is not met. The selected model does not represent a realistic leaching behaviour. There are a number of models on groundwater leaching of pesticides available, of which the PESTLA1.0 model was one of the earliest (Van der Linden and Boesten 1989). This model has been used up to now (2000) in the registration process for pesticides in the Netherlands, but will shortly be replaced by PEARL,

Table 14.3 Default settings of the module for groundwater

Parameter	Symbol	Unit	Value
Bulk density of fresh soil (not dry soil!)	$RHOsoil$	(kg m^{-3})	1 700
Density of soil solids	$RHOsolid_{soil}$	(kg m^{-3})	2 500
Fraction air in soil	$Fair_{soil}$	(m^3 m^{-3})	0.2
Fraction water in soil	$Fwater_{soil}$	(m^3 m^{-3})	0.2
Fraction solids in soil	$Fsolid_{soil}$	(m^3 m^{-3})	0.6
Weight fraction organic carbon in soil	Foc_{soil}	(kg kg^{-1})	0.02
Temperature at air-water interface	$TEMP$	(K)	285
Gas constant	R	(Pa m^3 mol^{-1} K^{-1})	8.314

Table 14.4. Results of PEC$_{soil}$ calculations ($\mu g\,kg^{-1}$ dwt) and of PEC$_{groundwater}$ ($\mu g\,l^{-1}$) for (oxy)tetracycline in grassland

| Animal | Sow | | Turkey in rearing 0–6 weeks | |
Formula set	Spaepen	Montforts	Spaepen	Montforts
PEC$_{soil}$ ($\mu g\,kg^{-1}$ dwt)	4	180	980	280
PEC$_{groundwater}$ ($\mu g\,l^{-1}$)	32	1 440	7 800	2 200

a more advanced version incorporating a.o. evaporation and fluctuating groundwater tables. A pleasant aspect of PESTLA is that one can use the meta-model: a set of graphs and tables. Using only the parameters DT$_{50,\,soil}$ and K_{oc}, the concentration in the upper meter of groundwater is calculated for a spring or an autumn scenario.

When applying PESTLA, no correction is made by the reviewer for transformation in the soil during the intervals between the four spreading events. This correction is already made by PESTLA, as this model incorporates transformation and leaching in the upper soil. The results for oxytetracycline are shown in Table 14.5.

One should be aware of the vulnerability of these model predictions: a factor of 2 in DT$_{50,\,soil}$ changes the PEC$_{groundwater}$ by a factor of 6. Furthermore, experimental K_{oc} are required, or more appropriate quantitative structure analogy relationships are needed. Because of the uncertainty in the modelling, the PEC$_{groundwater}$ > 0.001 $\mu g\,l^{-1}$ triggers the demand for lysimeter studies within the scope of the pesticide registration in the Netherlands. The leaching of most antibiotics would still be a point of concern.

This brings another point to attention: in the current method, the applicant of the veterinary medicinal product is not obliged to include studies on transformation routes in the animal, slurry, or soil in the dossier. However, metabolites are in general more hydrophilic than parent compounds. In case the parent compounds meet the trigger for groundwater, there is no Phase II on this aspect. The fate of metabolites is thus not examined.

14.2.2
Residues of Pharmaceuticals in Dung

All anthelmintics used on grazing animals (cattle, sheep) will be excreted, at least partially, in dung. One of the compounds that is dosed at the lowest rate is ivermectin: 0.2 $\mu g\,kg^{-1}$ body weight. Because the substance has to be active in the gut (colon), complete transformation before excretion is not likely (as opposed to substances to treat liver flukes). Table 14.6 shows measured concentrations of ivermectin in dung reported in public literature. The concentrations based on wet weight in the fourth column are recalculated using a moisture content of 85% for cattle dung and 80% for horse dung.

The exposure trigger level for further testing when the environment is exposed by dung from grazing animals is 10 $\mu g\,kg^{-1}$ wwt. This trigger will have no practical consequences for the pharmaceutical industry. Even substances with relatively low dosages (like ivermectin) will exceed this trigger 100 times. It is even more remarkable that ivermectin at concentrations of 0.5 $\mu g\,kg^{-1}$ wwt still induces aberrations in wings

Table 14.5. Results of the $PEC_{groundwater}$ ($\mu g\,l^{-1}$) calculations in grassland using the EMEA guidance and using PESTLA1.0 (spring scenario)

Animal Formula set	Sow Spaepen	Montforts	Turkey in rearing 0–6 weeks Spaepen	Montforts
$PEC_{groundwater}$ ($\mu g\,l^{-1}$) EMEA	32	1 440	7 800	2 200
$PEC_{groundwater}$ ($\mu g\,l^{-1}$) PESTLA 1.0	0.0002	0.011	0.057	0.016

Table 14.6. Measured ivermectin concentrations in dung. Abbreviations: *i.r.* = intra-ruminal; *s.c.* = subcutaneous; *o.* = oral; *p.* = pour-on; *dwt* = dry weight; *wwt* = wet weight; *bw* = body weight

Animal, body weight, dose (mg kg^{-1} bw) and route of administration	Highest concentra- tion in dung	Concentration recalculated to (mg kg^{-1} wwt)	Source
Cattle, 276 kg, 0.2 (s.c.)	0.42 mg kg^{-1} wwt	0.42	Lumaret et al. (1993)
Cattle, ca. 300 kg, 0.5 (p.)	9.0 mg kg^{-1} wwt	1.35	Sommer and Steffansen (1993)
Cattle, ca. 300 kg, 0.2 (s.c.)	3.9 mg kg^{-1} dwt	0.58	Sommer and Steffansen (1993)
Cattle, 278 kg, 12 mg d^{-1} (i.r.)	0.66 mg kg^{-1} wwt	0.66	Strong et al. (1996)
Horse, 0.2 (o.)	8.5 mg kg^{-1} dwt	1.70	Herd (1995)

of the dung fly *Scatophaga stercoraria* (Strong and James 1993). In this case the trigger is not even protective enough.

14.3
Human Pharmaceuticals in Surface Water

The German Ministry of Environment reported in 1996 a review of the available public literature on pharmaceuticals in the environment –both human and veterinary drugs (Römbke et al. 1996).

The measured concentrations that are reported in Römbke et al. (1996) are summarised below. Mostly maximum values are reported when ranges were available. The predicted environmental concentrations that were presented for the Lee River (UK), German surface waters and Dutch STP effluents are also presented. The overview presented here disregards the reliability of the measurements and models. All three models have the same approach: the estimated human consumption of the drug is divided by the water volume present. Table 14.7 presents an overview of the reported PEC_{sw} of drugs according to Römbke et al. (1996).

According to Römbke et al. (1996), the calculation for the Lee River is based on a water volume of only 1/10 of the general water volume used for the German surface water. These concentrations are therefore comparable to those from the Dutch STP effluents. Both data sets can be adjusted with a dilution factor of 10, the supposed dilution factor for STP effluent to surface water, to be compared to the German situation (Table 14.8).

Table 14.7. Overview of the reported PEC_{sw} of drugs according to Römbke et al. (1996)

PEC_{sw} (µg l^{-1})	Calculated 1 Lee River	Calculated 2 Germany	Calculated 3 NL STP effluent	Measured STP effluent	Measured River water	Measured Drinking water
Acetylcysteïne		1.83	75			
Acetylsalicylic acid	14.6	2.32		1.51	<0.01	
Acetylsalicylic acid	161					
Ambroxol		0.28				
Amitriptyline	0.88					
Ampicilline	7.9					
Androsteron				3.82		
Bacitracine		0.002				
Bezafibrate				6	0.38	0.027
Bleomycine				0.0158	0.0085	0.013
Broomhexine		0.01				
Chlormadinonacetate				0.08		
Chlortetracycline	0.15					
Clenbuterol-HCl		0.00003				
Clofibrate	6.3				0.04	
Clofibrinic acid		0.05		7.1	1.75	0.07
Clofibrinic acid				0.3	0.22	
Caffeine	0.29			292		>1
Cyclofosfamide		0.002		0.06		
Cyclofosfamide		0.0007	0.0067			
Dextropropoxyfen	3.2				1	
Diazepam	0.44		1.2	<1	0.01	0.01
Diclofenac		0.54		2	0.489	0.006
Dihydroandrosteron				0.64		
Dimethisteron				0.04		
Doxycycline		0.22	1			
Efedrine	0.44					
Erythromycine	2.2	3.69			1	
Ethinyloestradiol		0.0002		0.0005	0.0003	0.00006
Ethinyloestradiol				1.86	0.015	<0.005
Ethynodioldiacetate				0.55		
Etiocholanolon				2.37		
Eenofibrate					0.005	
Eenofibrinic acid				6	0.172	
Gemfibrozil				4	0.19	
Ibuprofen	9.5			12	0.139	0.003

Table 14.7. *Continued*

PEC_{sw} (µg l^{-1})	Calculated 1 Lee River	Calculated 2 Germany	Calculated 3 NL STP effluent	Measured STP effluent	Measured River water	Measured Drinking water
Indomethacine	1.32			0.52	0.121	
Ifosfamide		0.0008	0.0078	0.06		
Mebendazole			0.2			
Medroxyprogesteronacetate				0.16		
Meprobamate	2.6					
Methyldopa	17.5					
Metronidazol	0.29		0.2			
Minocycline			0.2			
Naproxen	2.3					
Nicotinamide	2					
Norethindron				0.6		
Norethindron acetate				0.2		
Norethynodrel				0.38		
Norethisteron		0.004		0.02	<0.017	<0.010
Oestradiol		0.01		0.35		
Oestradiol				0.01		
Oestriol		0.005		0.04		
Oestron				0.02		
Oxytetracycline	6.7	0.01				
Paracetamol	84.10	3.59				
Paracetamol	340					
Pentoxyverine		0.02				
Phenylpropanolamine	0.29					
Pregnanediol				4.09		
Progesteron				0.01		
Salicylic acid	0.29			28.8		
B-sitosterol		0.2		240		
Spironolacton		0.48				
Sulfamethoxazine	7.2				1	
Sulfasalazine	1.8					
Testosterone				0.02		
Tetracycline	2.9		4.5		1	
Theobromine	0.29					
Theophylline					1	
Tinidazol			0.1			
Tolbutamide	2.2					

Table 14.8. Comparison of the models (after correction)

PEC_{sw} ($\mu g\,l^{-1}$)	Corrected model 1	Corrected model 2	Corrected model 3	Difference
Acetylcysteïne		1.83	7.5	4
Acetylsalicylic acid	1.46	2.32		2
Acetylsalicylic acid	16.1	2.32		7
Cyclofosfamide		0.0007	0.00067	1
Diazepam	0.044		0.12	3
Doxycycline		0.22	0.1	4
Erythromycine	0.22	3.69		15
Ifosfamide		0.0008	0.00078	1
Metronidazol	0.029		0.02	1
Oxytetracycline	0.67	0.01		67
Paracetamol	8.41	3.59		2
Paracetamol	34	3.59		9
Tetracycline	0.29		0.45	2

The median difference amounts to 3, range 1–67. Therefore, with caution, one may conclude that the models are comparable to each other. The next question is whether the predicted concentrations are comparable to the measured concentrations. Table 14.9 shows the comparison for the STP effluents. The Dutch STP effluents and the Lee River values are the originally reported values; the German PEC_{sw} were multiplied with the supposed dilution factor for STP effluent to surface water of 10.

The median difference is 4–8, range 1–1 000. The outliers are caffeine, (acetyl)salicylic acid and ethinyloestradiol. The concentrations caffeine and (acetyl)salicylic acid are partly due to non-drug use (coffee and natural occurrence); (acetyl)salicylic acid and ethinyloestradiol are used privately a lot (aspirin and anticonception). The moment of measurement (time and what day of the week) and the location may have a rather large influence on the measured concentration. Table 14.10 shows the comparison for the surface waters. The Dutch STP effluents and the Lee River values are divided by the supposed dilution factor for STP effluent to surface water of 10; the German PEC_{sw} are the originally reported values.

The median difference is 4, range 1–>1 600. The outliers are acetylsalicylic acid and ethinyloestradiol. Acetylsalicylic acid and ethinyloestradiol are used privately a lot (aspirin and anticonception).

It can be concluded that the model predictions for surface water are comparable to the measurements. It can therefore be expected that many more drugs could be found in surface waters in Europe, if looked for.

In Table 14.11 one finds the measured concentrations in drinking water.

Caffeine was found in levels $>1\,\mu g\,l^{-1}$. Conclusion: pharmaceuticals may be present in drinking water, but probably in lower concentrations than in surface water.

Table 14.9. Comparison of the calculations for STP effluent with measured concentrations

	Corrected model 1 ($\mu g\,l^{-1}$)	Corrected model 2 ($\mu g\,l^{-1}$)	Corrected model 3 ($\mu g\,l^{-1}$)	STP effluent ($\mu g\,l^{-1}$)	Difference ($\mu g\,l^{-1}$)
Acetylsalicylic acid	14.6	23.2		1.51	9
Acetylsalicylic acid	161	23.2		1.51	100
Clofibrinic acid		0.5		7.1	14
Clofibrinic acid		0.5		0.3	2
Caffeïne	0.29			292	1 000
Cyclofosfamide		0.02		0.06	3
Diazepam	0.44		1.2	<1	1
Diclofenac		5.4		2	3
Ethinyloestradiol		0.002		0.0005	4
Ethinyloestradiol		0.002		1.86	930
Ibuprofen	9.5			12	1
Indomethacine	1.32			0.52	3
Ifosfamide		0.008	0.0078	0.06	8
Norethisteron		0.04		0.02	2
Oestradiol		0.1		0.35	4
Oestradiol		0.1		0.01	10
Oestriol		0.05		0.04	1
Phenylpropanolamine	0.29			4.09	12
Salicylic acid	0.29			240	800
Sulfasalazine	1.8			0.02	90

14.4
Results and Discussion

Evidently, many veterinary antibiotics intended for mass-treatment will enter a Phase II assessment for the soil compartment (because the PEC_{soil} are higher than the trigger) and for the groundwater compartment (because the K_{oc} will probably be $<500\,l\,kg^{-1}$, not discussed in this paper), unless the $DT_{50,\,slurry}$ is <30 days. This underlines the importance of a valid soil-slurry scenario and reliable test designs to determine the $DT_{50,\,slurry}$.

Predicted exposure concentrations may differ by a factor of forty, depending on the model and the substance properties. The availability of a $DT_{50,\,soil}$ can lower the $PIEC_{soil}$ for grassland substantially. The Dutch models give higher estimations for animals with long life cycles compared to the basic year-averaged model, whereas for animals with short life cycles (young turkeys, broilers) estimations can be lower, depending on the substance properties. These calculations show also that the choice of the trigger values ($DT_{50,\,slurry} < 30$ days, $PIEC_{soil} < 10\,\mu g\,kg^{-1}$, as made by the EMEA, are not harmonised.

Table 14.10. Comparison of the calculations for surface water with measured concentrations

	Corrected model 1 ($\mu g \, l^{-1}$)	Corrected model 2 ($\mu g \, l^{-1}$)	Corrected model 3 ($\mu g \, l^{-1}$)	River water ($\mu g \, l^{-1}$)	Difference ($\mu g \, l^{-1}$)
Acetylsalicylic acid	1.46	2.32		<0.01	>146
Acetylsalicylic acid	16.1	2.32		<0.01	>1616
Clofibrate	0.63			0.04	15
Clofibrinic acid		0.05		1.75	35
Clofibrinic acid		0.05		0.22	4
Dextropropoxyfen	0.32			1	3
Diazepam	0.044			0.01	4
Diazepam			0.12	0.01	12
Erythromycine	0.22	3.69		1	4
Ethinyloestradiol		0.0002		0.0003	2
Ethinyloestradiol		0.0002		0.015	75
Ibuprofen	0.95			0.139	2
Indomethacine	0.132			0.121	1
Norethisteron		0.004		<0.017	1
Spironolacton		0.48		1	2
Theobromine	0.029			1	30

Table 14.11. Measured concentrations in river water and drinking water (maximum values)

	River water ($\mu g \, l^{-1}$)	Drinking water ($\mu g \, l^{-1}$)
Bezafibrate	0.38	0.027
Bleomycine	0.0085	0.013
Clofibrinic acid	1.75	0.07
Diazepam	0.01	0.01
Diclofenac	0.489	0.006
Ethinyloestradiol	0.015	0.00006
Ibuprofen	0.139	0.003
Norethisteron	<0.017	<0.010

For example: with a DT_{50} of <30 days further assessment is not necessary, but $PIEC_{soil}$ may still be >10 $\mu g \, kg^{-1}$.

This exposure route is also of interest in regards to disinfectants (biocides) used for cleaning stables. Examples are trichlorfon, methomyl and diflubenzuron. Degradation of trichlorfon is highly pH-dependent: at pH 9 practically no residues will reach the soil; at pH 7 considerable amounts of parent compound and metabolites will reach the soil, and possibly the groundwater. Registration may therefore depend on the model parameters used (pH, redox potential, temperature in slurry basin) that determine the predicted environmental concentrations.

The concentration in groundwater depends on the concentration in the soil and the capacity of the substance to adsorb to the organic material in the soil. In Phase I the EU-approach is used, where the concentration in the groundwater is set equal to the concentration in the porewater. This model does not represent a realistic leaching behaviour. Suppose the concentration in soil is just below the soil trigger of 10 μg kg^{-1} dwt; the sorption coefficient (K_{oc}) has to be >5 600 l kg^{-1}, in order not to exceed the groundwater trigger of 0.1 μg l^{-1}. This high sorption coefficient does not apply for hydrophilic substances like most antibiotics. However, there are a number of (validated) models on groundwater leaching of pesticides available that can be applied in Phase II. One should be aware of the vulnerability of these model predictions: a factor 2 in DT$_{50, soil}$ or in K_{oc} changes the PIEC$_{groundwater}$ by a factor up to 10. Furthermore, experimental K_{oc} are required, or more appropriate QSARs for polar compounds are needed. Because of the uncertainty in the modelling, the PIEC$_{groundwater}$ > 0.001 μg l^{-1} should trigger the demand for lysimeter studies within the scope of the pesticide registration in the Netherlands. The leaching of most antibiotics would still be a point of concern.

This brings another point to the attention: in the current method, the applicant of the veterinary medicinal product is not obliged to perform transformation route studies in the animal, slurry, or soil. However, metabolites are in general more hydrophilic than parent compounds. In case the parent compounds meet the trigger for groundwater, there is no Phase II on this aspect. The fate of metabolites would thus never be examined.

The exposure trigger level for further testing when the environment is exposed by dung from grazing animals is 10 μg kg^{-1} wwt. This trigger will have no practical consequences for the pharmaceutical industry. Even substances with relatively low dosages (like ivermectin) will exceed this trigger 100 times. It is even more remarkable that ivermectin at concentrations of 0.5 μg kg^{-1} wwt still induces aberrations in wings of the dung fly *Scatophaga stercoraria* (Strong and James 1993). In this case the trigger is not even protective enough.

The testing in Phase II starts with laboratory tests. If these reveal >30% effect (which is very likely, given the nature of the substances), Phase II Tier B testing is required: investigations into the field effects. Pending the development of a method to assess population effects, will all anthelmintics be taken off the market? And will companies be willing to put so much effort into registration, regarding the costs these investigations bear?

The duration of exposure is not taken into account in Phase I. It was found that larvae of the dung fly *Neomyia cornicia* did not develop in dung from cattle collected up to 32 days after injection with ivermectin (Wardhaugh and Rodriguez-Menendez 1988), whereas after oral treatment, all ivermectin residues are excreted after one week (see Montforts et al. 1999). The Phase II assessment will eventually have to answer to the question whether field populations of insects will be reduced due to the use of the medicine. In view of this population-dynamic approach in Phase II (e.g. field testing), the Phase I assessment should at least take the expected distribution in space and time into account.

Currently over 70 pharmaceuticals have been found in groundwater, surface water and drinking water. Comparison could only be made between a dozen pharmaceuticals that were both measured and modelled. Comparison of measurements with model calculations indicate that the measurements represent the background-levels in surface water, rather than incidental high levels. It can therefore be expected that many more drugs could be found in surface waters in Europe, if looked for.

The next major question then is: what are the effects? Acute effects in the concentration range of several ng l^{-1} are not to be excluded for all substances. Furthermore, what are the chronic effects on environmental and human health (allergic reactions, resistance, changes in bacterial community structure)? What can be done to decrease the environmental contamination? Research into the behaviour of these compounds in sewage treatment plants is needed.

Summarising the above: a substantial amount of work has already been done in order to perform the environmental risk assessment for veterinary and human drugs. However, the implementation of the methodology for veterinary products has exposed several weaknesses that require adequate measures.

There is an urgent need for the validation of the slurry-soil-groundwater model, as the registration of many antibiotics will be endangered under the current methodology. The lack of knowledge on the behaviour of the polar antibiotics with respect to degradation in slurry and soil, and the sorption properties to organic matter and/or clay minerals hampers acceptable provisional assessments. Therefore, both the environmental conditions in slurry pits should be standardised for the calculations, the compound-specific behaviour should be investigated, and the fate of the residues in slurry and soil in field situations should be monitored, in an attempt to validate and standardise the slurry-soil exposure route.

There can be great differences in agricultural practice and environmental conditions from one country to another, while at the same time on the European scale there is a need for harmonised exposure models and realistic trigger values. This dilemma calls for an ongoing harmonisation process, preferably guided by a European technical guidance document on the environmental assessment of veterinary medicinal products.

With respect to antiparasitic and anthelmintic substances, the current dossier requirements regarding population effects on dung fauna give little hope for many applicants. Not only is little known of the dung fauna and its behaviour in many European countries, but also a test design that will satisfy the data requirements is not available.

The available information on the occurrence of human drugs in surface water, groundwater and drinking water is alarming: all drugs used should be traceable in surface water. The implementation of the methodology for the dossier evaluation of drugs should no longer be delayed. Further investigations into the (combined) effects of these compounds at these exposure levels are needed. Research into the behaviour of these compounds in sewage treatment plants is needed.

With respect to groundwater: given the nature of the antibiotics used as antimicrobial growth promoters and as veterinary products, groundwater under agricultural areas may contain high amounts of antibiotics. Systematic monitoring of surface waters and groundwater (especially in vulnerable areas, e.g. the combination of bio-industry in regions with sandy arable soils) should provide a better picture of the scope of the problem.

References

CBS (1996) De Landbouwtelling 1996 (in Dutch). Centraal Bureau voor de Statistiek, Misset uitgeverij B.V., Doetinchem

ECB (1996a) EUSES, the European Union system for the evaluation of substances. National Institute of Public Health and the Environment (RIVM), The Netherlands. (available from European Chemicals Bureau (ECB/DGXI), Ispra, Italy)

ECB (1996b) Technical guidance document in support of the commission directive 93/67/EEC on risk assessment for new notified substances and the commission regulation (EC) 1488/94 on risk assessment for existing substances. European Chemical Bureau, Ispra, Italy

EMEA (1997a) Note for guidance: environmental risk assessment for veterinary medicinal products other than GMO-containing and immunological products. European Agency for Evaluation of Medicinal Products, Committee for veterinary medicinal products (EMEA/CVMP/055/96, 1997)

EMEA (1997b) Human medicines evaluation unit. EMEA (Meeting: SWP 12 February 1997 Agenda point: VI.6. For discussion: FDA: Retrospective review of ecotoxicity data submitted in environmental assessment for public display, docket no. 96N-0057)

EU (1981) Directive 81/852/EEC of the Commission of September 28, 1981 as published in the Official Journal of the European Community of November 6, 1981, No. L317, page 16, amended by: Directive 92/18/EEC of the Commission of March 20, 1992 as published in the Official Journal of the European Community of April 10, 1992, No. L97, page 1; and Directive 93/40/EEC of the Council of June 14, 1993 as published in the Official Journal of the European Community of August 24, 1993, No. L214, page 31

EU (1997a) Directive 91/414/EEC of 15 July 1991 concerning the placing of plant protection products on the market. O.J. No L230, 19.8.1991 as lastly amended by: Directive 97/57/EC establishing Annex VI to Directive 91/414/EEC O.J. No. L265, 27.9.1997

EU (1997b) Directive of the European Parliament and of the Council concerning the placing of biocidal products on the market: joint text (doc. PE-CONS 3633/97 ENV394 ENT183 CODEC681) adopted by the Council on 18,19 December 1997

Herd R (1995) Endectocidal drugs: ecological risks and counter-measures. Int J Parasit 25:875–885

Leeuwen CJ Van (1995) General introduction. In: Leeuwen CJ Van, Hermens JLM (eds) Risk assessment of chemicals: an Introduction. Kluwer Academic Publishers, Dordrecht, Boston, London, pp 1–18

Linden AMA van der, Boesten JJTI (1989) Berekening van de mate van uitspoeling en accumulatie van bestrijdingsmiddelen als functie van hun sorptiecoefficient en omzettingssnelhed in bouwvoormateriaal (in Dutch). RIVM, Bilthoven, the Netherlands, (RIVM-Report No. 728800003)

Linders JBHJ, Jager DT (eds) (1997) USES 2.0 – The Uniform System for the Evaluation of Substances, version 2.0. The Netherlands' supplement to EUSES. RIVM, Bilthoven, the Netherlands (RIVM-Report No. 679102037)

Lumaret J, Galante E, Lumbreras C, Mena J, Bertrand M, Bernal JL, Cooper JF, Kadiri N, Crowe D (1993) Field effects of ivermectin residues on dung beetles. J Appl Ecol 30:428–436

Mensink BJWG, Montforts MHMM, Wijkhuizen-Maslankiewicz L, Tibosch H, Linders JBHJ (1995) Manual for summarising and evaluating the environmental aspects of pesticides. RIVM, Bilthoven, The Netherlands (RIVM-Report No. 679101022)

Montforts MHMM, Kalf DF, Vlaardingen PLA Van, Linders JBHJ (1999) The exposure assessment for veterinary medicinal products. Sci Total Environ 225:119–133

Rabølle M, Spliid NH (2000) Sorption and mobility of metronidazole, olaquindox, oxytetracycline and tylosin in soil. Chemosphere 40:715–722

Rekker RF (1977) The hydrophobic fragmental constant. Elsevier, Amsterdam

Roij ThAMJ, Vries PHU de (1980) Milieutoxicologische aspecten van het gebruik van veevoederadditieven en therapeutica. Persistentie in dierlijke excreta en milieu (in Dutch). Ministry of Housing, Spatial Planning and the Environment, The Hague, the Netherlands

Römbke J, Knacker T, Stahlschmidt-Allner P (1996) Umweltprobleme durch Arzneimittel – Literaturstudie (in German). Umweltbundesamt, Berlin (Report Nr. UBA-FB 96-060)

Sommer C, Steffansen B (1993) Changes with time after treatment in the concentrations of ivermectin in fresh cow dung and in cow pats aged in the field. Vet Parasit 48:67–73

Soulides DA, Pinck LA, Allison FE (1962) Antibiotics in soils. V. Stability and release of soil adsorbed antibiotics. Antib Soils 1962:239–244

Spaepen KRI, Leemput LJJ van, Wislocki PG, Verschueren C (1997) A uniform procedure to estimate the predicted environmental concentration of the residues of veterinary medicines in soil. Environ Toxicol Chem 16:1977–1982

Strong L, James S (1993) Some effects of ivermectin on the yellow dung fly Scatophaga stercoraria. Vet Parasit 48:181–191

Strong L, Wall R, Woolford A,Djeddour D (1996) The effect of faecally excreted ivermectin and fenbendazole on the insect colonisation of cattle dung following the oral administration of sustained-release bolus. Vet Parasit 2:253–266

Wardhaugh KG, Rodriguez-Menendez H (1988) The effect of the antiparasitic drug, ivermectin, on the development and survival of the dung breeding fly *Orthelia cornicia* and the scarabeine dung beetles, *Copris hispanus, Bubas bubalus* and *Onitis belial*. J Appl Entomol 106:381–389

A Data-based Perspective on the Environmental Risk Assessment of Human Pharmaceuticals I – Collation of Available Ecotoxicity Data

S. F. Webb

15.1
Introduction

There is a growing literature relating to observations of human pharmaceuticals in the environment. Discussions about the environmental consequences of the presence of such compounds have taken place in the general absence of a systematic analysis of the potential risk. This can partly be attributed to the lack of public domain information relating to the ecotoxicity of pharmaceuticals. The lack of such an analysis means that to date, decisions concerning environmental risk assessment criteria and/or regulatory thresholds have been somewhat arbitrary or based upon inappropriate groups of industrial chemicals such as pesticides. This study attempts to address that deficiency and collates examples of data relating to the ecotoxicity of existing human pharmaceuticals. The intention is to provide perspective that will prove useful during the further development of assessment criteria. The database may also prove useful in the context of the risk assessment of individual substances.

15.2
Methods

A review of available acute ecotoxicity data for macro-invertebrates, fish and algae was conducted. Results of studies from searches of the published scientific literature were supplemented with details of studies from the grey-literature or regulatory submissions secured via contacts with colleagues from industry and academia. In collating the data, attempts were made to ensure that the original sources of data were consulted. In many cases it was not always possible to establish if concentrations at the reported endpoints relate to nominal or measured concentrations. Inclusion of data does not imply endorsement – in terms of quality – of the study in question.

15.3
Results

15.3.1
Acute Ecotoxicity Data

The available acute ecotoxicity database for macro-invertebrates, fish and algae is presented in Table 15.1. There are over 360 endpoints for over 100 human pharmaceuticals.

Table 15.1. Acute ecotoxicity data for human pharmaceuticals

Compound	Category[a]	Value (mg l^{-1})	Endpoint/ Duration[b]	Species	Reference
Acarbose	Antidiabetic	>1 000	EC_{50}	Unspecified fish	FDA-CDER (1996)
Acarbose	Antidiabetic	>1 000	EC_{50}	*Daphnia* spp.	FDA-CDER (1996)
Acriflavine	Anti-infective	5	96h LC_{50}	*Morone saxatilis* (larvae)	Hughes (1973)
Acriflavine	Anti-infective	30.0	48h LC_{50}	*Morone saxatilis* (fingerling)	Hughes (1973)
Acriflavine	Anti-infective	28.0	72h LC_{50}	*Morone saxatilis* (fingerling)	Hughes (1973)
Acriflavine	Anti-infective	27.5	96h LC_{50}	*Morone saxatilis* (fingerling)	Hughes (1973)
Acriflavine	Anti-infective	30.1	24h LC_{50}	*Oncorhynchus mykiss*	Wilford (1966)
Acriflavine	Anti-infective	19.9	48h LC_{50}	*Oncorhynchus mykiss*	Wilford (1966)
Acriflavine	Anti-infective	37.5	24h LC_{50}	*Salvelinus namaycush*	Wilford (1966)
Acriflavine	Anti-infective	28.0	48h LC_{50}	*Salvelinus namaycush*	Wilford (1966)
Acriflavine	Anti-infective	40.0	24h LC_{50}	*Salmo trutta*	Wilford (1966)
Acriflavine	Anti-infective	27.0	48h LC_{50}	*Salmo trutta*	Wilford (1966)
Acriflavine	Anti-infective	43.5	24h LC_{50}	*Ictalurus punctatus*	Wilford (1966)
Acriflavine	Anti-infective	33.2	48h LC_{50}	*Ictalurus punctatus*	Wilford (1966)
Acriflavine	Anti-infective	48.0	24h LC_{50}	*Salvelinus fontinalis*	Wilford (1966)
Acriflavine	Anti-infective	14.8	48h LC_{50}	*Salvelinus fontinalis*	Wilford (1966)
Acriflavine	Anti-infective	18.0	24h LC_{50}	*Lepomis macrochirus*	Wilford (1966)
Acriflavine	Anti-infective	13.5	48h LC_{50}	*Lepomis macrochirus*	Wilford (1966)
Alendronate sodium	Metabolic bone disease	1 450	LC_{50}	*Pimephales promelas*	FDA-CDER (1996)
Alendronate sodium	Metabolic bone disease	>1 000	LC_{50}	*Oncorhynchus mykiss*	FDA-CDER (1996)
Alendronate sodium	Metabolic bone disease	22	LC_{50}	*Daphnia* spp.	FDA-CDER (1996)
Alendronate sodium	Metabolic bone disease	>0.5	MIC	Green algae	FDA-CDER (1996)
Aminosidine	Antibacterial; antiamebic	2 220	48h EC_{50}	*Artemia*	Migliore et al. (1997)
Aminosidine	Antibacterial; antiamebic	847	72h EC_{50}	*Artemia*	Migliore et al. (1997)
Aminosidine sulfate (Neomycin E)	Antibacterial; antiamebic	1 055	24h LC_{50}	*D. magna*	Di Delupis et al. (1992)
Aminosidine sulfate (Neomycin E)	Antibacterial; antiamebic	503	48h LC_{50}	*D. magna*	Di Delupis et al. (1992)
Amitriptyline	Antidepressant	1.2	24h EC_{50}	*D. magna*	Lilius et al. (1994)
Amitriptyline	Antidepressant	36.9	24h LC_{50}	*Artemia salina*	Calleja et al. (1994b)

Table 15.1. *Continued*

Compound	Category[a]	Value (mg l^{-1})	Endpoint/ Duration[b]	Species	Reference
Amitriptyline	Antidepressant	0.78	24h LC$_{50}$	*Streptocephalus proboscideus*	Calleja et al. (1994b)
Amitriptyline	Antidepressant	5.55	24h EC$_{50}$	*D. magna*	Calleja et al. (1994b)
Amitriptyline	Antidepressant	0.80	24h LC$_{50}$	*Brachionus calyciflorus*	Calleja et al. (1994b)
Amobarbital	Sedative; hypnotic	85.4	96h EC$_{50}$	*Pimephales promelas*	Russom et al. (1997)
Amopyroquin dihydrochloride	Antimalarial	47.0	24h LC$_{50}$	*Oncorhynchus mykiss*	Willford (1966)
Amopyroquin dihydrochloride	Antimalarial	35.3	48h LC$_{50}$	*Oncorhynchus mykiss*	Willford (1966)
Amopyroquin dihydrochloride	Antimalarial	15.5	24h LC$_{50}$	*Salvelinus namaycush*	Willford (1966)
Amopyroquin dihydrochloride	Antimalarial	14.0	48h LC$_{50}$	*Salvelinus namaycush*	Willford (1966)
Amopyroquin dihydrochloride	Antimalarial	42.0	24h LC$_{50}$	*Salmo trutta*	Willford (1966)
Amopyroquin dihydrochloride	Antimalarial	36.0	48h LC$_{50}$	*Salmo trutta*	Willford (1966)
Amopyroquin dihydrochloride	Antimalarial	19.8	24h LC$_{50}$	*Ictalurus punctatus*	Willford (1966)
Amopyroquin dihydrochloride	Antimalarial	12.5	48h LC$_{50}$	*Ictalurus punctatus*	Willford (1966)
Amopyroquin dihydrochloride	Antimalarial	52.0	24h LC$_{50}$	*Salvelinus fontinalis*	Willford (1966)
Amopyroquin dihydrochloride	Antimalarial	40.0	48h LC$_{50}$	*Salvelinus fontinalis*	Willford (1966)
Amopyroquin dihydrochloride	Antimalarial	33.0	24h LC$_{50}$	*Lepomis macrochirus*	Willford (1966)
Amopyroquin dihydrochloride	Antimalarial	18.5	48h LC$_{50}$	*Lepomis macrochirus*	Willford (1966)
Amphetamine sulfate	CNS stimulant; anorexic	28.8	96h EC$_{50}$	*Pimephales promelas*	Russom et al. (1997)
Amphetamine sulfate	CNS stimulant; anorexic	60	24h EC$_{50}$	*D. magna*	Lilius et al. (1994)
Amphetamine sulfate	CNS stimulant; anorexic	1 515	24h LC$_{50}$	*Artemia salina*	Calleja et al. (1994b)
Amphetamine sulfate	CNS stimulant; anorexic	55	24h LC$_{50}$	*Streptocephalus proboscideus*	Calleja et al. (1994b)
Amphetamine sulfate	CNS stimulant; anorexic	270	24h EC$_{50}$	*D. magna*	Calleja et al. (1994b)
Amphetamine sulfate	CNS stimulant; anorexic	4.90	24h LC$_{50}$	*Brachionus calyciflorus*	Calleja et al. (1994b)
Aprotinin	Enzyme inhibitor (protease)	>1 000	EC$_{50}$	*Daphnia* spp.	FDA-CDER (1996)

Table 15.1. *Continued*

Compound	Category[a]	Value (mg l^{-1})	Endpoint/ Duration[b]	Species	Reference
Aspirin	Analgesic; antipyretic; anti-inflammatory	1468	24h EC_{50}	*D. magna*	Lilius et al. (1994)
Aspirin	Analgesic; antipyretic; anti-inflammatory	382	24h LC_{50}	*Artemia salina*	Calleja et al. (1994b)
Aspirin	Analgesic; antipyretic; anti-inflammatory	178	24h LC_{50}	*Streptocephalus proboscideus*	Calleja et al. (1994b)
Aspirin	Analgesic; antipyretic; anti-inflammatory	168	24h EC_{50}	*D. magna*	Calleja et al. (1994b)
Aspirin	Analgesic; antipyretic; anti-inflammatory	141	24h LC_{50}	*Brachionus calyciflorus*	Calleja et al. (1994b)
Atropine sulfate	Anticholinergic; mydriatic	258	24h EC_{50}	*D. magna*	Lilius et al. (1994)
Atropine sulfate	Anticholinergic; mydriatic	15773	24h LC_{50}	*Artemia salina*	Calleja et al. (1994b)
Atropine sulfate	Anticholinergic; mydriatic	661	24h LC_{50}	*Streptocephalus proboscideus*	Calleja et al. (1994b)
Atropine sulfate	Anticholinergic; mydriatic	356	24h EC_{50}	*D. magna*	Calleja et al. (1994b)
Atropine sulfate	Anticholinergic; mydriatic	334	24h LC_{50}	*Brachionus calyciflorus*	Calleja et al. (1994b)
Azithromycin	Antibacterial	>120	LC_{50}	Unspecified amphipod	FDA-CDER (1996)
Azithromycin	Antibacterial	120	EC_{50}	*Daphnia* spp.	FDA-CDER (1996)
Bacitracin	Antibacterial	34.1	24h EC_{50}	*Artemia salina* (nauplii)	Migliore et al. (1997)
Bacitracin	Antibacterial	21.8	48h EC_{50}	*Artemia salina* (nauplii)	Migliore et al. (1997)
Bacitracin	Antibacterial	34.1	24h LC_{50}	*Artemia salina* (nauplii)	Brambilla et al. (1994)
Bacitracin	Antibacterial	21.8	48h LC_{50}	*Artemia salina* (nauplii)	Brambilla et al. (1994)
Bacitracin	Antibacterial	126.4	24h LC_{50}	*D.magna*	Brambilla et al. (1994)
Bacitracin	Antibacterial	30.5	48h LC_{50}	*D.magna*	Brambilla et al. (1994)
Bacitracin	Antibacterial	126.4	24h LC_{50}	*D.magna*	Di Delupis et al. (1992)
Bacitracin	Antibacterial	30.5	48h LC_{50}	*D.magna*	Di Delupis et al. (1992)
Bicalutamide	Non-steroidal antiandrogen	>5	EC_{50}	*Daphnia* spp.	FDA-CDER (1996)
Bicalutamide	Non-steroidal antiandrogen	>1	EC_{50}	Unspecified green algae	FDA-CDER (1996)

Table 15.1. *Continued*

Compound	Category[a]	Value (mg l^{-1})	Endpoint/ Duration[b]	Species	Reference
Bicalutamide	Non-steroidal antiandrogen	>1	EC$_{50}$	Unspecified blue-green algae	FDA-CDER (1996)
Budesonide	Anti-inflammatory	20	EC$_{50}$	*Daphnia* spp.	FDA-CDER (1996)
Budesonide	Anti-inflammatory	>19	LC$_{50}$	Unspecified fish	FDA-CDER (1996)
Caffeine	CNS stimulant	151	96h EC$_{50}$	*Pimephales promelas*	Russom et al. (1997)
Caffeine	CNS stimulant	684	24h EC$_{50}$	*D. magna*	Lilius et al. (1994)
Caffeine	CNS stimulant	3 457	24h LC$_{50}$	*Artemia salina*	Calleja et al. (1994b)
Caffeine	CNS stimulant	410	24h LC$_{50}$	*S. proboscideus*	Calleja et al. (1994b)
Caffeine	CNS stimulant	160	24h EC$_{50}$	*D. magna*	Calleja et al. (1994b)
Caffeine	CNS stimulant	4 661	24h LC$_{50}$	*Brachionus calyciflorus*	Calleja et al. (1994b)
Carvedilol	Antihypertensive; antianginal	>3	EC$_{50}$	*Daphnia* spp.	FDA-CDER (1996)
Carvedilol	Antihypertensive; antianginal	1	LC$_{50}$	Unspecified fish	FDA-CDER (1996)
Cefprozil	Antibacterial	>642	EC$_{50}$	*Daphnia* spp.	FDA-CDER (1996)
Ceftibuten	Antibacterial	>600	EC$_{50}$	*Daphnia* spp.	FDA-CDER (1996)
Ceftibuten	Antibacterial	>520	LC$_{50}$	Amphipod	FDA-CDER (1996)
Cetirizine HCl	Antihistaminic	330	EC$_{50}$	*Daphnia* spp.	FDA-CDER (1996)
Chloramine T	Antibacterial	23.6	24h LC$_{50}$	*Penaeus setiferus*	Johnson (1976)
Chloramine T	Antibacterial	22	96h LC$_{50}$	*Rasbora heteromorpha*	Tooby et al. (1975)
Chloramphenicol	Antibacterial; antirickettsial	543	24h EC$_{50}$	*D. magna*	Lilius et al. (1994)
Chloramphenicol	Antibacterial; antirickettsial	2 042	24h LC$_{50}$	*Artemia salina*	Calleja et al. (1994b)
Chloramphenicol	Antibacterial; antirickettsial	305	24h LC$_{50}$	*Streptocephalus proboscideus*	Calleja et al. (1994b)
Chloramphenicol	Antibacterial; antirickettsial	1 086	24h EC$_{50}$	*D. magna*	Calleja et al. (1994b)
Chloramphenicol	Antibacterial; antirickettsial	2 074	24h LC$_{50}$	*Brachionus calyciflorus*	Calleja et al. (1994b)
Chloroquine phosphate	Antimalarial; antiamebic; antirheumatic	50	24h EC$_{50}$	*D. magna*	Lilius et al. (1994)
Chloroquine phosphate	Antimalarial; antiamebic; antirheumatic	2 043	24h LC$_{50}$	*Artemia salina*	Calleja et al. (1994b)
Chloroquine phosphate	Antimalarial; antiamebic; antirheumatic	11.7	24h LC$_{50}$	*Streptocephalus proboscideus*	Calleja et al. (1994b)
Chloroquine phosphate	Antimalarial; antiamebic; antirheumatic	43.5	24h EC$_{50}$	*D. magna*	Calleja et al. (1994b)

Table 15.1. *Continued*

Compound	Category[a]	Value (mg l^{-1})	Endpoint/ Duration[b]	Species	Reference
Chloroquine phosphate	Antimalarial; antiamebic; antirheumatic	4.39	24h LC$_{50}$	*Brachionus calyciflorus*	Calleja et al. (1994b)
Cimetidine	Anti-ulcerative	740	EC$_{50}$	*Daphnia* spp.	FDA-CDER (1996)
Cimetidine	Anti-ulcerative	>1 000	LC$_{50}$	*Lepomis macrochirus*	FDA-CDER (1996)
Cisapride	Peristaltic stimulant	>1 000	EC$_{50}$	*Daphnia* spp.	FDA-CDER (1996)
Cisapride	Peristaltic stimulant	>1 000	LC$_{50}$	*Lepomis macrochirus*	FDA-CDER (1996)
Cladribine	Antineoplastic	233	EC$_{50}$	*Daphnia* spp.	FDA-CDER (1996)
Clofibrate	Antihyperlipo-proteinemic	28.2	24h EC$_{50}$	*D. magna*	Köpf (1995)
Clofibrate	Antihyperlipo-proteinemic	12.0	EC$_{50}$	Unspecified algae	Köpf (1995)
Clofibrinic acid	Antihyperlipo-proteinemic	106	EC$_{50}$	*D. magna*	Henschel et al. (1997)
Clofibrinic acid	Antihyperlipo-proteinemic	86.0	48h EC$_{50}$	*Brachydanio rerio* (embryos)	Henschel et al. (1997)
Clofibrinic acid	Antihyperlipo-proteinemic	89	72h EC$_{50}$	*Scenedesmus subspicatus*	Henschel et al. (1997)
Cyclosporine	Immunosuppressant	>100	LC$_{50}$	*Oncorhynchus mykiss*	FDA-CDER (1996)
Cyclosporine	Immunosuppressant	20	EC$_{50}$	*Daphnia* spp.	FDA-CDER (1996)
Dextroproproxyphene HCl	Narcotic analgesic	14.6	24h EC$_{50}$	*D. magna*	Lilius et al. (1994)
Dextroproproxyphene HCl	Narcotic analgesic	308	24h LC$_{50}$	*Artemia salina*	Calleja et al. (1994b)
Dextroproproxyphene HCl	Narcotic analgesic	7.6	24h LC$_{50}$	*Streptocephalus proboscideus*	Calleja et al. (1994b)
Dextroproproxyphene HCl	Narcotic analgesic	19	24h EC$_{50}$	*D. magna*	Calleja et al. (1994b)
Dextroproproxyphene HCl	Narcotic analgesic	4.2	24h LC$_{50}$	*Brachionus calyciflorus*	Calleja et al. (1994b)
Diazepam	Anxiolytic; muscle relaxant	65.4	24h LC$_{50}$	*Artemia salina*	Calleja et al. (1994b)
Diazepam	Anxiolytic; muscle relaxant	103	24h LC$_{50}$	*Streptocephalus proboscideus*	Calleja et al. (1994b)
Diazepam	Anxiolytic; muscle relaxant	14.1	24h EC$_{50}$	*D. magna*	Calleja et al. (1994b)
Diazepam	Anxiolytic; muscle relaxant	>10 000	24h LC$_{50}$	*Brachionus calyciflorus*	Calleja et al. (1994b)
Diazepam	Anxiolytic; muscle relaxant	4.3	24h EC$_{50}$	*D. magna*	Lilius et al. (1994)
Didanosine	Anti(retro)viral	>1 020	EC$_{50}$	*D. magna*	FDA-CDER (1996)
Diethylstilbestrol	Oestrogen	4.0	LC$_{50}$	*D. magna*	Coats et al. (1976)
Diethylstilbestrol	Oestrogen	>10	LC$_{50}$	*Physa* spp.	Coats et al. (1976)
Diethylstilbestrol	Oestrogen	>1	48h LC$_{50}$	*Gambusia affinis*	Coats et al. (1976)

Table 15.1. *Continued*

Compound	Category[a]	Value (mg l^{-1})	Endpoint/ Duration[b]	Species	Reference
Diethylstilbestrol	Oestrogen	1.09	48h LC$_{50}$	*D. magna*	Zou and Fingerman (1997)
Diethylstilbestrol	Oestrogen	1.2	48h LC$_{50}$	*D. magna*	Baldwin et al. (1995)
Diethylstilbestrol	Oestrogen	316	14d LC$_{50}$	*Pimephales promelas*	Panter et al. (1999)
Digoxin	Cardiotonic	24	24h EC$_{50}$	*D. magna*	Lilius et al. (1994)
Dirithromycin	Antibacterial	>2880	LC$_{50}$	*Oncorhynchus mykiss*	FDA-CDER (1996)
Dirithromycin	Antibacterial	>48	EC$_{50}$	*D. magna*	FDA-CDER (1996)
Dorzolamide HCl	Carbonic anhydrase inhibitor, treatment of glaucoma	>1000	LC$_{50}$	*Pimephales promelas*	FDA-CDER (1996)
Dorzolamide HCl	Carbonic anhydrase inhibitor, treatment of glaucoma	699	EC$_{50}$	*D. magna*	FDA-CDER (1996)
Erythromycin	Antibacterial	388	24h LC$_{50}$	*D.magna*	Di Delupis et al. (1992)
Erythromycin	Antibacterial	211	48h LC$_{50}$	*D.magna*	Di Delupis et al. (1992)
Erythromycin phosphate	Antibacterial	818	24h LC$_{50}$	*Salvelinus namaycush*	Marking et al. (1988)
Erythromycin phosphate	Antibacterial	410	96h LC$_{50}$	*Salvelinus namaycush*	Marking et al. (1988)
Erythromycin thiocyanate	Antibacterial	>80	48h LC$_{50}$	*Oncorhynchus mykiss, Salmo trutta, Salvelinus fontinalis, Ictalurus punctatus, Lepomis macrochirus* and *Salvelinus namaycush*	Wilford (1966)
Ethinyloestradiol	Oestrogen	5.7	24h EC$_{50}$	*D. magna*	Köpf (1995)
Ethinyloestradiol	Oestrogen	0.84	EC$_{50}$	Unspecified algae	Köpf (1995)
Ethinyloestradiol	Oestrogen	6.4	48h EC$_{50}$	*D. magna*	Schweinfurth et al. (1996b)
Ethinyloestradiol	Oestrogen	1.6	96h EC$_{50}$	*Oncorhynchus mykiss*	Schweinfurth et al. (1996b)
Etidronic acid	Metabolic bone Disease	200	96h LC$_{50}$	*Oncorhynchus mykiss*	Gledhill and Feijtel (1992)
Etidronic acid	Metabolic bone disease	868	96h LC$_{50}$	*Lepomis macrochirus*	Gledhill and Feijtel (1992)
Etidronic acid	Metabolic bone disease	695	48h LC$_{50}$	*Ictalurus punctatus*	Gledhill and Feijtel (1992)
Etidronic acid	Metabolic bone disease	3.0	96h EC$_{50}$	Unspecified algae	Gledhill and Feijtel (1992)
Etidronic acid	Metabolic bone disease	527	48h EC$_{50}$	*D. magna*	Gledhill and Feijtel (1992)
Famciclovir	Antiviral	>986	LC$_{50}$	*Lepomis macrochirus*	FDA-CDER (1996)
Famciclovir	Antiviral	820	EC$_{50}$	*D. magna*	FDA-CDER (1996)

Table 15.1. *Continued*

Compound	Category[a]	Value (mg l^{-1})	Endpoint/ Duration[b]	Species	Reference
Famotidine	Anti-ulcerative	>680	LC$_{50}$	*Pimephales promelas*	FDA-CDER (1996)
Famotidine	Anti-ulcerative	398	EC$_{50}$	*D. magna*	FDA-CDER (1996)
Finasteride	Treatment of benign prostatic hypertrophy	21	EC$_{50}$	*Daphnia* spp.	FDA-CDER (1996)
Finasteride	Treatment of benign prostatic hypertrophy	20	LC$_{50}$	*Oncorhynchus mykiss*	FDA-CDER (1996)
Flumazenil	Benzodiazepine antagonist	>500	EC$_{50}$	*D. magna*	FDA-CDER (1996)
Flumequine	Antibacterial	476.8	24h EC$_{50}$	*Artemia salina* (nauplii)	Migliore et al. (1997)
Flumequine	Antibacterial	307.7	48h EC$_{50}$	*Artemia salina* (nauplii)	Migliore et al. (1997)
Flumequine	Antibacterial	96.4	72h EC$_{50}$	*Artemia salina* (nauplii)	Migliore et al. (1997)
Flumequine	Antibacterial	477	24h LC$_{50}$	*Artemia salina* (nauplii)	Brambilla et al. (1994)
Flumequine	Antibacterial	308	48h LC$_{50}$	*Artemia salina* (nauplii)	Brambilla et al. (1994)
Flumequine	Antibacterial	96.4	72h LC$_{50}$	*Artemia salina* (nauplii)	Brambilla et al. (1994)
Flutamide	Androgen	>1 000	14d LC$_{50}$	*Pimephales promelas*	Panter et al. (1999)
Fluticasone propionate	Corticosteroid antiasthmatic	0.55	EC$_{50}$	*Daphnia* spp.	FDA-CDER (1996)
Fluoxetine HCl	Antidepressant	0.94	EC$_{50}$	*Daphnia* spp.	FDA-CDER (1996)
Fluoxetine HCl	Antidepressant	2.0	LC$_{50}$	*Oncorhynchus mykiss*	FDA-CDER (1996)
Fluoxetine HCl	Antidepressant	0.031	EC$_{50}$	Unspecified green algae	FDA-CDER (1996)
Fluoxetine	Antidepressant	1.55	4h LOEC	*Sphaerium* spp.	Fong et al. (1998)
Fluvoxamine maleate	Antidepressant	63	MIC	Unspecified algae	FDA-CDER (1996)
Fluvoxamine	Antidepressant	0.003	4h LOEC	*Sphaerium striatinum*	Fong et al. (1998)
Gabapentin	Antiepileptic adjunctive	>1 100	EC$_{50}$	*Daphnia* spp.	FDA-CDER (1996)
Ibuprofen	Analgesic; anti-inflammatory	7.1	96h EC$_{50}$	*Skeletonema costatum*	Knoll/BASF (1995)
Ibuprofen	Analgesic; anti-inflammatory	9.06	48h EC$_{50}$	*D. magna*	Knoll/BASF (1995)
Ibuprofen	Analgesic; anti-inflammatory	173	96h LC$_{50}$	*Lepomis macrochirus*	Knoll/BASF (1995)
Iopromide	Diagnostic aid (radiopaque medium)	>962	LC$_{50}$	*Oncorhynchus mykiss*	FDA-CDER (1996)
Iopromide	Diagnostic aid (radiopaque medium)	>973	LC$_{50}$	*Lepomis macrochirus*	FDA-CDER (1996)

Table 15.1. *Continued*

Compound	Category[a]	Value (mg l^{-1})	Endpoint/ Duration[b]	Species	Reference
Iopromide	Diagnostic aid (radiopaque medium)	137	MIC	Unspecified green algae	FDA-CDER (1996)
Iopromide	Diagnostic aid (radiopaque medium)	>1016	EC$_{50}$	*Daphnia*	FDA-CDER (1996)
Iopromide	Diagnostic aid (radiopaque medium)	>10000	24h EC$_{50}$	*D. magna*	Schweinfurth et al. (1996a)
Iopromide	Diagnostic aid (radiopaque medium)	>10000	48h EC$_{50}$	Unspecified fish	Schweinfurth et al. (1996a)
Isoniazid	Antibacterial	85	24h EC$_{50}$	*D. magna*	Lilius et al. (1994)
Isoniazid	Antibacterial	322	24h LC$_{50}$	*Artemia salina*	Calleja et al. (1994b)
Isoniazid	Antibacterial	24.4	24h LC$_{50}$	*Streptocephalus proboscideus*	Calleja et al. (1994b)
Isoniazid	Antibacterial	125.5	24h EC$_{50}$	*D. magna*	Calleja et al. (1994b)
Isoniazid	Antibacterial	3045	24h LC$_{50}$	*Brachionus calyciflorus*	Calleja et al. (1994b)
Ketorolac tromethamine	Analgesic; anti-inflammatory	1480	96h LC$_{50}$	*Lepomis macrochirus*	Anon (1993)
Lansoprazole	Proton pump inhibitor (Anti-ulcerative)	>22	EC$_{50}$	*Daphnia* spp.	FDA-CDER (1996)
Lansoprazole	Proton pump inhibitor (Anti-ulcerative)	18	LC$_{50}$	*Oncorhynchus mykiss*	FDA-CDER (1996)
Lincomys(c)in	Antibacterial	283.1	72h EC$_{50}$	*Artemia*	Migliore et al. (1997)
Lincomys(c)in	Antibacterial	379.39	72h LC$_{50}$	*D.magna*	Di Delupis et al. (1992)
Lithium sulfate	Antidepressant	197	24h EC$_{50}$	*D. magna*	Lilius et al. (1994)
Lithium sulfate	Antidepressant	4318	24h LC$_{50}$	*Artemia salina*	Calleja et al. (1994b)
Lithium sulfate	Antidepressant	112	24h LC$_{50}$	*Streptocephalus proboscideus*	Calleja et al. (1994b)
Lithium sulfate	Antidepressant	33.1	24h EC$_{50}$	*D. magna*	Calleja et al. (1994b)
Lithium sulfate	Antidepressant	712	24h LC$_{50}$	*Brachionus calyciflorus*	Calleja et al. (1994b)
Lomefloxacin	Antibacterial	130	EC$_{50}$	*Daphnia* spp.	FDA-CDER (1996)
Lomefloxacin	Antibacterial	170	LC$_{50}$	*Oncorhynchus mykiss*	FDA-CDER (1996)
Lomefloxacin	Antibacterial	2.4	EC$_{50}$	Unspecified green algae	FDA-CDER (1996)
Loracarbef	Anti-infective	>963	EC$_{50}$	*Daphnia* spp.	FDA-CDER (1996)
Losartan K	Antihypertensive	331	EC$_{50}$	*Daphnia* spp.	FDA-CDER (1996)
Losartan K	Antihypertensive	>929	LC$_{50}$	*Oncorhynchus mykiss*	FDA-CDER (1996)
Losartan K	Antihypertensive	>1000	LC$_{50}$	*Pimephales promelas*	FDA-CDER (1996)
Losartan K	Antihypertensive	245	MIC	Unspecified green algae	FDA-CDER (1996)

Table 15.1. *Continued*

Compound	Category[a]	Value (mg l^{-1})	Endpoint/ Duration[b]	Species	Reference
Losartan K	Antihypertensive	949	MIC	Unspecified blue-green alage	FDA-CDER (1996)
Merthiolate (Thimerosal)	Anti-infective	60.5	24h LC$_{50}$	*Oncorhynchus mykiss*	Wilford (1966)
Merthiolate (Thimerosal)	Anti-infective	21.2	48h LC$_{50}$	*Oncorhynchus mykiss*	Wilford (1966)
Merthiolate (Thimerosal)	Anti-infective	13.0	24h LC$_{50}$	*Salvelinus namaycush*	Wilford (1966)
Merthiolate (Thimerosal)	Anti-infective	2.13	48h LC$_{50}$	*Salvelinus namaycush*	Wilford (1966)
Merthiolate (Thimerosal)	Anti-infective	110	24h LC$_{50}$	*Salmo trutta*	Wilford (1966)
Merthiolate (Thimerosal)	Anti-infective	54.0	48h LC$_{50}$	*Salmo trutta*	Wilford (1966)
Merthiolate (Thimerosal)	Anti-infective	7.50	24h LC$_{50}$	*Ictalurus punctatus*	Wilford (1966)
Merthiolate (Thimerosal)	Anti-infective	5.65	48h LC$_{50}$	*Ictalurus punctatus*	Wilford (1966)
Merthiolate (Thimerosal)	Anti-infective	89.5	24h LC$_{50}$	*Salvelinus fontinalis*	Wilford (1966)
Merthiolate (Thimerosal)	Anti-infective	74.5	48h LC$_{50}$	*Salvelinus fontinalis*	Wilford (1966)
Merthiolate (Thimerosal)	Anti-infective	110	24h LC$_{50}$	*Lepomis macrochirus*	Wilford (1966)
Merthiolate (Thimerosal)	Anti-infective	64.5	48h LC$_{50}$	*Lepomis macrochirus*	Wilford (1966)
Metformin HCl	Antidiabetic	>982	LC$_{50}$	*Lepomis macrochirus*	FDA-CDER (1996)
Metformin HCl	Antidiabetic	130	EC$_{50}$	*Daphnia* spp.	FDA-CDER (1996)
Methotrexate	Antineoplastic; antirheumatic	>1000	EC$_{50}$	*D. magna*	Henschel et al. (1997)
Methotrexate	Antineoplastic; antirheumatic	85.0	48h EC$_{50}$	*Brachydanio rerio* (embryos)	Henschel et al. (1997)
Methotrexate	Antineoplastic; antirheumatic	260	72h EC$_{50}$	*Scenedesmus subspicatus*	Henschel et al. (1997)
Metronidazole	Antiprotozoal	>100	72h EC$_{50}$	*Acartia tonsa*	Lanzky and Halling-Sørenson (1997)
Metronidazole	Antiprotozoal	>500	96h EC$_{50}$	*Brachydanio rerio*	Lanzky and Halling-Sørenson (1997)
Metronidazole	Antiprotozoal	39.1	72h EC$_{50}$	*Selenastrum capricornutum*	Lanzky and Halling-Sørenson (1997)
Metronidazole	Antiprotozoal	12.5	72h EC$_{50}$	*Chlorella* spp.	Lanzky and Halling-Sørenson (1997)
Metronidazole	Antiprotozoal	>100	48h LC$_{50}$	*Oncorhynchus mykiss, Salmo trutta, Salvelinus fontinalis, Ictalurus punctatus, Lepomis macrochirus* and *Salvelinus namaycush*	Wilford (1966)
Midazolam	Anesthetic (intravenous)	0.2	EC$_{50}$	*D. magna*	FDA-CDER (1996)
Milrinone lactate	Cardiotonic	414	EC$_{50}$	*Daphnia* spp.	FDA-CDER (1996)
Moexipril HCl (pro-drug)	Antihypertensive	800	EC$_{50}$	*Daphnia* spp.	FDA-CDER (1996)

Table 15.1. *Continued*

Compound	Category[a]	Value (mg l^{-1})	Endpoint/ Duration[b]	Species	Reference
Moexiprilat (active metabolite)	Antihypertensive	>1 000	EC$_{50}$	*Daphnia* spp.	FDA-CDER (1996)
Naproxen sodium	Anti-inflammatory; analgesic; antipyretic	140	24h EC$_{50}$	*D. magna*	Rodriguez et al. (1992)
Naproxen sodium	Anti-inflammatory; analgesic; antipyretic	383	96h LC$_{50}$	*Hyalella azteca*	Rodriguez et al. (1992)
Naproxen sodium	Anti-inflammatory; analgesic; antipyretic	560	96h LC$_{50}$	*Lepomis macrochirus*	Rodriguez et al. (1992)
Naproxen sodium	Anti-inflammatory; analgesic; antipyretic	690	96h LC$_{50}$	*Oncorhynchus mykiss*	Rodriguez et al. (1992)
Nefazodone HCl	Antidepressant	7	EC$_{50}$	*Daphnia* spp.	FDA-CDER (1996)
Nicotine sulfate	Cholinergic agonist	13.8	96h EC$_{50}$	*Pimephales promelas*	Russom et al. (1997)
Nicotine	Cholinergic agonist	3.0	EC$_{50}$	*D. magna*	FDA-CDER (1996)
Nicotine	Cholinergic agonist	7.0	LC$_{50}$	*Oncorhynchus mykiss*	FDA-CDER (1996)
Nicotine	Cholinergic agonist	20.0	LC$_{50}$	*Pimephales promelas*	FDA-CDER (1996)
Nicotine	Cholinergic agonist	4.0	LC$_{50}$	*Lepomis macrochirus*	FDA-CDER (1996)
Nicotine	Cholinergic agonist	13	LC$_{50}$	"Goldfish"	FDA-CDER (1996)
Nisoldipine	Antihypertensive; antianginal	33	EC$_{50}$	*Daphnia* spp.	FDA-CDER (1996)
Nisoldipine	Antihypertensive; antianginal	3	EC$_{50}$	Unspecified fish	FDA-CDER (1996)
Nitrofurazone	Topical anti-infective	1.45	EC$_{50}$	*Selenastrum capricornutum*	Macrì and Sbardella (1984)
Nitrofurazone	Topical anti-infective	28.7	LC$_{50}$	*D. magna*	Macrì and Sbardella (1984)
Nitrofurazone	Topical anti-infective	10	96h LC$_{50}$	*Morone saxatilis* (larvae)	Hughes (1973)
Nitrofurazone	Topical anti-infective	>5	24h LC$_{50}$	*Penaeus setiferus*	Johnson (1976)
Omeprazole	Anti-ulcerative	88	EC$_{50}$	*Daphnia* spp.	FDA-CDER (1996)
Ondansetron HCl	Antiemetic	28	EC$_{50}$	*Daphnia* spp.	FDA-CDER (1996)
Orphenadrine HCl (mephenamin)	Relaxant; antihistaminic	8.9	24h EC$_{50}$	*D. magna*	Lilius et al. (1994)
Orphenadrine HCl (mephenamin)	Relaxant; antihistaminic	45	24h LC$_{50}$	*Artemia salina*	Calleja et al. (1994b)
Orphenadrine HCl (mephenamin)	Relaxant; antihistaminic	4.3	24h LC$_{50}$	*Streptocephalus proboscideus*	Calleja et al. (1994b)
Orphenadrine HCl (mephenamin)	Relaxant; antihistaminic	10.6	24h EC$_{50}$	*D. magna*	Calleja et al. (1994b)
Orphenadrine HCl (mephenamin)	Relaxant; antihistaminic	5.4	24h LC$_{50}$	*Brachionus calyciflorus*	Calleja et al. (1994b)
Oxytetracycline	Antibacterial	>5	24h LC$_{50}$	*Penaeus setiferus*	Johnson (1976)
Oxytetracycline HCl	Antibacterial	62.5	24/48/72/96h LC$_{50}$	*Morone saxatilis* (larvae)	Hughes (1973)

Table 15.1. *Continued*

Compound	Category[a]	Value (mg l^{-1})	Endpoint/ Duration[b]	Species	Reference
Oxytetracycline HCl	Antibacterial	150	24h LC$_{50}$	*Morone saxatilis* (fingerling)	Hughes (1973)
Oxytetracycline HCl	Antibacterial	125	48h LC$_{50}$	*Morone saxatilis* (fingerling)	Hughes (1973)
Oxytetracycline HCl	Antibacterial	100	72h LC$_{50}$	*Morone saxatilis* (fingerling)	Hughes (1973)
Oxytetracycline HCl	Antibacterial	75	96h LC$_{50}$	*Morone saxatilis* (fingerling)	Hughes (1973)
Oxytetracycline HCl	Antibacterial	<200	24/96h LC$_{50}$	*Salvelinus namaycush*	Marking et al. (1988)
Oxytetracycline	Antibacterial	0.231	EC$_{50}$	*Microcystis aeruginosa*	Holten Lützhøft et al. (1998)
Oxytetracycline	Antibacterial	5.0	EC$_{50}$	*Selenastrum capricornutum*	Holten Lützhøft et al. (1998)
Oxytetracycline	Antibacterial	1.7	EC$_{50}$	*Rhodomonas*	Holten Lützhøft et al. (1998)
Paclitaxel	Antineoplastic	>0.74	LC$_{50}$	*Daphnia* spp.	FDA-CDER (1996)
Paracetamol/ Acetaminophen	Analgesic; antipyretic	577	24h LC$_{50}$	*Artemia salina*	Calleja et al. (1994b)
Paracetamol/ Acetaminophen	Analgesic; antipyretic	29.6	24h LC$_{50}$	*Streptocephalus proboscideus*	Calleja et al. (1994b)
Paracetamol/ Acetaminophen	Analgesic; antipyretic	55.5	24h EC$_{50}$	*D. magna*	Calleja et al. (1994b)
Paracetamol/ Acetaminophen	Analgesic; antipyretic	5306	24h LC$_{50}$	*Brachionus calyciflorus*	Calleja et al. (1994b)
Paracetamol/ Acetaminophen	Analgesic; antipyretic	13	24h EC$_{50}$	*D. magna*	Kühn et al. (1989)
Paracetamol/ Acetaminophen	Analgesic; antipyretic	9.2	48h EC$_{50}$	*D. magna*	Kühn et al. (1989)
Paracetamol/ Acetaminophen	Analgesic; antipyretic	293	24 EC$_{50}$	*D. magna*	Henschel et al. (1997)
Paracetamol/ Acetaminophen	Analgesic; antipyretic	50.0	48 EC$_{50}$	*D. magna*	Henschel et al. (1997)
Paracetamol/ Acetaminophen	Analgesic; antipyretic	378	48h EC$_{50}$	*Brachydanio rerio* (embryos)	Henschel et al. (1997)
Paracetamol/ Acetaminophen	Analgesic; antipyretic	134	72h EC$_{50}$	*Scenedesmus subspicatus*	Henschel et al. (1997)
Paroxetine HCl	Antidepressant	3.0	EC$_{50}$	*Daphnia* spp.	FDA-CDER (1996)
Paroxetine HCl	Antidepressant	2.0	LC$_{50}$	*Lepomis macrochirus*	FDA-CDER (1996)
Paroxetine HCl	Antidepressant	3.29	4h LOEC	*Sphaerium* spp.	Fong et al. (1998)
Perindopril Erbumine	Antihypertensive	>1000	EC$_{50}$	*Daphnia* spp.	FDA-CDER (1996)
Perindopril Erbumine	Antihypertensive	>990	LC$_{50}$	*Lepomis macrochirus*	FDA-CDER (1996)
Pentobarbital	Sedative; hypnotic	49.5	96h EC$_{50}$	*Pimephales promelas*	Russom et al. (1997)

Table 15.1. *Continued*

Compound	Category[a]	Value (mg l^{-1})	Endpoint/ Duration[b]	Species	Reference
Phenobarbital	Anticonvulsant; sedative; hypnotic	484	96h EC$_{50}$	*Pimephales promelas*	Russom et al. (1997)
Phenobarbital (phenobarbitone)	Anticonvulsant; sedative; hypnotic	>10 000	24h LC$_{50}$	*Artemia salina*	Calleja et al. (1994b)
Phenobarbital (phenobarbitone)	Anticonvulsant; sedative; hypnotic	1 212	24h LC$_{50}$	*Streptocephalus proboscideus*	Calleja et al. (1994b)
Phenobarbital (phenobarbitone)	Anticonvulsant; sedative; hypnotic	1 463	24h EC$_{50}$	*D. magna*	Calleja et al. (1994b)
Phenobarbital (phenobarbitone)	Anticonvulsant; sedative; hypnotic	5 179	24h LC$_{50}$	*Brachionus calyciflorus*	Calleja et al. (1994b)
Porfirmer sodium	Photosensitiser	>994	EC$_{50}$	*Daphnia* spp.	FDA-CDER (1996)
Propranolol HCl	Antihypertensive; antianginal; antiarrhythmic	2.7	24h EC$_{50}$	*D. magna*	Lilius et al. (1994)
R-(±) Propranolol	Antihypertensive; antianginal; antiarrhythmic	407	24h LC$_{50}$	*Artemia salina*	Calleja et al. (1994b)
R-(±) Propranolol	Antihypertensive; antianginal; antiarrhythmic	1.87	24h LC$_{50}$	*Streptocephalus proboscideus*	Calleja et al. (1994b)
R-(±) Propranolol	Antihypertensive; antianginal; antiarrhythmic	15.87	24h EC$_{50}$	*D. magna*	Calleja et al. (1994b)
R-(±) Propranolol	Antihypertensive; antianginal; antiarrhythmic	2.59	24h LC$_{50}$	*Brachionus calyciflorus*	Calleja et al. (1994b)
Quinacrine HCl	Anthelminthic; antimalarial	122	48h LC$_{50}$	*Oncorhynchus mykiss*	Willford (1966)
Quinacrine HCl	Anthelminthic; antimalarial	25.0	24h LC$_{50}$	*Salvelinus namaycush*	Willford (1966)
Quinacrine HCl	Anthelminthic; antimalarial	21.0	48h LC$_{50}$	*Salvelinus namaycush*	Willford (1966)
Quinacrine HCl	Anthelminthic; antimalarial	300	24h LC$_{50}$	*Salmo trutta*	Willford (1966)
Quinacrine HCl	Anthelminthic; antimalarial	230	48h LC$_{50}$	*Salmo trutta*	Willford (1966)
Quinacrine HCl	Anthelminthic; antimalarial	196	24h LC$_{50}$	*Ictalurus punctatus*	Willford (1966)
Quinacrine HCl	Anthelminthic; antimalarial	70	48h LC$_{50}$	*Ictalurus punctatus*	Willford (1966)
Quinacrine HCl	Anthelminthic; antimalarial	230	48h LC$_{50}$	*Salvelinus fontinalis*	Willford (1966)
Quinacrine HCl	Anthelminthic; antimalarial	120	24h LC$_{50}$	*Lepomis macrochirus*	Willford (1966)

Table 15.1. *Continued*

Compound	Category[a]	Value (mg l^{-1})	Endpoint/ Duration[b]	Species	Reference
Quinacrine HCl	Anthelminthic; antimalarial	79	48h LC$_{50}$	Lepomis macrochirus	Willford (1966)
Quinacrine HCl	Anthelminthic; antimalarial	7.7	24h LC$_{50}$	Penaeus setiferus	Johnson (1976)
Quinidine sulfate	Cardiac depressant (antiarrhythmic)	60	24h EC$_{50}$	D. magna	Lilius et al. (1994)
Quinidine sulfate	Cardiac depressant (antiarrhythmic)	274	24h LC$_{50}$	Artemia salina	Calleja et al. (1994b)
Quinidine sulfate	Cardiac depressant (antiarrhythmic)	8.3	24h LC$_{50}$	Streptocephalus proboscideus	Calleja et al. (1994b)
Quinidine sulfate	Cardiac depressant (antiarrhythmic)	60	24h EC$_{50}$	D. magna	Calleja et al. (1994b)
Quinidine sulfate	Cardiac depressant (antiarrhythmic)	8.7	24h LC$_{50}$	Brachionus calyciflorus	Calleja et al. (1994b)
Quinine bisulfate	Antimalarial; oral sclerosing agent	13.1	24h LC$_{50}$	Penaeus setiferus	Johnson (1976)
Quinine HCl	Antimalarial	>100	48h LC$_{50}$	Oncorhynchus mykiss, Salmo trutta, Salvelinus fontinalis, Ictalurus punctatus, Lepomis macrochirus and Salvelinus namaycush	Willford (1966)
Quinine sulfate	Antimalarial; muscle relaxant	13.8	24h LC$_{50}$	Penaeus setiferus	Johnson (1976)
Ranitidine HCl	Anti-ulcerative	650	EC$_{50}$	Daphnia spp.	FDA-CDER (1996)
Risperidone	Antipsychotic	6.0	LC$_{50}$	Lepomis macrochirus	FDA-CDER (1996)
Risperidone	Antipsychotic	6.0	EC$_{50}$	Daphnia spp.	FDA-CDER (1996)
Salicylic acid	Topical keratolytic	>1 440	24h EC$_{50}$	D. magna	Bringmann and Kühn (1982)
Salicylic acid	Topical keratolytic	230	24h EC$_{50}$	D. magna	Wang and Lay (1989)
Salicylic acid	Topical keratolytic	118	EC$_{50}$	D. magna	Henschel et al. (1997)
Salicylic acid	Topical keratolytic	37.0	48h EC$_{50}$	Brachydanio rerio (embryos)	Henschel et al. (1997)
Salicylic acid	Topical keratolytic	>100	72h EC$_{50}$	Scenedesmus subspicatus	Henschel et al. (1997)
Simethicone	Antiflatulent	44.5	48h TL$_{50}$	D.magna	Hobbs (1975)
Salmeterol	Antiasthmatic?	20	EC$_{50}$	Daphnia spp.	FDA-CDER (1996)
Secobarbital, sodium salt	Sedative; hypnotic	23.6	96h EC$_{50}$	Pimephales promelas	Russom et al. (1997)
Spirapril HCl	Antihypertensive	>930	EC$_{50}$	Daphnia spp.	FDA-CDER (1996)
Spirapril HCl	Antihypertensive	>970	LC$_{50}$	Lepomis macrochirus	FDA-CDER (1996)
Stavudine	Anti(retro)viral	>980	EC$_{50}$	Daphnia spp.	FDA-CDER (1996)
Sulfadimethoxine	Antibacterial	1 866	24h LC$_{50}$	Artemia salina (nauplii)	Brambilla et al. (1994)

Table 15.1. *Continued*

Compound	Category[a]	Value (mg l^{-1})	Endpoint/ Duration[b]	Species	Reference
Sulfadimethoxine	Antibacterial	851	48h LC$_{50}$	*Artemia salina* (nauplii)	Brambilla et al. (1994)
Sulfadimethoxine	Antibacterial	537	72h LC$_{50}$	*Artemia salina* (nauplii)	Brambilla et al. (1994)
Sulfadimethoxine	Antibacterial	19.5	96h LC$_{50}$	*Artemia salina* (nauplii)	Brambilla et al. (1994
Sulfadimethoxine	Antibacterial	1 866	24h LC$_{50}$	*Artemia salina* (nauplii)	Migliore et al. (1993)
Sulfadimethoxine	Antibacterial	851	48h LC$_{50}$	*Artemia salina* (nauplii)	Migliore et al. (1993)
Sulfadimethoxine	Antibacterial	537	72h LC$_{50}$	*Artemia salina* (nauplii)	Migliore et al. (1993)
Sulfadimethoxine	Antibacterial	19.5	96h LC$_{50}$	*Artemia salina* (nauplii)	Migliore et al. (1993)
Sulfamerazine	Antibacterial	>100	48h LC$_{50}$	*Oncorhynchus mykiss, Salmo trutta, Salvelinus fontinalis, Ictalurus punctatus, Lepomis macrochirus* and *Salvelinus namaycush*	Willford (1966)
Sulfamethazine	Antibacterial	>100	48h LC$_{50}$	*Oncorhynchus mykiss, Salmo trutta, Salvelinus fontinalis, Ictalurus punctatus, Lepomis macrochirus* and *Salvelinus namaycush*	Willford (1966)
Sulfisoxazole	Antibacterial	>100	48h LC$_{50}$	*Oncorhynchus mykiss, Salmo trutta, Salvelinus fontinalis, Ictalurus punctatus, Lepomis macrochirus* and *Salvelinus namaycush*	Willford (1966)
Sumatriptan succinate	Antimigraine	290	EC$_{50}$	*Daphnia* spp.	FDA-CDER (1996)
Tetracycline	Antiamebic; antibacterial; antiricketettsial	16	72h EC$_{50}$	*Nitzschia closterium*	Peterson et al. (1993)
Tetracycline HCl	Antiamebic; antibacterial; antiricketettsial	220	24/96h LC$_{50}$	*Salvelinus namaycush*	Marking et al. (1988)
Tetracycline HCl	Antiamebic; antibacterial; antiricketettsial	>182	24/48/96h LC$_{50}$	*Morone saxatilis*	Welborn (1969)
Theophylline	Bronchodilator	155	24h EC$_{50}$	*D. magna*	Lilius et al. (1994)
Theophylline	Bronchodilator	8 247	24h LC$_{50}$	*Artemia salina*	Calleja et al. (1994b)
Theophylline	Bronchodilator	425	24h LC$_{50}$	*Streptocephalus proboscideus*	Calleja et al. (1994b)
Theophylline	Bronchodilator	483	24h EC$_{50}$	*D. magna*	Calleja et al. (1994b)
Theophylline	Bronchodilator	3 926	24h LC$_{50}$	*Brachionus calyciflorus*	Calleja et al. (1994b)
Thiopental, sodium salt	Anesthetic	26.2	96h EC$_{50}$	*Pimephales promelas*	Russom et al. (1997)
Thiotepa	Antineoplastic	546	EC$_{50}$	*Daphnia* spp.	FDA-CDER (1996)
Thioridazine HCl	Antipsychotic	0.69	24h EC$_{50}$	*D. magna*	Lilius et al. (1994)

Table 15.1. *Continued*

Compound	Category[a]	Value (mg l^{-1})	Endpoint/ Duration[b]	Species	Reference
Thioridazine HCl	Antipsychotic	14.5	24h LC$_{50}$	*Artemia salina*	Calleja et al. (1994b)
Thioridazine HCl	Antipsychotic	0.33	24h LC$_{50}$	*Streptocephalus proboscideus*	Calleja et al. (1994b)
Thioridazine HCl	Antipsychotic	4.56	24h EC$_{50}$	*D. magna*	Calleja et al. (1994b)
Thioridazine HCl	Antipsychotic	0.30	24h LC$_{50}$	*Brachionus calyciflorus*	Calleja et al. (1994b)
Tiludronate disodium	Metabolic Bone Disease	562	24h EC$_{50}$	*D. magna*	Sanofi (1996)
Tiludronate disodium	Metabolic Bone Disease	320	48h EC$_{50}$	*D. magna*	Sanofi (1996)
Tolazoline HCl	Antiadrenergic	354	96h EC$_{50}$	*Pimephales promelas*	Russom et al. (1997)
Tramadol HCl	Analgesic	130	LC$_{50}$	Unspecified fish	FDA-CDER (1996)
Tramadol HCl	Analgesic	73	EC$_{50}$	*Daphnia spp*	FDA-CDER (1996)
Verapamil HCl	Antianginal; antiarrhythmic	327	24h EC$_{50}$	*D. magna*	Lilius et al. (1994)
Verapamil HCl	Antianginal; antiarrhythmic	356	24h LC$_{50}$	*Artemia salina*	Calleja et al. (1994b)
Verapamil HCl	Antianginal; antiarrhythmic	6.24	24h LC$_{50}$	*Streptocephalus proboscideus*	Calleja et al. (1994b)
Verapamil HCl	Antianginal; antiarrhythmic	55.5	24h EC$_{50}$	*D. magna*	Calleja et al. (1994b)
Verapamil HCl	Antianginal; antiarrhythmic	10.90	24h LC$_{50}$	*Brachionus calyciflorus*	Calleja et al. (1994b)
Warfarin	Anticoagulant	12	96h LC$_{50}$	*Rasbora heteromorpha*	Tooby et al. (1975)
Warfarin	Anticoagulant	89	24h EC$_{50}$	*D. magna*	Lilius et al. (1994)
Warfarin	Anticoagulant	3 638	24h LC$_{50}$	*Artemia salina*	Calleja et al. (1994b)
Warfarin	Anticoagulant	342	24h LC$_{50}$	*Streptocephalus proboscideus*	Calleja et al. (1994b)
Warfarin	Anticoagulant	475	24h EC$_{50}$	*D. magna*	Calleja et al. (1994b)
Warfarin	Anticoagulant	444	24h LC$_{50}$	*Brachionus calyciflorus*	Calleja et al. (1994b)
Zalcitabine	Anti(retro)viral	>1 790	EC$_{50}$	*Daphnia* spp.	FDA-CDER (1996)

[a] Therapeutic category is as detailed in the Merck Index (Budavari 1989).
[b] LC$_{50}$ values relate to lethality in all organisms. EC$_{50}$ values in Daphnia typically relate to immobilisation. In the case of algae, EC$_{50}$ values relate to effects upon growth (i.e. biomass or cell number). US FDA test guidelines include: 4.01 Algal assay, 4.08 *Daphnia* acute toxicity (48 h), 4.09 *Daphnia* chronic testing, 4.10 *Hyalella azteca* acute toxicity, and 4.11 Freshwater fish acute toxicity.

The distribution of the acute data is presented in Table 15.2. In collating and summarising the data, the most sensitive species/endpoint and most toxic salt were chosen for any given drug active.

Comparisons of taxa sensitivities (in terms of acute responses) are presented in Table 15.3 and Fig. 15.1a–c. Fish, *Daphnia magna* and algae were chosen as representa-

Table 15.2. Summary of available acute ecotoxicity data for human pharmaceuticals

Ecotoxicity range	Number	Frequency (%)	Cumulative (%)
<0.1 mg l^{-1}	2	1.9	1.9
>0.1–1 mg l^{-1}	8	7.5	9.3
>1–10 mg l^{-1}	22	20.3	29.9
>10–100 mg l^{-1}	31	29.0	58.9
>100–1 000 mg l^{-1}	37	34.6	93.5
>1 000 mg l^{-1}	7	6.5	100
Total	107	–	–

Table 15.3. Paired comparison of relative taxa sensitivity

Comparison	Regression	r
Fish vs. *Daphnia magna* (n = 40)	Fish LogEC$_{50}$ (µg l^{-1}) = *Daphnia magna* EC$_{50}$ (µg l^{-1}) × 0.84 + 0.37	0.76
Fish vs. Algae (n = 15)	Fish LogEC$_{50}$ (µg l^{-1}) = Algae EC$_{50}$ (µg l^{-1}) × 0.71 + 0.33	0.53
Daphnia magna vs. Algae (n = 12)	*Daphnia magna* LogEC$_{50}$ (µg l^{-1}) = Algae EC$_{50}$ (µg l^{-1}) × 0.87 – 0.24	0.66

$p < 0.05$ in all cases. NB: Some algal endpoints are MIC rather than EC$_{50}$.

tive of different trophic levels. Significant ($p < 0.05$) correlations were observed between all taxa pairs with r values in the range 0.53–0.76. A sensitivity order algae > *Daphnia magna* > fish is consistent with the results of the regressions.

The median and range of acute endpoints for selected therapeutic categories for which there are two or more different compounds are presented in Fig. 15.2. This allows some interpretation of the relative ecotoxicity of different classes of pharmaceuticals. The most ecotoxic of the various therapeutic classes of pharmaceuticals (in terms of observed minima) were antidepressants, antibacterials and antipsychotics, although the range of reported responses within each of these categories (and indeed most the other categories) was large, i.e. typically over several orders of magnitude.

15.3.2
Chronic Ecotoxicity Data

The available chronic ecotoxicity database is presented in Table 15.4. Most endpoints were determined via standard tests with *D. magna* and algae. Other more sensitive endpoints for ethinyloestradiol relate to the induction of plasma vitellogenin, gonadosomatic index (GSI) and spermatogenesis in roach (*Rutilus rutilus*) and/or rainbow trout (*Oncorhynchus mykiss*) (FWR 1992; Purdom et al. 1994; FWR 1995; Jobling et al. 1996).

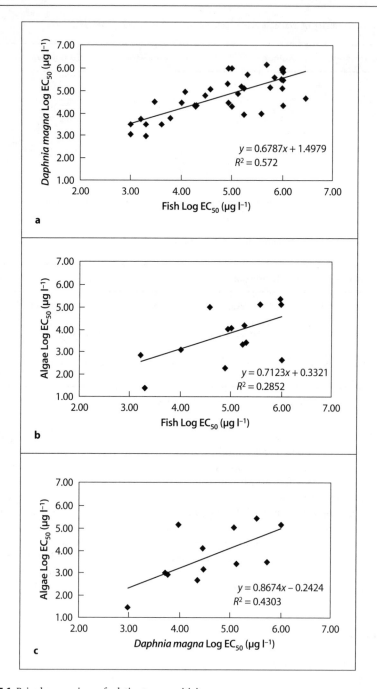

Fig. 15.1. Paired comparison of relative taxa sensitivity

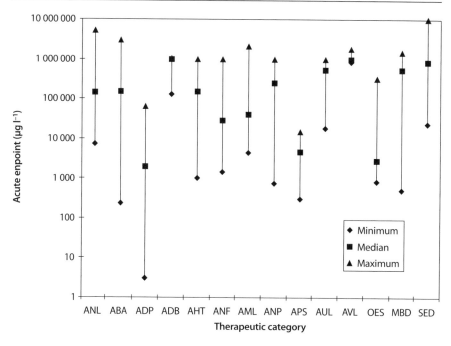

Fig. 15.2. Median and range of acute endpoints for selected therapeutic categories. *ANL* = analgesic, anti-inflammatory, antipyretic (7); *ABA* = antibacterial (18); *ADP* = antidepressant (5, excluding lithium); *ADB* = antidiabetic (2); *AHT* = antihypertensive, antianginal, antiarrhythmic (9); *ANF* = anti-infective (4); *AML* = antimalarial (4); *ANP* = antineoplastic (4); *APS* = antipsychoitc (2); *AUL* = anit-ulcerative (5); *AVL* = antiviral (4); *OES* = oestrogen (2); *MDB* = Metabolic Bone Disease (3); *SED* = sedative/hypnotic (4). Numbers in brackets denote the number of compounds

15.4
Discussion

Acute ecotoxicity data are available for a large number of pharmaceuticals (i.e. >100). The results presented here possibly represent the most comprehensive dataset yet collated. Most of the data relates to acute ecotoxicity endpoints, although some chronic data are available. The range of reported acute ecotoxicity endpoints varied from >15 000 mg l^{-1} for atropine sulfate (anticholinergic/mydriatic) in a standard 24 hour LC$_{50}$ *Artemia salina* test (Calleja et al. 1994b) down to 0.003 mg l^{-1} for fluvoxamine (an antidepressant) in a (non-standard) study examining the effects of selective serotonin re-uptake inhibitors (SSRIs) upon parturition (release of juveniles) in fingernail clams (Fong et al. 1998). This corresponds to a difference of 6 orders of magnitude. Ten of the compounds had acute endpoints of ≤1 mg l^{-1}. They were alendronate (a biphosphonate used in the treatment of metabolic bone disease), amitriptyline (an antidepressant), carvedilol (an antihypertensive and antianginal), ethinyloestradiol (an oestrogen), fluticasone (a corticosteroid antiasthmatic), fluoxetine (an antidepressant),

Table 15.4. Chronic ecotoxicity data for human pharmaceuticals

Compound	Category	Value (mg l⁻¹)	Endpoint/Duration	Species	Reference
Alendronate sodium	Metabolic bone disease	0.5	NOEC	Unspecified green algae	FDA-CDER (1996)
Bicalutamide	Non-steroidal antiandrogen	1	NOEC	Unspecified blue-green algae	FDA-CDER (1996)
Bicalutamide	Non-steroidal antiandrogen	1	NOEC	Unspecified green algae	FDA-CDER (1996)
Budenoside	Anti-inflammatory	10	NOEC	Unspecified green algae	FDA-CDER (1996)
Cisapride	Peristaltic stimulant	100	"*Effects*"	Unspecified blue-green algae	FDA-CDER (1996)
Cisapride	Peristaltic stimulant	320	"*Effects*"	Unspecified green algae	FDA-CDER (1996)
Clofibrate	Antihyper-lipoproteinemic	0.01 (A/C 1428)	21d reproduction NOEC	*D. magna*	Köpf (1995)
Clofibrate	Antihyper-lipoproteinemic	0.0084	21d reproduction EC$_{10}$	*D. magna*	Köpf (1995)
Clofibrate	Antihyper-lipoproteinemic	0.106	21d reproduction EC$_{50}$	*D. magna*	Köpf (1995)
Clofibrate	Antihyper-lipoproteinemic	5.4	EC$_{10}$	Unspecified algae	Köpf (1995)
Diethylstilbestrol	Oestrogen	0.25/0.5	F$_1$ 21d molt frequency NOEC/LOEC	*D. magna*	Baldwin et al. (1995)
Diethylstilbestrol	Oestrogen	0.062/0.5 (A/C 17.6)	F$_2$ 21d brood size NOEC/ LOEC	*D. magna*	Baldwin et al. (1995)
Ethinyloestradiol	Oestrogen	1 ng l⁻¹	10d plasma vitello-genin NOEC (9.5°C)	*Rutilus rutilus*	FWR (1992)
Ethinyloestradiol	Oestrogen	1 ng l⁻¹	10d plasma vitello-genin NOEC (9.5°C)	*Oncorhynchus mykiss*	FWR (1992)
Ethinyloestradiol	Oestrogen	0.3 ng l⁻¹	28wk plasma vitello-genin LOEC	*Oncorhynchus mykiss*	Sheahan et al. (1994)
Ethinyloestradiol	Oestrogen	0.1 ng l⁻¹	10d plasma vitello-genin LOEC (16.5°C)	*Oncorhynchus mykiss*	Purdom et al. (1994)
Ethinyloestradiol	Oestrogen	0.01 (A/C 570)	21d reproduction NOEC	*D. magna*	Köpf (1995)
Ethinyloestradiol	Oestrogen	0.0125	21d reproduction EC$_{10}$	*D. magna*	Köpf (1995)
Ethinyloestradiol	Oestrogen	0.105	21d reproduction EC$_{50}$	*D. magna*	Köpf (1995)
Ethinyloestradiol	Oestrogen	0.054	EC$_{10}$	Unspecified algae	Köpf (1995)
Ethinyloestradiol	Oestrogen	2 ng l⁻¹ (A/C 800 000)	21d spermatogenesis, GSI and plasma vitello-genin LOEC	*Oncorhynchus mykiss*	FWR (1995)
Ethinyloestradiol	Oestrogen	1 ng l⁻¹	21d plasma vitello-genin (positive control for AP)	*Rutilus rutilus*	FWR (1995)

Table 15.4. *Continued*

Compound	Category	Value (mg l^{-1})	Endpoint/Duration	Species	Reference
Ethinyloestradiol	Oestrogen	2 ng l^{-1}	21d spermatogenesis, GSI and plasma vitellogenin (positive control for AP)	*Oncorhynchus mykiss*	Jobling et al. (1996)
Ethinyloestradiol	Oestrogen	0.387	21d reproduction LOEC	*D. magna*	Schweinfurth et al. (1996)
Ethinyloestradiol	Oestrogen	10 ng l^{-1}	28d reproduction LOEC	*Pimephales promelas*	Schweinfurth et al. (1996)
Ethinyloestradiol	Oestrogen	1.25 ng l^{-1}	50–60d LOEC (growth)	*Lymnaea stagnalis*	Belfroid and Leonards (1996)
Ethinyloestradiol	Oestrogen	0.125 ng l^{-1}	50–60d LOEC (growth)	*Bithynia tentaculata*	Belfroid and Leonards (1996)
Ethinyloestradiol	Oestrogen	1 ng l^{-1}	9month reproduction NOEC (growth retardation LOEC 4 ng l^{-1})	*Pimephales promelas*	Länge et al. (1997)
Etidronic acid	Metabolic Bone Disease	>12 (A/C 43.9)	28d NOEC	*D. magna*	Gledhill and Feijtel (1992)
Etidronic acid	Metabolic Bone Disease	1.3	96h NOEC	*Selenastrum* spp.	Gledhill and Feijtel (1992)
Etidronic acid	Metabolic Bone Disease	13.2	14d NOEC	*Selenastrum* spp.	Gledhill and Feijtel (1992)
Finasteride	Treatment of benign prostatic hypertrophy	≥49	NOEC	Unspecified green algae	FDA-CDER (1996)
Fluoxetine HCl	Antidepressant	0.001	NOEC	Unspecified green algae	FDA-CDER (1996)
Fluvoxamine maleate	Antidepressant	31	NOEC	Unspecified green algae	FDA-CDER (1996)
Iopromide	Diagnostic aid (radiopaque medium)	>1 000 (A/C 1.0)	21d reproduction NOEC	*D. magna*	Schweinfurth et al. (1996a)
Iopromide	Diagnostic aid (radiopaque medium)	68	NOEC	Unspecified blue-green algae	FDA-CDER (1996)
Lomefloxacin	Antibacterial	2	NOEC	Unspecified green algae	FDA-CDER (1996)
Lorcarbef	Anti-infective	13	NOEC	Unspecified green algae	FDA-CDER (1996)
Losartan K	Antihypertensive	556	NOEC	Unspecified blue-green algae	FDA-CDER (1996)
Losartan K	Antihypertensive	143	NOEC	Unspecified green algae	FDA-CDER (1996)
Metronidazole	Antiprotozoal	19.9	72h EC$_{10}$	*Selenastrum capricornutum*	Lanzky and Halling-Sørenson (1997)
Metronidazole	Antiprotozoal	2.03	72h EC$_{10}$	*Chlorella* spp.	Lanzky and Halling-Sørenson (1997)

Table 15.4. *Continued*

Compound	Category	Value (mg l⁻¹)	Endpoint/Duration	Species	Reference
Nicotine	Cholinergic agonist	0.07 (A/C 42.9)	LOEC (length)	*D. pulex*	FDA-CDER (1996)
Riseperidone	Antipsychotic	100	"*Effects*"	Unspecified blue-green algae	FDA-CDER (1996)
Riseperidone	Antipsychotic	10	"*Effects*"	Unspecified green algae	FDA-CDER (1996)
Salicylic acid	Topical keratolytic	<20.0 (A/C 5.9)	21d reproduction NOEC	*D. magna*	Wang and Lay (1989)
Tiludronate disodium	Metabolic bone disease	36.6	14d EC$_{50}$	*Selenastrum capricornutum*	Sanofi (1996)
Tiludronate disodium	Metabolic bone disease	13.3	21d EC$_{50}$	*Microcystis aeruginosa*	Sanofi (1996)

fluvoxamine (an antidepressant), midazolam (an anesthetic), paclitaxel (an antine-oplastic) and thioridazine (an antipsychotic).

In a similar review exercise, the US FDA Center for Drug Evaluation and Research (CDER) has performed a retrospective review of toxicity information available in Environmental Assessments (EA) previously submitted in support of New Drug Applications (NDA) (FDA-CDER 1996). The data showed no observed effects on relevant standard environmental test organisms at drug concentrations below 1 µg l⁻¹ (based on both acute and chronic data from approximately 60 compounds). The results of the FDA-CDER review provided the justification for the 1 µg l⁻¹ cut-off threshold employed in the US FDA environmental risk assessment framework for pharmaceuticals (Federal Register 29/07/97, vol. 62, p. 40569). All acute ecotoxicity endpoints considered in this study (which includes the data from the FDA-CDER review) were similarly also >1 µg l⁻¹. That the majority of the pharmaceuticals examined are limited (90th-percentile > 1 mg l⁻¹) in their acute ecotoxicity is not surprising, given the generally limited mammalian toxicity required of pharmaceuticals. A relationship between mammalian toxicity and invertebrate ecotoxicity has similarly been noted elsewhere (e.g. Enslein et al. 1987; Enslein et al. 1989; Calleja et al. 1993; Calleja et al. 1994a). For perspective, the EU classification criteria for risk phrases (67/548/EEC) defines compounds with an L(E)C$_{50}$ ≤ 1 mg l⁻¹ as "very toxic to aquatic organisms" (R-50), 1–10 mg l⁻¹ as "toxic to aquatic organisms" (R-51) and 10–100 mg l⁻¹ as "harmful to aquatic organisms" (R-52).

The comparisons of paired taxa in terms of responses to acute ecotoxicity testing suggests a general hierarchy of sensitivity corresponding to algae > *Daphnia magna* > fish. Nevertheless, where differences in responses are observed, they are typically limited to one order of magnitude. The average difference between fish and *Daphnia magna* is <0.5 log units, between fish and algae 1.2 log units and between *Daphnia magna* and algae 1.0 log units. Relative algal sensitivity may have resulted in part from the effects of anti-infectives and antibacterials (such as oxytetracycline) upon algae.

The most ecotoxic of the various therapeutic classes of pharmaceuticals (in terms of observed minima) were antidepressants, antibacterials and antipsychotics. The lowest endpoint ($3 \mu g \, l^{-1}$) for antidepressants relates to a test in a freshwater bivalve (Fong et al. 1998). Even without the inclusion of this non-standard endpoint, antidepressants would remain the most potent therapeutic class in terms of acute ecotoxicity by virtue of an algal EC_{50} of $31 \mu g \, l^{-1}$ for fluoxetine (FDA-CDER 1996). As indicated above, the effects of antibacterials upon algae and in particular blue-green algae (cyanobacteria) accounts for the extension of the (lower) range of reported responses for antibacterials. After antibacterials, the next lowest minima of any category is that of antipsychotics. In addition, it is also worth noting that the potency of oestrogens in the acute tests reviewed here is reflected in the relatively low median value for this category. Variation within each of these categories (and indeed most the other categories) was large, i.e. typically over several orders of magnitude. This presumably reflects the variation in responses of the differing taxa/trophic levels (i.e. fish, invertebrates or algae) when exposed to representative compounds from the various differing therapeutic classes.

The overall applicability of acute ecotoxicity data in general for environmental risk assessment purposes has been criticised (Halling-Sørensen et al. 1998). Standard acute bioassays with their focus on immediate endpoints such as lethality may not be the most appropriate basis for risk assessment given the intended narrow scope of biological activity/effect and general potency of pharmaceuticals in general. It has consequently been suggested that chronic bioassays performed over the life-cycle of various organisms from different trophic levels may be more appropriate (Halling-Sørensen et al. 1998).

Within this study, chronic ecotoxicity data for aquatic organisms were secured for 20 compounds. The chronic database itself is dominated by data relating to ethinyloestradiol. The various endpoints reported for ethinyloestradiol demonstrate the exquisite potency of this compound. The ecological significance of some of the various biomarker responses reported for ethinyloestradiol is not known, and they are less readily employed in risk characterisation. This contrasts with the more integrative fathead minnow reproduction LOEC/NOEC endpoints for ethinyloestradiol reported by Schweinfurth et al. (1996b) and Länge et al. (1997).

The chronic database for the remaining compounds is dominated by algal endpoints (i.e. NOEC or EC_{10} values). Chronic toxicity studies relating to fauna (namely *Daphnia magna* or *pulex*) are limited to clofibrate, diethylstilbestrol, etidronic acid, iopromide, nicotine, and salicylic acid. Acute EC_{50}/chronic NOEC (A/C) ratios have been calculated for *Daphnia* spp. (Table 15.4). Acute/chronic ratios varied from 1 for iopromide to 1 428 for clofibrate with a median of 43 ($n = 7$). This does not contrast markedly with A/C ratios in the range of 1.6 to 1 030 (median = 22.1) previously reported for invertebrates for industrial chemicals (ECETOC 1993). Whilst not normally considered, A/C ratios can also be calculated for algae. In this study, values were typically approximately 2 and were limited in all cases to one order of magnitude.

Only one example of an acute/chronic ratio was available for a fish species (*Oncorhynchus mykiss*) and pertains to ethinyloestradiol. The A/C ratio was 800 000 and reflects the marked difference in the magnitude of the observed endpoints in the respective acute and chronic bioassays that results from the endocrine modality of this compound. Such an observation could be employed as the basis of an argument that would preclude the use of short-term ecotoxicity testing for the purposes of risk assessment of endocrinologically active compounds and oblige chronic testing preferably with vertebrates (i.e. fish). The lack of comparative acute and chronic data relating to fish for other (non-oestrogenic) pharmaceuticals precludes the calculation of A/C ratios for such compounds.

15.5
Conclusions

Data relating to the effects of human pharmaceuticals upon aquatic organisms are available, although the majority relates to short-term acute responses such as lethality. A review revealed over 360 endpoints in macro-invertebrates, fish and algae for 107 compounds. Over 90% of the observations were at concentrations >1 mg l^{-1}, suggesting the relative limited acute ecotoxicity of pharmaceuticals in general. All values were >1 μg l^{-1}. It is interesting to note that the majority of compounds with endpoints in acute bioassays of <1 mg l^{-1} are pharmaceuticals intended to impact the human nervous system (i.e. antidepressants, antipsychotics or anesthetics). The relative sensitivity of tested taxa to pharmaceuticals was algae > *Daphnia magna* > fish, although this trend may reflect the impact of some compounds with intended biocidal modes of action (e.g. antibiotics) when tested upon algae. Differences in the responses of different taxa to the same compound were typically limited to one order of magnitude.

The applicability of the acute ecotoxicity database for environmental risk assessment purposes has been criticised on the basis of the appropriateness of the focus upon immediate endpoints such as lethality. Pharmaceuticals are intended to have a narrow scope of biological effect, and it has been suggested that chronic testing may therefore be more appropriate. The available chronic ecotoxicity database is more limited, and data for only 20 compounds are available. The chronic database was dominated by studies upon ethinyloestradiol. The remaining endpoints were mostly concerned with algae or *Daphnia* spp. Acute/chronic ratios for *Daphnia magna* and algae were calculated and do not differ markedly from those reported elsewhere for industrial chemicals. Whilst the scientific basis for the use of application factors in risk assessment to derive the PNEC (predicted no-effect concentration) from acute ecotoxicity data is not contraindicated by the A/C ratios observed for *Daphnia* or algae for pharmaceuticals, the absence of relevant chronic data precludes the derivation of A/C ratios for fish and a categorical conclusion vis-à-vis the applicability of current risk assessment practice to pharmaceuticals. More work relating to the potential chronic effects of pharmaceuticals in general and upon fish in particular is required.

References

Anon (1993) Acute toxicity to bluegill (*Lepomis macrochirus*) of the test substance ketorolac tromethamine from Radian Corporation in a 96-hr static non-renewal test. Performed for Radian Corporation by AnaltiKEM Environmental Lab, Houston, USA (AnalytiKEM Test Number 01628)

Baldwin WS, Milam DL, Leblanc GA (1995) Physiological and biochemical perturbations in *Daphnia magna* following exposure to the model environmental estrogen diethylstilbestrol. Environ. Toxicol Chem 14(6):945–952

Belfroid A, Leonards P (1996) Effect of ethinyl oestradiol on the development of snails and amphibians. SETAC 17th Annual Meeting November 1996, Washington DC (Abstract PO/508)

Brambilla G, Civitareale C, Migliore L (1994) Experimental toxicity and analysis of bacitracin, flumequine and sulphadimethoxine in terrestrial and aquatic organisms as a predictive model for ecosystem damage. Qumica Analitica 13(Suppl 1):S73–S77

Bringmann G, Kühn R (1982) Ergebnisse der Schadwirkung wassergefährdender Stoffe gegen *Daphnia magna* in einem weiterentwickelten standardisierten Testverfahren. Z Wasser Abwasser Forsch 15(1):1–6 (Results of the harmful effects of water pollutants to *Daphnia magna* in a further developed standardized test procedure)

Budavari S (ed) (1989) The Merck Index – An Encyclopedia of Chemicals, Drugs and Biologicals (11th edn). Merck & Co. Inc. Rahway, N.J., USA

Calleja MC, Personne G, Geladi P (1993) The predictive potential of a battery of ecotoxicological tests for human acute toxicity, as evaluated with the first 50 MEIC chemicals. ATLA 21:330–349

Calleja MC, Geladi P, Personne G (1994a) Modelling of human acute toxicity from physicochemical properties and non-vertebrate acute toxicity of the 38 organic chemicals of the MEIC priority list by PLS regression and neural network. Fd Chem Toxic 32(10):923–941

Calleja MC, Personne G, Geladi P (1994b) Comparative acute toxicity of the first 50 Multicentre Evaluation of in vitro cytotoxicity chemicals to aquatic non-vertebrates. Arch Environ Contam Toxicol 26:69–78

Coats JR, Metcalf RL, Lu P-Y, Brown DD, Williams JF, Hansen LG (1976) Model ecosystem evaluation of the environmental impacts of the veterinary drugs phenothiazine, sulfametazine, clopidol and diethylstibestrol. Environ Health Perspect 1:167–197

Di Delupis GD, Macri A, Civitareale C, Migliore L (1992) Antibiotics of zootechnical use: effects of acute high and low dose contamination on *Daphnia magna* Straus. Aquatic Toxicology 22:53–60

ECETOC (1993). Aquatic toxicity data evaluation. European Centre for Ecotoxicology and Toxicity of Chemicals, Brussels (Technical Report 56)

Enslein K, Tuzzeo TM, Borgstedt HH, Blake BW, Hart JB (1987) Prediction of rat oral LD50 from *Daphnia magna* LC50 and chemical structure. In: Kaiser KLE (ed) QSAR in environmental toxicology, vol II. D.D. Reidel Publishing Company, Dordrecht, pp 91–106

Enslein K, Tuzzeo TM, Blake BW, Hart JB, Landis WG (1989) Prediction of *Daphnia magna* EC50 values from rat oral LD50 and structural parameters. In: Suter GW, Lewis MA (eds) Aquatic toxicology and environmental fate, vol XI. American Society for Testing and Materials, Philadelphia (ASTM STP 1007, pp 397–409)

FDA-CDER (1996) Retrospective review of ecotoxicity data submitted in environmental assessments. FDA Center for Drug Evaluation and Research, Rockville, MD, USA (Docket No. 96N-0057)

Fong PP, Huminski PT, D'Urso LM (1998) Induction and potentiation of parturition in fingernail clams (*Sphaerium striatinum*) by selective serotonin re-uptake inhibitors (SSRIs). J Exper Zool 280:260–264

FWR (1992) Effects of trace organics on fish. Foundation for Water Research, Marlow (Bucks.), UK (October 1992 FR/D 0008)

FWR (1995) Effects of trace organics on fish – Phase 2. Foundation for Water Research, Marlow (Bucks.), UK (July 1995 FR/D 0022)

Gledhill WE, Feijtel, TCJ (1992) Environmental properties and safety assessment of organic phosphonates used for detergent and water treatment. In: Oude NT de (ed) Detergents – Handbook of environmental chemistry, vol III. Springer-Verlag, New York, Berlin, Heidelberg (Part F: Anthropogenic compounds, pp 261–285)

Halling-Sørensen B, Nors Nielsen S, Lanzky PF, Ingerslev F, Holten-Lützhøft HC, Jørgensen SE (1998) Occurrence, fate and effects of pharmaceutical substances in the environment – a review. Chemosphere 36(2):357–393

Henschel KP, Wenzel A, Diederich M, Fliedner A (1997) Environmental hazard assessment of pharmaceuticals. Reg Toxicol Pharmacol 25:220–225

Hobbs EJ (1975) Toxicity of polydimethylsiloxanes in certain environmental systems. Environ Res 10:397–406

Holten Lützhøft HC, Halling-Sørensen B, Jørgensen SE (1998). Algal testing of antibiotics applied in Danish fish farming. SETAC-Europe 8th Annual Meeting 14th–18th April 1998, Bordeaux (Abstract 4I/004)

Hughes JS (1973) Acute toxicity of thirty chemicals to stripped bass (*Morone saxatilis*). Presented at the Western Association of State Game and Fish Commissioners in Salt Lake City, Utah July 1973

Jobling S, Sheahan D, Osborne J, Matthiessen P, Sumpter JP (1996) Inhibition of testicular growth in rainbow trout (*Oncorhynchus mykiss*) exposed to estrogenic alkylphenolic chemicals. Environ Toxicol Chem 15(2):194–202

Johnson SK (1976) Twenty-four hour toxicity tests of six chemicals to mysis larvae of *Penaeus setiferus*. Texas A and M University Extension, Disease Laboratory (Publication No. FDDL-S8)

Knoll/BASF (1995) Pharmaceutical safety data sheet (Issue/Revision 06/04/94). Knoll Pharmaceuticals, Nottingham, UK (quoted in Halling-Sørensen et al. 1998)

Köpf W (1995) Wirkung endokriner Stoffe in Biotests mit Wasserorganismen. Vortag bei der 50. Fachtagung des Bayerisches Landesamt für Wasserwirtschaft: Stoffe mit endokriner Wirkung im Wasser (Abstract). (Effects of endocrine substances in bioassays with aquatic organisms. Presentation at the 50th Seminar of the Bavarian Association for Waters Supply. Substances with endocrine effects in water) (quoted in Römbke et al. 1995)

Kühn R, Pattard, M, Pernak KD, Winter A (1989) Results of the harmful effects of selected water pollutants (anilines, phenols, aliphatic compounds) to *Daphnia magna*. Wat Res 23(4):495–499

Länge R, Schweinfurth H, Croudace C, Panther G (1997) Growth and reproduction of fathead minnow (*Pimephales promelas*) exposed to the synthetic steroid hormone ethinylestradiol in a life cycle test (Abstract). Seventh Annual Meeting of SETAC – Europe, April 6–10, 1997, Amsterdam, the Netherlands

Lanzky PF, Halling-Sørensen B, (1997) The toxic effect of the antibiotic metronidazole on aquatic organisms. Chemosphere 35(11):2553–2561

Lilius H, Isomaa B, Holmström T (1994) A comparison of the toxicity of 50 reference chemicals to freshly isolated rainbow trout hepatocytes and *Daphnia magna*. Aquatic Toxicology 30:47–60

Macrì A, Sbardella E (1984) Toxicological evaluation of Nitrofurazone and Furazolidone on *Selenastrum capricornutum*, *Daphnia magna* and *Musca domestica*. Ecotoxicol Environ Safety 8:115–105

Marking L, Howe GE, Crowther JR (1988) Toxicity of erythromycin, oxytetracycline and tetracycline administered to Lake Trout in water baths, by injection or by feeding. The Progressive Fish-Culturist 50:197–201

Migliore L, Brambilla G, Grassitellis A, Di Delupis GD (1993) Toxicity and bioaccumulation of sulphadimethoxine in *Artemia* (Crustacea, Anostraca). Int J Salt Lake Res 2(2):141–152

Migliore L, Civitareale C, Brambilla G, Di Delupis GD (1997) Toxicity of several important agricultural antibiotics to *Artemia*. Wat. Res. 31(7):1801–1806

Panter GH, Thompson RS, Beresford N, Sumpter JP (1999) Transformation of a non-oestrogenic steroid metabolite to an oestrogenically active substance by minimal bacterial activity. Chemosphere 38(15):3579–3596

Peterson SM, Batley GE, Scammell, MS (1993) Tetracycline in antifouling paints. Mar Pollut Bull 26(2):96–100

Purdom CE, Hardiman PA, Bye VJ, Eno NC, Tyler CR, Sumpter JP (1994) Estrogenic effects of effluents from sewage treatment works. Chem Ecol 8:275–285

Rodriguez C, Chellman K, Gomez S, Marple L (1992) Environmental assessment report pursuant to 21 CFR 25.31(a) submitted to the US FDA in support of the New Drug Application (NDA) for naproxen for over-the-counter use. Hamilton Pharmaceuticals Limited, Puerto Rico

Römbke J et al. (1996) Minutes of the round table discussion: medicines in the environment held at the Federal German Bureau of the Environment (Berlin) on 15th December 1995 on behalf of the Federal German Bureau of the Environment (UBA)

Russom CL, Bradbury SP, Broderius SJ, Hammermeister DE, Drummond RA (1997) Predicting modes of toxic action from chemical structure: acute toxicity in the fathead minnow (*Pimephales promelas*). Environ Toxicol Chem 16(5):948–967

Sanofi (1996) Tiludronate disodium material safety data sheet SR 41319B. Sanofi Research

Schweinfurth H, Länge R, Schneider PW (1996a) Environmental risk assessment in the pharmaceutical industry. Presentation at the 3rd Eurolab Symposium – Testing and Analysis for Industrial Competitiveness and Sustainability, 5–7th June, 1996, Berlin

Schweinfurth H, Länge R, Günzel P (1996b) Environmental fate and ecological effects of steroidal estrogens. Presentation at the Oestrogenic Chemicals in the Environment conference organised by IBC Technical Services Ltd in London on 9th and 10th May, 1996

Sheahan DA, Bucke D, Matthiessen P, Sumpter JP, Kirby MF, Neall P, Waldock M (1994) The effects of low levels of 17α-ethynylestradiol upon plasma vitellogenin levels in male and female rainbow trout, *Oncorhynchus mykiss*, held at two acclimation temperatures. In: Müller R, Lloyd R (eds) Sublethal and chronic effects of pollutants on freshwater fish. Blackwell Science, Oxford (Fishing News Books, pp 99–112)

Tooby TE, Hursey PA, Alabaster JS (1975) The acute toxicity of 102 pesticides and miscellaneous substances to fish. Chemistry and Industry 6/1975:523–526

Wang WH, Lay JP (1989) Fate and effects of salicylic acid compounds in freshwater systems. Ecotoxicol Environ Safety 17(3):308–316

Welborn TL (1969) The toxicity of nine therapeutic and herbicidal compounds to stripped bass. The Progressive Fish Culturist 31(1):27–32

Wilford WA (1966) Toxicity of 22 therapeutic compounds to six fishes. US Dept. of the Interior, Fish and Wildlife Service, Bureau of Sports Fisheries and Wildlife, Washington DC (Resource Publication 35)

Zou E, Fingerman (1997) Synthetic estrogenic agents do not interfere with sex differentiation but do inhibit molting of the cladoceran *Daphnia magna*. Bull Environ Contam Toxicol 58:596–602

Appendix

A
Fish

- *Brachyderio (= Danio) rerio* – zebrafish
- *Gambusia affinis* – mosquito fish
- *Ictalurus punctatus* – channel catfish
- *Lepomis macrochirus* – bluegill sunfish
- *Morone saxatilis* – striped bass
- *Oncorhynchus mykiss* – rainbow trout
- *Pimephales promelas* – fathead minnow
- *Rasbora heteromorpha* – harlequin fish
- *Rutilus rutilus* – roach
- *Salmo trutta* – brown trout
- *Salvelinus fontinalis* – brook trout
- *Salvelinus namaycush* – lake trout

B
Invertebrates

- *Acartia tonsa* – copepod crustacean
- *Artemia salina* – anostracan crustacean
- *Brachionus calyciflorus* – rotifer
- *Bithynia tentaculata* – gastropod mollusc
- *Daphnia magna* – cladoceran crustacean (water flea)
- *Hyalella azteca* – amphipod crustacean
- *Lymnaea stagnalis* – gastropod mollusc (pond snail)
- *Panaeus setiferus* – decapod crustacean (white shrimp)
- *Sphaerium striatinum* – bivalve mollusc (fingernail clam)
- *Physa* spp. – gastropod mollusc (bladder snail)
- *Streptocephalus proboscideus* – anostracan crustacean

C
Algae

- *Scenedesmus subspicatus* – green algae
- *Selenastrum capricornutum* – green algae
- *Nitzschia closterium* – marine diatom
- *Skeletonema costatum* – marine diatom
- *Chlorella* spp. – green algae
- *Microcystis aeruginosa* – blue-green algae

A Data Based Perspective on the Environmental Risk Assessment of Human Pharmaceuticals II – Aquatic Risk Characterisation

S. F. Webb

16.1
Introduction

Environmental risk assessment (ERA) evaluates the likelihood that adverse ecological effects result from exposure to a substance. It therefore requires a consideration of both exposure and effects in relevant environmental compartments. The exposure assessment considers the fate of a substance released to the environment and predicts the environmental concentration or PEC ("predicted environmental concentration"). The effects assessment considers data relating to the effects of the substance upon representative biota and uses such data to predict the no-effect concentration or PNEC ("predicted no-effect concentration") for the various environmental compartments (i.e. surface waters, sediment, soil, etc.). The PEC and PNEC are combined in order to characterise the risk, i.e. calculation of the PEC/PNEC ratio (see Fig. 16.1). Decisions regarding the safety of the substance depend upon the value of this quotient.

Risk assessment conventionally proceeds in an iterative/tiered process, employing simple and conservative assumptions to estimate PEC and PNEC at initial tiers and progressing through subsequent tiers by employing more realistic or representative assumptions when estimating PEC and PNEC. Conservatism is incorporated into both the PEC (via the assumptions used to estimate the exposure) and PNEC (via use of assessment factors to extrapolate from laboratory derived-data to the ecosystem). The exposure and effects assessments do not have to simultaneously progress to successive tiers, and effort can be focused on those data that potentially have the largest impact upon the risk quotient or will reduce uncertainties.

If the environmental concentration in a compartment is less than the concentration causing "no effect" to that compartment, i.e. PEC/PNEC < 1, then it is assumed that use of the substance carries little risk of an adverse environmental effect. If the PEC/PNEC > 1, then a decision must be made either to further refine the data upon which the risk characterisation is based (i.e. progress to a subsequent tier), to manage the risk by limiting the amount of the substance released to the environment or to accept the level of risk following risk-benefit analysis. This latter option may be particularly pertinent to pharmaceuticals. Environmental (and human) risk assessment of both new and existing industrial substances in the European Union are conducted according to the Technical Guidance Document or TGD (CEC 1996).

By means of a new directive (93/39/EEC), the Council of the European Union amended 65/65/EEC ("Council Directive 65/65/EEC of 26 January 1965 on the approximation of provisions laid down by law, regulation or administration action relating to medicinal products"). Article 4.6 of the amendment states "If applicable, reasons for any precautionary and safety measures to be taken for the storage of the medicinal

Fig. 16.1. Risk assessment framework for the aquatic environment of pharmaceuticals

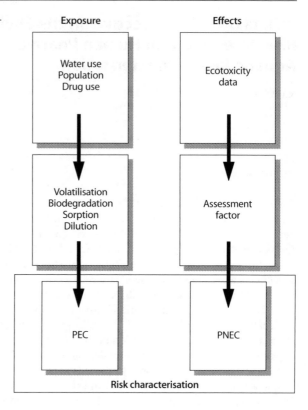

product, its administration to patients and for the disposal of waste products, together with an indication of any potential risks presented by the medicinal product for the environment." The amendment effectively requires an environmental risk assessment (ERA) be submitted with marketing authorisation applications (MAA) for pharmaceutical products containing novel compounds. EU member states were required to implement necessary regulations by January 1, 1995. However, technical guidelines for the environmental risk assessment (ERA) of pharmaceutical products for human use have yet to be finalised and are still subject to change. Drafts were prepared under the aegis of several technical committees, including a task force under DGIII (the European Commission's Industry Directorate) providing comment to the CPMP ("Committee for Proprietary Medicinal Products"). The nature and implications of the draft European guidelines are more fully reviewed elsewhere (see Hussain and Hennessy 1995; Olejniczak 1995; Webb 1995). Development of the guidelines was halted pending clarification and further information from the US Food and Drug Administration (FDA) with respect to their experience of the value of environmental assessments (EAs). This followed the FDA's declaration that EA requirements for pharmaceuticals were to be simplified and that the number of EAs required to be submitted to the FDA for review would be reduced (FDA 1995). This conclusion was based on the fact that virtually all EAs submitted to the FDA have been issued with a "Finding Of No Significant Impact" (FONSI). Following finalisation of the FDA's EA requirements, there is now a categorical exclusion for New Drug Actives (NDA) if the estimated concentration of the substance at the point of entry into the aquatic environment (i.e. in sewage effluent) is below 1 μg l^{-1} (US FDA Final Rule – Federal Register 29/07/97, vol. 62, no. 145, pp 40569–40600). This corresponds to a de facto threshold of ~41 t yr^{-1} in the USA. Guidance on the FDA's EA requirements can be found in an FDA-CDER publication entitled: "Guidance for Industry – Environmental Assessment of Human Drugs and Biologics Applications" (FDA-CDER 1998).

This study brings together collated data relating to the usage and ecotoxicity of existing pharmaceuticals. Where possible, these data were employed in preliminary ERAs of compounds in the aquatic compartment (which is assumed to be predominantly relevant) in a fashion consistent with that prescribed by the draft European Guidelines. The intention is to provide perspective that will prove useful during the further development of any assessment criteria.

16.2
Methodology

In general, there is a paucity of readily accessible data relating to the consumption of pharmaceuticals. This has hitherto precluded attempts at the systematic analysis of the potential impacts of pharmaceuticals upon the environment. The most comprehensive survey of drug usage to date was conducted by Richardson and Bowron (1985), who examined drug prescription patterns in the UK for the years 1975–76. Of a total of 1 600 compounds considered, approximately 170 were used at >1 t yr^{-1}. Of these 170, it is possible to derive consumption values for 141 compounds from the publication. The distribution of the data is summarised in Table 16.1. The corresponding overall consumption totals <6 700 t yr^{-1}. Usage data for 10 drugs in Germany (1995) is presented in Ternes (1998). Some limited drug consumption data for Sweden, the Netherlands and Denmark is presented in Eckerman and Martineus (1997), Van Der Heide and Hueck-Van Der Plas (1984) and Halling-Sørensen et al. (1998).

Given the absence of recently published usage data, an audit of 1995 UK pharmaceutical usage was commissioned from IMS (Intercontinental Medical Statistics – UK and Ireland Ltd). Approximately 60 compounds were selected for audit on the basis of the availability of ecotoxicity data (thereby allowing risk characterisation). The results of the audit are presented in Table 16.4 and reflect sales of all products containing these compounds (irrespective of salt and including combination products) into retail pharmacies, dispensing general practitioners and hospital pharmacies. Data relating to the UK usage of OTC analgesics were obtained from the Paracetamol Information Centre (Brandon, pers. comm.) and the European Aspirin Foundation (Hopkins, pers. comm.). Data are summarised in Table 16.2.

Where data are available for both drug consumption and ecotoxicity, an aquatic risk characterisation was undertaken for human pharmaceuticals. A review of short-term/acute ecotoxicity data for macro-invertebrates, fish and algae for over 100 human pharmaceuticals is presented in Chap. 15. Although the results of the risk characterisation are specific to the United Kingdom, they are probably equally applicable to other countries with similarly developed healthcare provisions and wastewater treatment infrastructure. Sewage influent concentrations are calculated throughout on the basis of a UK population of 57.6 million and a specific water consumption of 259 l capita^{-1} day^{-1} (WSA 1994). The

Table 16.1. Summary of UK consumption data (derived from Richardson and Bowron 1985)

| | Tonnes per year | | | | | | | |
	1–<10	10–<20	20–<30	30–<40	40–<50	50–<100	>100	Total ≥1
Number	115	13	3	0	3	4	3	141
Frequency (%)	82	9	2	0	2	3	2	100

Table 16.2. Summary of 1995 UK consumption data (commissioned from IMS)

| | Tonnes per year | | | | | | | |
	<1	1–<10	10–<20	20–<30	30–<40	40–<50	50–<100	>100
Number	38	14	3	3	1	1	4	3
Frequency (%)	57	21	4.5	4.5	1.5	1.5	6	4.5

assumptions of no human metabolism, passage of all material to drain, no removal during wastewater treatment (via biodegradation, sorption or volatilisation) and no surface water dilution of effluent that were used to calculate the PEC are all conservative. Collectively, they can be thought of as "worst-case" (see Fig. 16.2). The PNEC values are derived using an assessment factor of 1 000 with the relevant acute data. This is consistent with the approach employed for other chemical compounds in the EU Technical Guidance Document (CEC 1996).

16.3
Results

The results of the preliminary assessment for over 60 compounds are presented in Table 16.3 and summarised in Fig. 16.3[1]. Together, these compounds will probably account for over half of all known pharmaceuticals consumption in tonnage terms. The PEC/PNEC ratio was <1 in all but eight cases. PEC/PNEC ratios less than unity are taken as indicative of a negligible risk of an adverse environmental effect. The exceptions were paracetamol (acetaminophen), aspirin, dextropropoxyphene, fluoxetine, oxytetracycline, propranolol, amitriptyline and thioridazine. It is notable that paracetamol and aspirin are the two most commonly consumed pharmaceutical compounds. One possible caveat to the approach adopted is the implicit assumption of homogenous distribution of use in the UK. Certain drugs such as antineoplastics may only be used in hospitals on an in-patient basis.

Further refinement of the risk assessment is therefore required for paracetamol, aspirin, dextropropoxyphene, fluoxetine, oxytetracycline, propranolol, amitriptyline,

---

[1] These results were originally presented at SETAC-Europe 1998 (Webb 1998).

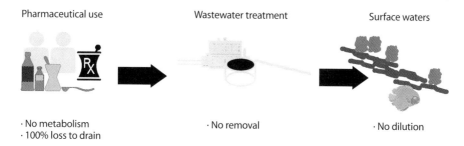

Pharmaceutical use   Wastewater treatment   Surface waters

· No metabolism   · No removal   · No dilution
· 100% loss to drain

Fig. 16.2. "Worst-case" PEC estimation for pharmaceuticals

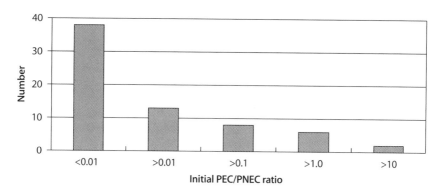

Fig. 16.3. Initial preliminary risk characterisation

and thioridazine. Chronic ecotoxicity data – which would have allowed use of an alternative assessment factor to calculate the PNEC – are not available for most of the drugs and the initial effects assessments were therefore retained. Refinement was consequently confined to the exposure assessments (i.e. PECs). This required a consideration of the likely degree of removal during wastewater treatment (via biodegradation[2], adsorption or volatilisation) and/or surface water dilution of sewage effluent. From a regulatory perspective, any further discussion of removal during wastewater treatment of aspirin, dextropropoxyphene, propranolol, amitriptyline and thioridazine is academic as a consideration of surface water dilution alone is sufficient to ensure a PEC/PNEC < 1. This assumes a dilution factor 10, which is the default from the EU Technical Guidance Document (CEC 1996).

---

[2] Biodegradation data were available for five of the compounds (or a closely related analogue in the case of oxytetraceycline). The likely biodegradation profile of all the compounds was also predicted using the group contribution method of Boethling et al. (1994). Biodegradation of paracetamol, aspirin, oxytetracycline and amitriptyline as predicted via the group contribution method was comparable with that reported by Richardson and Bowron (1985). Only in the case of dextro-propoxyphene did reported biodegradation differ from the predicted profile. The group contribution algorithm suggests that dextropropoxyphene is not recalcitrant and may even be readily biodegradable.

Table 16.3. Initial aquatic risk assessment for selected pharmaceuticals in the UK

Name	UK use (t yr^{-1})[a]	PEC (µg l^{-1})	PNEC (µg l^{-1})	PEC/PNEC
Paracetamol	~2000	367.3	9.2	39.92
Aspirin	770	141.4	141	1.00
Metformin	106.1	19.49	101[b]	0.19
Cimetidine	72.0	13.22	740	0.02
Ranitidine	69.0	12.67	582[b]	0.02
Erythromycin	67.7	12.43	>74	<0.17
Naproxen	60.6	11.13	128[b]	0.09
Dextropropoxyphene	42.5	7.81	3.79[b]	2.06
Oxytetracycline	33.7	6.19	0.23	26.8
Quinine	29.7	5.45	10.1[b]	0.54
Theophylline	21	3.86	155	0.02
Lithium Salts	20.5[c]	0.35 (Li)	4.18 (Li)	0.08
Metronidazole	15.5	2.85	12.5	0.23
Iopromide	11.9	2.19	>92	<0.01
Propranolol	11.8	2.17	1.87	1.16
Verapamil	9.9	1.82	5.78[b]	0.31
Amitriptyline	5.5	1.01	0.78	1.29
Tetracycline	4.7	0.86	16.0	0.05
Omeprazole	3.9	0.72	88	<0.01
Thioridazine	3.8	0.70	0.27[b]	2.59
Chloroquine	2.9	0.53	2.72[b]	0.20
Gabapentin	2.6	0.48	>1100	<0.01
Etidronic acid	2.1	0.39	3.0	0.13
Fluoxetine	2.0	0.37	0.026[b]	14.19
Phenobarbital	1.7	0.31	484	<0.01
Tramadol	1.7	0.31	64[b]	<0.01
Clofibrate	1.5	0.28	12.0	0.02
Paroxetine	1.3	0.24	1.8[b]	0.13
Orphenadrine	1.1	0.20	3.82[b]	0.05
Diazepam	0.957	0.18	4.3	0.04
Acarbose	0.918	0.17	>1000	<0.01
Isoniazid	0.690	0.13	24.4	<0.01
Nefazodone	0.618	0.11	6.5[b]	0.02
Quinidine	0.601	0.11	7.2[b]	0.02
Sumatriptan	0.521	0.10	207[b]	<0.01
Aminosidin/Neomycin E	0.487	0.09	340[b]	<0.01
Warfarin	0.476	0.09	12.0	<0.01

Table 16.3. *Continued*

Name	UK use (t yr^{-1})^a	PEC (µg l^{-1})	PNEC (µg l^{-1})	PEC/PNEC
Lansoprazole	0.434	0.08	18.0	<0.01
Cisapride	0.413	0.08	1 000	<0.01
Chloramphenicol	0.377	0.07	305	<0.01
Famciclovir	0.286	0.05	820	<0.01
Azithromycin	0.276	0.05	120	<0.01
Cetirizine	0.273	0.05	278^b	<0.01
Famotidine	0.246	0.05	398	<0.01
Ceftibuten	0.095	0.017	>520	<0.01
Lorsatan	0.087	0.016	331	<0.01
Budesonide	0.081	0.015	>19	<0.01
Finasteride	0.067	0.012	20	<0.01
Perindopril	0.047	0.009	>990^b	<0.01
Didanosine	0.039	0.007	>1 021	<0.01
Midazolam	0.037	0.007	0.2	0.04
Fluticasone	0.034	0.006	0.48^b	0.01
Digoxin	0.031	0.006	24	<0.01
Ethinyloestradiol	0.029	0.005	0.84	<0.01
Risperidone	0.021	0.004	6	<0.01
Atropine	0.016	0.003	221^b	<0.01
Carvedilol	0.008	0.001	1	<0.01
Salmeterol	0.007	0.001	20	<0.01
Bicalutamide	0.007	0.001	>1	<0.01
Alendronic acid	0.007	0.001	0.46^b	<0.01
Dorzolamide	0.004	0.001	604^b	<0.01
Diethystilbestrol	0.002	<0.001	1.09	<0.01
Paclitaxel	0.001	<0.001	0.74	<0.01
Zalcitabine	<0.001	<0.001	>1 790	<0.01
Thiotepa	<0.001	<0.001	546	<0.01
Flumazenil	<0.001	<0.001	>500	<0.01
Milrinone	<0.001	<0.001	223^b	<0.01

^{a} Quoted figures are all assumed to refer to the organic parent molecule (although in some cases the active will actually be the salt and the values will therefore be overestimates).
^{b} Adjustment for molar equivalent of organic parent molecule.
^{c} Includes 16.89 t yr^{-1} lithium citrate and 3.54 t yr^{-1} lithium carbonate. PEC and PNEC values are adjusted to the lithium ion.

Paracetamol: A high degree of elimination (98%) of paracetamol during activated sludge wastewater treatment has been reported by Ternes (1998). This is not surprising given the biodegradation profile of paracetamol (Richardson and Bowron 1985). An estimated paracetamol "worst-case" (i.e. no human metabolism) sewage influent concentration of 367 µg l^{-1} would therefore be reduced to an effluent concentration of 7.3 µg l^{-1} following activated sludge treatment. The corresponding PEC after 1:10 dilution of effluent in surface water would be 0.7 µg l^{-1}. A PNEC of 9.2 µg l^{-1} can be derived for paracetamol by the application of an assessment factor of 1 000 to the lowest of 3 acute endpoints in algae, fish and *Daphnia* (Henschel et al. 1997; Kühn et al. 1989). The resultant PEC/PNEC ratio is 0.08 and environmental safety is assumed (even without any consideration of human metabolism). It is notable that paracetamol was not detected in the environmental matrices examined by Richardson and Bowron (1985) or in German surface waters (LOD = 0.15 µg l^{-1}) by Ternes (1998). Concentrations in treated sewage effluents in Germany were similarly less than the detection limit (LOD = 0.5 µg l^{-1}) at the 90th-percentile (Ternes 1998). Risk characterisation based the measured (rather than predicted) environmental concentrations (MEC) from Ternes (1998) would yield MEC/PNEC ratios <0.02.

Fluoxetine: The likely biodegradation profile of fluoxetine can be predicted using the group contribution method of Boethling et al. (1994). The linear model predicts rapid biodegradation. A degree of elimination via biodegradation of fluoxetine during wastewater treatment is therefore likely. A removal of ≥91% can be predicted for readily biodegradable substances (regardless of K_{ow}) from the WWTP removal defaults in the appendices of the TGD (CEC 1996). Incorporation of such an elimination rate and a consideration of surface water dilution of effluent (dilution factor 10) would yield a revised PEC for fluoxetine of 0.003 µg l^{-1}. The initial PNEC for fluoxetine of 0.026 µg l^{-1} is derived from an application of an assessment factor to the lowest (algae) of three acute endpoints (FDA-CDER 1996). A revised PEC/PNEC based upon the above exposure and effects scenarios would be 0.12.

Oxytetracycline: Human metabolism of oxytetracycline is limited (Dollery 1991). Biodegradation is also likely to be limited (based on observations for tetracycline from Richardson and Bowron 1985). As such the initial assumptions of 100% loss to drain (i.e. no metabolism) and 0% removal during wastewater treatment is retained. The estimated sewage influent and effluent concentrations remain at 6.2 µg l^{-1}. With surface water dilution of effluent (dilution factor 10) this corresponds to a PEC of 0.62 µg l^{-1}. A PNEC of 0.23 µg l^{-1} can be derived from the use of an application factor of 1 000 on an algal EC$_{50}$ (Holten Lützhøft et al. 1998). The revised PEC/PNEC is 2.7 and nominally requires further refinement. It is notable that tetracycline is photodegradable in surface waters with a half-life in terms of hours (Peterson et al. 1993). Photodegradation may help to explain why oxytetracycline was not detected (90th-percentile < LOD = 0.05 µg l^{-1}) in German rivers by Hirsch et al. (1999). Similarly, the complexing properties of tetracyclines with calcium and other similar ions have also been highlighted as a possible reason to explain their absence from the water column (Hirsch et al. 1999). Risk characterisation based on measured concentrations from Hirsch et al. (1999) yield MEC/PNEC ratios <0.22.

Ethinyloestradiol: Although initial risk characterisation of ethinyloestradiol yielded PEC/PNEC ratios <1, specific concerns have been raised around the possible effects of this compound following observations in environmental matrices. These concerns can also be addressed via risk characterisation based on *(i)* actual monitoring data rather than predicted concentrations and *(ii)* a PNEC derived from chronic endpoints. Acute/short term ecotoxicity endpoints for ethinyloestradiol initially employed to derive a PNEC are *(i)* algal $EC_{50} = 0.84$ mg l^{-1} (Köpf 1995) *(ii)* *Oncorhynchus mykiss* LC_{50} 1.6 mg l^{-1} (Schweinfurth et al. 1996) and *(iii)* *Daphnia magna* EC_{50} 6.4 mg l^{-1} (Schweinfurth et al. 1996). In contrast, sub-lethal responses in *Daphnia* and algae (Köpf 1995) were at concentrations 1–3 orders of magnitude less. Even more sensitive endpoints for ethinyloestradiol exist for fish. They include plasma vitellogenin bioassay effect concentrations of <1 ng l^{-1} in rainbow trout (*Oncorhynchus mykiss*) and a spermatogenesis/gonadosomatic index (GSI) effect concentration of 2 ng l^{-1} in roach (*Rutilus rutilus*) and rainbow trout (Purdom et al. 1994; FWR 1995). Although the ecological significance of responses in these biomarkers is unclear, other more readily interpretable endpoints are available. For example, Schweinfurth et al. (1996) also detail preliminary chronic test data from studies conducted with fathead minnows (*Pimephales promelas*). These include a 28 d LOEC of 10 ng l^{-1} for inhibited egg production. A subsequent study revealed a 9-month reproduction NOEC of 1 ng l^{-1} (Länge et al. 1997). With an appropriate assessment factor (i.e. 10), the corresponding PNEC is therefore 0.1 ng l^{-1}.

At a consumption figure of 29 kg yr^{-1} in the UK – equivalent to ~2.65 million daily doses of 30 μg – the predicted influent concentration is ~5 ng l^{-1}. This excludes human metabolism. Less than 1% of ethinyloestradiol is excreted unchanged. The major pathway of metabolism is 2-hydroxylation. Hydroxylated metabolites have little oestrogenic activity. Up to 30% is excreted unoxidised as glucuronide or sulfate conjugates in urine and bile (Dollery 1991). However, this assumption of no human metabolism is somewhat vindicated by the recent observation that non-oestrogenic steroids metabolites (i.e. oestradiol-3-glucuronide) can be readily biotransformed into biologically active oestrogens via microbial activity (Panter et al. 1999).

Incorporation of a consideration of removal during wastewater treatment (78% by activated sludge treatment and 64% by trickling filter treatment, Ternes et al. 1999) and effluent dilution in surface water (1:10) results in a surface water PEC of 0.03–0.05 ng l^{-1}. This can be compared with values of 2–15 ng l^{-1} reported in UK rivers by Aherne and Briggs (1989). However, other authorities have doubted the veracity of such observations following subsequent monitoring studies (FWR 1995). This is supported by the most recent observations from studies detailing *(i)* German surface water concentrations where values were all <0.2 ng l^{-1} (Kalbfus 1995) and *(ii)* how ethinyloestradiol was undetectable (<0.2 ng l^{-1}) in more than half of UK sewage effluents sampled and where detectable was usually below 1 ng l^{-1} (Desbrow et al. 1996). With sufficient surface water dilution of the effluent (i.e. 1:10), the PEC would typically range from <0.02 ng l^{-1} to <0.1 ng l^{-1}, and the environmental safety of ethinyloestradiol could be assumed. Only under low dilution scenarios (i.e. <1:2, where effluent concentrations are above the detection limit of 0.2 ng l^{-1}) will risk characterisation yield PEC/PNEC ratios >1.

However, it should also be noted that Desbrow et al. (1996) also details how the majority (90%) of oestrogenic activity in sewage effluent in the UK is accounted for by the presence of the natural oestrogens, oestrone and 17β-oestradiol. The source of these natural oestrogens appears to be excretion from women, particularly pregnant women. It is suspected that the conjugated forms of oestrone and 17β-oestradiol that are excreted by women are metabolised by bacterial β-glucuronidase enzymes to produce active hormones. Desbrow et al. (1996) therefore concluded that although ethinyloestradiol may contribute to the overall oestrogenicity of sewage effluents, it appears likely that natural oestrogens are responsible for the majority of the feminised responses observed in fish populations exposed to sewage effluents.

Clofibrate/Clofibric acid: Acute/short term ecotoxicity endpoints for clofibrate/clofibric acid ranged from 12 mg l^{-1} to 89 mg l^{-1} (Köpf 1995). The initial PNEC value was 12 μg l^{-1} (based on algal EC$_{50}$ from Köpf 1995) and the PEC was 0.28 μg l^{-1}. Risk characterisation yielded a PEC/PNEC ratio of 0.02. For comparison, the PNEC value that can be derived from chronic data is 0.2 μg l^{-1}. This is based on a 21 d NOEC in *Daphnia magna* of 10 μg l^{-1} (Köpf 1995) with an assessment factor of 50 (algal and *Daphnia* chronic endpoints). The PEC could be further refined by an incorporation of the reported degree of elimination (51%) of clofibric acid during wastewater treatment (Ternes 1998) and surface water dilution of effluent (dilution factor 10). This would yield a PEC of 0.014 μg l^{-1}. The maximum reported environmental concentrations (MEC) of clofibric acid in surface waters in Germany is 1.75 μg l^{-1} with a 90th-percentile of 0.72 μg l^{-1} (Ternes 1998). MEC/PNEC ratios are therefore 8.75 and 3.6, respectively. Further revision of the effects assessment to generate a third chronic endpoint for fish would allow an assessment factor of 10. This may improve the MEC/PNEC ratio at the 90th-percentile. Differences between the PECs for the UK and reported concentrations of clofibric acid in German surface waters in part reflect differing use patterns in the two countries, i.e. 1.5 t yr^{-1} in the UK compared with 16 t yr^{-1} reported for Germany by Ternes (1998).

Other drugs: Observations of surface water concentrations are available for several other pharmaceuticals (see Table 16.4). Maximal measured environmental concentrations (MECs) for most compounds were generally less than the corresponding "worst-case" PECs from Table 16.3. Although in several cases, the difference was less than one order of magnitude. Whilst many of the measured observations relate to German surface waters, they may be considered indicative of the conservatism employed in this study when deriving the PECs. The surface water concentrations can also be compared with a PNEC to derive MEC/PNEC ratios. In all cases, MEC/PNEC ratios are <1. It is notable that aspirin, dextropropoxyphene and propranolol were also amongst those compounds highlighted for further refinement of the risk assessment following initial characterisation under the "worst-case" exposure assessment assumptions (see Table 16.3).

16.4
Discussion

The general lack of public domain usage data had previously precluded estimates of the environmental concentrations of pharmaceuticals. Data presented in this study allowed the aquatic exposure assessment of a large number of compounds from across a wide variety of therapeutic classes. Initial risk characterisation utilising acute ecotoxicity data and conservative fate assumptions (including no human metabolism, no removal during wastewater treatment and no surface water dilution of effluent) demonstrated the nominal environmental safety (i.e. PEC/PNEC < 1) of all but eight of the greater than 60 pharmaceutical compounds considered. The exceptions were paracetamol, aspirin, dextropropoxyphene, fluoxetine, oxytetracycline, propranolol, amitriptyline, and thioridazine. Incorporation of their likely fate following use

Table 16.4. Comparison of maximal measured environmental concentrations (MEC) with predicted no-effect concentrations (PNEC)

Drug/Metabolite	MEC (ng l^{-1})	PNEC (ng l^{-1})	MEC/PNEC ratio
Aspirin	340[b]	141 000	<0.01
Chloroamphenicol	60[c]	305 000	<0.01
Dextroproproxyphene	1 000[d]	3 790	0.26
Diazepam	<30[b]	4 300	<0.01
Erythromycin	1 700[c]	>74 000	<0.02
Ibuprofen	530[b]	7 100[a]	0.07
Methotrexate	<6.25[e]	85 000[a]	<0.01
Naproxen	390[b]	128 000	<0.01
Oxytetracycline	<50[c]	230	<0.22
Propranolol	590[b]	1 870	0.32
Sulfamethazine	<20[c]	>100 000[a]	<0.01
Tetracycline	1 000[f]	16 000	0.06
Theophylline	1 000[f]	155 000	<0.01

[a] See Chap. 15 for ecotoxicological data.
[b] Ternes (1998).
[c] Hirsch et al. (1999).
[d] Richardson and Bowron (1995).
[e] Aherne et al. (1985).
[f] Watts et al. (1983).

(i.e. removal during wastewater treatment and/or surface water dilution of effluent) yielded a marked reduction in the surface water PEC values, and the resultant PEC/PNEC ratios were generally less than unity when the PNEC was based on acute data. This use of acute ecotoxicity data for risk assessment purposes for pharmaceuticals has been criticised (Halling-Sørensen et al. 1998). Standard acute bioassays with their focus on immediate endpoints such as lethality may not be the most appropriate basis for risk assessment given the intended narrow scope of biological activity/effect and general potency of pharmaceuticals in general. It has consequently been suggested that chronic bioassays performed over the life-cycle of various organisms from different trophic levels may be more appropriate (Halling-Sørensen et al. 1998). A limited amount of data relating to the effects of pharmaceuticals upon chronic ecotoxicity endpoints was available. It is interesting to note that in this study when PNECs were derived from this chronic data set, values were less than the corresponding values derived from acute data (i.e. in the case of ethinyloestradiol and clofibrate). MEC/PNEC ratios based on maximal measured surface water concentrations rather than PECs were similarly less than unity. In general, these maximal MECs were less than the "worst-case" PECs and this was interpreted as confirmation of the conservative nature of the underlying assumptions used to derive the PECs.

Following use, most human drugs (or their metabolites) will tend to enter the environment by excretion (via urine and/or faeces) from patients. Incorporation of a consideration of human metabolism during the exposure assessment would therefore have the potential to reduce PEC values. Even though it has not proven necessary to include a consideration of metabolism to demonstrate nominal environmental safety of parent compounds, reported metabolism of many drugs is known to be considerable. Where metabolism does take place, metabolites in general will tend to be more polar and water soluble. Metabolism is also often associated with a loss of pharmacological action and detoxification. For example, Richardson and Bowron (1985) noted that a significant number of pharmaceuticals undergo mammalian metabolism to yield conjugates, and that the toxicity and pharmacological activity of these conjugates is likely to be much lower than that of the parent compounds. However, any effects on solubility may also have a concomitant influence on removal via adsorption during wastewater treatment. A full consideration of the fate and effects of all the metabolites of each drug considered in this study would clearly be prohibitive. Risk characterisation was therefore exclusively conducted on the parent drug substance as representative of substances potentially entering the environment. Alternative practices may need to be applied for drugs where there are clear indications that the fate of the metabolites differ from the parent compound or that the metabolites could adversely effect the environment to a greater extent than the parent drug substance. In some cases, incorporation of a consideration of metabolism when estimating exposure may even be inadvisable, as there is a suggestion that some drug conjugates have the potential to be reactivated during biological wastewater treatment (FWR 1995). Similarly, Henschel et al. (1997) speculate whether paracetamol and salicylic acid conjugates can be reactivated via microbial β-gluconidase or sulfatase. Most recently, Panter et al. (1999) demonstrated the transformation of a non-oestrogenic steroid metabolite to an oestrogenically active substance via bacterial activity. It is interesting to note that both clofibrate and ethinyloestradiol – two pharmaceuticals that have attracted particular attention following observations in environmental samples – are excreted in considerable amounts as conjugates in the urine or faeces (Dollery 1991). Some 50–85% of dosed clofibrate is excreted in the urine as the glucuronic conjugate of clofibric acid. In the case of ethinyloestradiol, considerable amounts (~30%) are excreted in urine and bile as the primary glucuronide and sulfate conjugates.

One potential issue that has not been directly addressed is that of bioaccumulation. The potential to bioaccumulate is driven by lipophilicity. Octanol/water partition coefficient (K_{ow}) is a surrogate measure of lipophilicity and has frequently been correlated with bioaccumulation in non-polar/non-ionisable substances, e.g. Mackay (1982) and Veith and Kosian (1983). A quantitative inclusion of a consideration of bioaccumulation into the risk assessment process is described by Cowan et al. (1995). One important aspect of the integrated assessment framework relating to bioaccumulation was whether the duration of ecotoxicity tests are sufficient to achieve maximal body burdens and elicit potential ecotoxic effects upon test organisms. Based on a consideration of such an issue, the study also proposed an initial action threshold for a tiered bioaccumulation assessment of a fish bioconcentration factor (BCF) of 1 000. Both Mackay (1982) and Veith and Kosian (1983) predict a BCF of 1 000 at $\log K_{ow} \sim 4.3$. Such models typically overestimate actual bioaccumulation and may trigger unjustifiable concerns (ECETOC 1995). Deviations from predicted bioaccumulation will occur with *(i)* substances of molecular weight greater than ~700, thereby inhibiting or excluding penetration of biological membranes, *(ii)* substances that are ionisable, surface active or polar or *(iii)* where active biotransformation of the substance to a more hydrophilic derivative occurs (ECETOC 1995).

Of particular importance in reducing the bioconcentration and bioaccumulation of substances within aquatic organisms is biotransformation (ECETOC 1995). Two types of biotransformation reactions are observed in aquatic organisms and these have been classified as Phase I and Phase II reactions. Phase I reactions are the primary phase of metabolism involving oxidation, reduction or hydrolysis of functional groups. Phase II reactions involve conjugation, whereby substances or their metabolites are bound to other substances such as sulfate or glucuronic acid. Several cases of the influence of metabolism on measured BCFs have been reported, and it is evident that biotransformation is crucial in reducing the bioconcentration and bioaccumulation of substances within aquatic organisms (see ECETOC 1995). Significant discrepancies can exist between measured and calculated BCF values, and these become more pronounced with increasing $\log K_{ow}$ (ECETOC 1995). Therefore, where biotransformation is known to occur, $\log K_{ow}$ cannot be reliably used to predict actual potential to bioconcentrate.

$\log K_{ow}$ data are available for a large number of pharmaceuticals (e.g. Bowman and Rand 1980; Dollery 1991; Hansch et al. 1995; Hoekman 1997). Of those considered in this study, only four compounds had $\log K_{ow}$ values >4.3. These were amitriptyline, chloroquine, diethylstilbestrol and thioridazine. All have molecular weights <700. It is known that lower vertebrates and invertebrates maintain many of the same systems to biotransform xenobiotics which are present in mammals (ECETOC 1995). Mammalian metabolism studies may therefore have some value as a first indication of the potential of fish to metabolise a substance. Mammalian metabolism of diethylstilbestrol, amitriptyline and thioridazine is similarly reported by Dollery (1991). Only in the case of chloroquine ($K_{ow} = 4.63$) is mammalian metabolism limited. Excretion is slow with a plasma half-life of 30–60 days and chloroquine may persist in tissues for months or even years after discontinuation of therapy (Reynolds 1996). Substantial amounts (35%) are excreted unchanged in the urine (Dollery 1991). However, bioconcentration of chloroquine is unlikely to be an issue. With pK_a values of 8.4 and 10.8 it will be mainly present as the ionised di-cation moiety at ambient pH in surface waters, and this is likely to limit bioconcentration.

Given that *(i)* few pharmaceuticals appear to have $\log K_{ow}$ values >4.3, *(ii)* many pharmaceuticals are weak acids/bases and exist as the ionised moiety under conditions of ambient pH, *(iii)* many pharmaceuticals are readily metabolised to more polar metabolites such as conjugates, *(iv)* the relatively low levels of pharmaceuticals likely to occur in the environment and *(v)* the lack of reported examples, it is suggested that the bioaccumulation of human pharmaceuticals will generally not be an issue. This stance is supported by explicit statements from the US FDA that similarly suggest bioaccumulation is not an issue for human pharmaceuticals, i.e.:

- "In general, pharmaceuticals tend not to be very lipophilic and are produced/used in relatively low quantities compared to industrial chemicals. In humans, the majority of pharmaceuticals are metabolised to some extent in humans to SRSs (structurally related substances) that are more polar, less toxic and less pharmacologically active than the parent compound. This suggests that there is a low potential for bioaccumulation or bioconcentration of pharmaceuticals ..." (FDA-CDER 1998).

- "The vast majority of drugs do not have the physical or chemical characteristics that would allow them to bioaccumulate in tissue because this would raise safety concerns for use in humans. If a drug does have the physical or chemical characteristics that would allow it to bioaccumulate, there has to be some mechanism for the human body to metabolize the compound to a substance that has lower bioaccumulation potential so that it is cleared from the body. In the environmental assessments that CDER reviewed, bioaccumulation has not been an issue." (FDA 1996).

Many pharmaceuticals are weak acids or bases and therefore subject to ionisation (Newton and Kluza 1978; Raymond and Born 1986). The degree of ionisation can greatly affect both their fate and the effects as the hydrophobicity, adsorption, volatilisation, bioconcentration, and ecotoxicity of the ionised moiety may differ markedly from the unionised or neutral moiety. These processes will be particularly sensitive to changes in pH in the case of substances with pK_a values within the range of environmentally relevant pH values (i.e. 5–9). This therefore necessitates that due attention be given to the role of ionisation in determining the effects and fate behaviour of pharmaceuticals subject to ERA. The general lack of empirical study in this respect needs to be rectified.

Environmental risk assessment in this study has focused upon the water column and has ignored other compartments such as soil and sediment. Most pharmaceuticals tend to have low K_{ow} values and are often metabolised to more polar (and hence more water soluble) moieties. As such, the soil and sediment compartments may be less important, although they should not and indeed cannot be ignored.

Given the increasing number of observations of pharmaceutical compounds in sewage, surface waters and drinking water, the environmental fate of pharmaceuticals cannot be ignored and should be considered in the development process. Whilst relative metabolic recalcitrance in humans may be necessary for the pharmacological effect of some compounds (e.g. ethinyl substitution in the case of ethinyloestradiol), it will likely correspond to a poorer biodegradation profile in the environment. As such it may not always be possible to design "biodegradable" pharmaceuticals. Under such circumstances, other degradation mechanisms could perhaps be considered. For example, it may be possible to develop photolabile analogues of compounds which otherwise resist metabolism as well as biodegradation per se. One example of a drug where photodegradation is known to be the major elimination pathway in surface waters is diclofenac (Buser et al. 1998). Kümmerer et al. (2000) similarly highlight how it is potentially feasible to reduce the impact of pharmaceuticals on the aquatic environment by the development of biodegradable structural analogues of existing antineoplastic compounds.

16.5
Conclusions

There are a growing number of observations of pharmaceuticals in environmental matrices such as sewage influent, effluent, surface waters and potable water. This implies exposure of aquatic biota and necessitates risk assessment. The general lack of public domain usage data had previously precluded estimates of the environmental concentrations of pharmaceutical. Data presented in this study allowed the aquatic exposure assessment of a large number of compounds (>60) from across a wide variety of therapeutic classes. Risk characterisation based on acute ecotoxicity data and "worst-case" conservative fate assumptions demonstrated the nominal environmental safety (i.e. PEC/PNEC < 1) of the large majority of pharmaceuticals considered. For the remainder, the incorporation of their likely fate following use (i.e. likely removal during wastewater treatment and/or surface water dilution of effluent), yielded a marked reduction in the surface water PEC values, and the resultant PEC/PNEC ratios were generally less than unity for most of the compounds. Further refinement of the risk assessment is required for relatively few drugs. An important caveat to this conclusion relates to the assumption that the standard ecotoxicity tests that constitute the acute aquatic database are appropriate to the assessment of compounds with specific modes of action. Risk characterisation was exclusively conducted on the parent drug substance as representative of substances entering the environment. Whilst human metabolism is a mechanism that will potentially reduce environmental exposure, Phase II human metabolism of pharmaceuticals to produce conjugates may be reversible if the metabolites are exposed to microbial activity (i.e. in sewage). This potential re-release of biologically active parent compounds has to be considered in any exposure assessment. Metabolites per se should also not be ignored if their fate or effects differ markedly from that of the parent compound. The potential bioaccumulation/bioconcentration of pharmaceuticals was also considered, although it was deemed not to be a general issue.

References

Aherne GW, Briggs R (1989) The relevance of the presence of certain synthetic steroids in the aquatic environment. J Pharm Pharmacol 41:735–736

Aherne GW, English J, Marks V (1985) The role of immunoassay in the analysis of micro-contaminants in water samples. Ecotoxicol Environ Safety 9:79–83

Boethling RS, Howard PH, Meylan W, Stitler W, Beuman, J, Tirado N (1994) Group contribution method for predicting probability and rate of aerobic biodegradation. Environ Sci Technol 28:459–465

Bowman WC, Rand MJ (1980) Textbook of Pharmacology, 2nd edn. Blackwell Scientific Publications, Oxford

Buser H-R, Poiger T, Müller D (1998) Occurrence and fate of the pharmaceutical drug diclofenac in surface waters: rapid photodegradation in a lake. Environ Sci Technol 32:3449–3456

CEC (1996) Technical guidance document in support of the Commission Directive 93/67/EEC on risk assessment for new notified substances and Commission Regulation (EEC) No. 1488/94 on risk assessment for existing substances. Commission of the European Communities, European Chemicals Bureau, Ispra, Italy

Cowan CE, Versteeg DJ, Larson RJ, Kloepper-Sams PJ (1995) Integrated approach for environmental assessment of new and existing substances. Reg Toxicol Pharmacol 21:3–31

Desbrow C, Routledge E, Sheahan D, Waldock M, Sumpter JP (1996) The identification of oestrogenic substances in sewage treatment effluents. Environment Agency, Bristol, UK

Dollery CT (ed) (1991) Therapeutic drugs, vol I and II. Churchill Livingstone, Edinburgh

ECETOC (1995) The role of bioaccumulation in environmental risk assessment: the aquatic environment and related food webs. European Centre for Ecotoxicology and Toxicity of Chemicals, Brussels (Technical Report 67)

Eckerman I, Martineus JC (1997) Medicines and the environment: what do we know today? Swedish Association of Physicians for the Environment (SLFM), Stockholm

FDA (1995) Streamlining food and drug administration – environmental assessments. FDA Backgrounder BG95-9 (March 16, 1995)

FDA (1996) 21 CFR Part 25 – National Environmental Policy Act: proposed revision of policies and procedures; proposed rule. Federal Register 61(65):14922–14942

FDA-CDER (1996) Retrospective review of ecotoxicity data submitted in environmental assessments. FDA Center for Drug Evaluation and Research, Rockville (MD), USA (Docket No. 96N-0057)

FDA-CDER (1998) Guidance for industry – environmental assessment of human drugs and biologics applications. FDA Center for Drug Evaluation and Research, Rockville MD, USA (CMC6 Revision 1, http://www.fda.gov/cder/guidance/index.htm)

FWR (1995) Effects of trace organics on fish – Phase 2. Foundation for Water Research, Marlow (Bucks.), UK (FR/D 0022)

Halling-Sørensen B, Nielsen SN, Lanzky PF, Ingerslev F, Holten Lützhøft HC, Jørgensen SE (1998) Occurrence, fate and effects of pharmaceutical substances in the environment – a review. Chemosphere 36(2):357–393

Hansch C, Leo A, Hoekman D (1995) Exploring QSAR – hydrophobic, electronic and steric constants. American Chemical Society, Washington DC, USA (ACS Professional Reference Book)

Heide EF Van Der, Hueck Van Der Plas EH (1984) Genessmiddelen en milieu. Pharmaceutisch Weekblad 119:936–947

Henschel KP, Wenzel A, Diederich M, Fliedner A (1997) Environmental hazard assessment of pharmaceuticals. Reg Toxicol Pharmacol 25:220–225

Hirsch R, Ternes T, Haberer K, Kratz KL (1999) Occurrence of antibiotics in the aquatic environment. Sci Total Environ 225:109–118

Hoekman D (1997) http://clogp.edu/medchem/chem/clogp/drugs/html (Internet site)

Holten Lützhøft HC, Halling-Sørensen B, Jørgensen SE (1998) Algal testing of antibiotics applied in Danish fish farming. SETAC-Europe 8th Annual Meeting 14–18th April 1998, Bordeaux (Abstract 4I/004)

Hussain Z, Hennessy T (1995) EC environmental risk assessment (1). The Regulatory Affairs Journal 6(8):634–640

Kalbfus W (1995) Belastung bayerischer Gewässer durch synthetische Östrogene. Vortag bei der 50. Fachtagung des Bayerischen Landesamtes für Wasserwirtschaft "Stoffe mit endokriner Wirkung im Wasser" (Abstract). (Effects in Bavarian watercourses through synthetic oestrogens. Presentation at the 50th Seminar of the Bavarian Association for Waters Supply "Substances with endocrine effects in water")

Köpf W (1995) Wirkung endokriner Stoffe in Biotests mit Wasserorganismen. Vortag bei der 50. Fachtagung des Bayerisches Landesamt für Wasserwirtschaft "Stoffe mit endokriner Wirkung im Wasser" (Abstract). (Effects of endocrine substances in bioassays with aquatic organisms. Presentation at the 50th Seminar of the Bavarian Association for Waters Supply "Substances with endocrine effects in water")

Kühn R, Pattard M, Pernak KD, Winter A (1989) Results of the harmful effects of selected water pollutants (anilines, phenols, aliphatic compounds) to *Daphnia magna*. Wat Res 23(4):495–499

Kümmerer K, Al-Ahmad A, Betram B, Wießler M (2000) Biodegradability of antineoplastic compounds in screening tests: influence of glucosidation and of stereochemistry. Chemosphere 40: 767–773

Länge R, Schweinfurth H, Croudace C, Panther G (1997) Growth and reproduction of fathead minnow (*Pimephales promelas*) exposed to the synthetic steroid hormone ethinylestradiol in a life cycle test (Abstract). 7th Annual Meeting of SETAC-Europe April 6–10, 1997, Amsterdam, the Netherlands

Mackay D (1982) Correlation of bioconcentration factors. Environ Sci Technol 16:274–276

Newton DW, Kluza RB (1978) pKa values of medicinal compounds in pharmacy practice. Drug Intell Clin Pharm 12:546–554

Olejniczak K (1995) Environmental risk assessment for medicinal products in the EU, Phase I. In: Wolf PU (ed) Environmental risk assessment for pharmaceuticals and veterinary medicines. RCC Group, Itingen, CH (Proceedings of the International RCC Workshop held in Basel, Switzerland, February 1, 1995, pp 58–66)

Panter GH, Thompson RS, Beresford N, Sumpter JP (1999) Transformation of a non-oestrogenic steroid metabolite to an oestrogenically active substance by minimal bacterial activity. Chemosphere 38(15):3579–3596

Peterson SM, Batley GE, Scammell MS (1993) Tetracycline in antifouling paints. Mar Pollut Bull 26(2):96–100

Purdom CE, Hardiman PA, Bye VJ, Eno NC, Tyler CR, Sumpter JP (1994) Estrogenic effects of effluents from sewage treatment works. Chem Ecol 8:275–285

Raymond GG, Born JL (1986) An updated pKa listing of medicinal compounds. Drug Intell Clin Pharm 20:683–686

Reynolds JEF (ed) (1996) Martindale – the extra pharmacopoeia (electronic version). The Royal Pharmaceutical Society of Great Britain. Micromedex Inc., Engelwood, CO, USA

Richardson ML, Bowron JM (1985) The fate of pharmaceutical chemicals in the aquatic environment. J Pharm Pharmacol 37:1–12

Schweinfurth H, Länge R, Günzel P (1996) Environmental fate and ecological effects of steroidal estrogens. Presentation at the Oestrogenic Chemicals in the Environment conference organised by IBC Technical Services Ltd in London on the 9th and 10th May, 1996

Ternes TA (1998) Occurrence of drugs in German sewage treatment plants and rivers. Chemosphere 32(11):3245–3260

Ternes TA, Stumpf M, Mueller J, Haberer K, Wilken R-D, Servos M (1999) Behaviour and occurrence of estrogens in municipal sewage treatment plants – I. Investigations in Germany, Canada and Brazil. Sci Total Environ 225:81–90

Veith GD, Kosian P (1983) Estimating bioconcentration potential from octanol/water partition coefficients. In: Mackay D, Paterson R, Eisenreich S, Simmons M (eds) PCBs in the Great Lakes. Ann Arbor Science, Ann Arbor, MI, USA (Chap 15)

Watts CD, Crathorne B, Fielding M, Steel CP (1983) Identification of non-volatile organics in water using field desorption mass spectrometry and high performance liquid chromatography. In: Angeletti G, Bjørseth A (eds) Analysis of organic micropollutants in water. D.D. Reidel Publishing Company, Dordrecht, pp 120–131

Webb SF (1995) Current status of the European guidelines on environmental risk assessment. ESRA Rapporteur 2(3):27

Webb SF (1998) A data-based perspective on the environmental risk assessment (ERA) of human pharmaceuticals (Abstract). SETAC-Europe 8th Annual Meeting Interfaces in Environmental Chemistry and Toxicology: from the global to the molecular level (April 14–18, 1998), Bordeaux, France

WSA (1994) Waterfacts '94. Water Services Association, London

A Data Based Perspective on the Environmental Risk Assessment of Human Pharmaceuticals III – Indirect Human Exposure

S. F. Webb

17.1
Introduction

Concerns have previously been expressed over the possibility of adverse human effects arising from indirect exposure to pharmaceuticals via drinking water supplies (e.g. Richardson and Bowron 1985; Christensen 1998). This follows numerous observations of pharmaceuticals (or their metabolites) as contaminants in wastewater, surface water and groundwater following normal usage (e.g. Rurainski et al. 1977; Aherne et al. 1985; Aherne and Briggs 1989; Aherne et al. 1990; Stan et al. 1994; Stumpf et al. 1996; Ternes 1998; Hirsch et al. 1999). At present there is no regulatory guidance as to how the significance of the potential presence of pharmaceuticals at trace concentrations in drinking water supplies may be assessed. Risk assessment of pharmaceuticals for marketing authorisation purposes within both the United States and European Union do not address this point (Olejniczak 1995; FDA-CDER 1998). In order to provide some perspective on this issue, quantitative estimates of potential worse case indirect exposure to pharmaceuticals via drinking water have been undertaken. Potential effects endpoints against which to benchmark such exposure include daily therapeutic dosage.

17.2
Methodology

I_{70} values based on the lifetime (i.e. 70 years) ingestion of $2 \, l \, d^{-1}$ of water were calculated using the "worst-case" predictions for UK surface water concentrations from Chap. 16 with the additional assumption of no drug removal during drinking water treatment (Fig. 17.1). In the absence of a readily available comparable mammalian no-effects endpoints database, the I_{70} values were compared with minimum adult or pae-

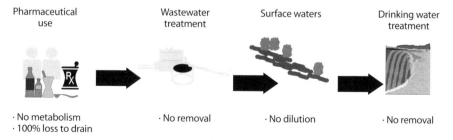

Pharmaceutical use   Wastewater treatment   Surface waters   Drinking water treatment

· No metabolism
· 100% loss to drain   · No removal   · No dilution   · No removal

Fig. 17.1. "Worst-case" estimation of indirect pharmaceutical exposure via drinking water

diatric daily therapeutic doses (Dollery 1991; Reynolds 1996). The I_{70} concept was first employed by Richardson and Bowron (1985).

17.3
Results

Details of the analysis are presented in Table 17.1 and summarised in Table 17.2[1]. The calculated "worst-case" lifetime ingestion of a pharmaceutical compound via potable water is of the order of <1 days therapeutic dose for at least for 80% of the compounds assessed. For illustration, the calculated "worst-case" I_{70} values for paracetamol, diazepam and clofibrate were nine times the daily dose, one and half times the daily dose and one-hundredth of the daily dose respectively. ethinyloestradiol represented the extreme case with a "worst-case" I_{70} of 26 times the daily dose.

17.4
Discussion

Within the European Union, the quality of water for human consumption is determined by the Drinking Water Directive (Council Directive 98/93/EC on the quality of water intended for human consumption). None of the 48 parameters within the directive relate to pharmaceuticals. The most comprehensive consideration of the potential long-term public health risk of the ingestion of drinking water contaminated with human pharmaceuticals was undertaken by Richardson and Bowron (1985). I_{70} values based on the lifetime (i.e. 70 years) ingestion of $2 \, l \, d^{-1}$ of water were similarly calculated using "worst-case" predictions for surface water concentrations. These I_{70} values were also similarly compared with typical adult and paediatric therapeutic doses. The calculated ingested quantities were small and a lifetime ingestion of a pharmaceutical compound via potable water would typically be of the order of one day's recommended therapeutic dose. The calculated I_{70} values for paracetamol, diazepam and clofibrate were four times the daily dose, one daily dose and one-sixth the daily dose respectively. Similar results for I_{70} were observed in this study with large differences between I_{70} values and therapeutic doses. More recently, Christensen (1998) estimated "worst-case" environmental fate and human exposure of ethinyloestradiol (oestrogen), phenoxymethylpenicillin (antibiotic) and cyclophosphamide (antineoplastic) employing the EUSES software. The results yielded a "negligible" human risk connected to predicted human exposure based on diffuse emissions from the use phase via drinking water and diet (vegetables, fish, meat and dairy produce). The effects benchmarks were male endogenous oestrogen production, tolerable food residues based an allergic reactions and genotoxic carcinogenicity thresholds respectively.

Relatively few attempts have been made to detect pharmaceuticals in potable water supplies. Data for a number of compounds are presented in Table 17.3. These include observations for bleomycin (Aherne et al. 1990), clofibric acid (Stan et al. 1994; Heberer et al. 1997), diazepam (Waggott 1981), diethylstilbestrol (Rurainski et al. 1977),

---

[1] These results were originally presented at SETAC 1998 (Webb 1998).

Table 17.1. "Worst-case" lifetime drinking water exposure

Compound	UK use (t yr^{-1})	PEC (µg l^{-1})	Dose (mg d^{-1})	I$_{70}$ (mg)	I$_{70}$ (daily dose)
Paracetamol	~2 000	367.3	2 000 (analgesia)	18 769	9.38
Aspirin	770	141.4	1 200 (analgesia)	7 226	6.02
Metformin	106.1	19.49	500 (type 2 diabetes)	996	1.99
Cimetidine	72	13.22	800 (gastric/duodenal ulceration)	676	0.84
Ranitidine	69	12.67	300 (gastric/duodenal/stomal ulceration)	647	2.16
Erythromycin	67.7	12.43	1 000 (bacterial infection)	635	0.64
Naproxen	60.6	11.13	500 (analgesia)	569	1.14
Dextroproproxyphene	42.5	7.81	175 (analgesia)	399	2.28
Oxytetracycline	33.7	6.19	1 000 (microbial infection)	316	0.32
Quinine	29.7	5.45	1 500 (malaria)	279	0.18
Theophylline	21	3.86	240 (bronchospasm in asthma)	197	0.82
Lithium salts	20.5	0.35 (Li)	75 (manic depression)	17.9	0.23
Metronidazole	15.5	2.85	1 200 (protozoal infections)	146	0.12
Iopromide	11.9	2.19	20 000 (angiography/urography/ arthrography contrast medium)	112	<0.01
Propranolol	11.8	2.17	80 (hypertension/angina)	111	1.39
Verapamil	9.9	1.82	120 (supraventricular arrhythmia)	93	0.78
Amitriptyline	5.5	1.01	75 (depression)	52	0.69
Tetracycline	4.7	0.86	1 000 (bacterial infection)	44	0.04
Omeprazole	3.9	0.72	20 (duodenal/gastric ulceration)	37	1.84
Thioridazine	3.8	0.7	150 (schizophrenia)	36	0.24
Chloroquine	2.9	0.53	40 (malarial prophylaxis)	27	0.68
Gabapentin	2.6	0.48	<2 400 (treatment of partial epileptic seizures)	25	0.01
Etidronic acid	2.1	0.39	275 (Paget's disease)	20	0.07
Fluoxetine	2	0.37	20 (depressive disorder)	19	0.95
Phenobarbital	1.7	0.31	60 (antiepileptic)	16	0.26
Tramadol	1.7	0.31	50 (analgesia)	15.84	0.32
Clofibrate	1.5	0.28	2 000 (type III hyperlipoproteinaemia)	14.31	0.01
Paroxetine	1.3	0.24	20 (depression)	12.26	0.61
Orphenadrine	1.1	0.2	150 (parkinsonism)	10.22	0.07
Diazepam	0.957	0.18	6 (insomnia/anxiety)	9.20	1.53
Acarbose	0.918	0.17	300 (type I/II diabetes)	8.69	0.03
Isoniazid	0.69	0.13	300 (tuberculosis)	6.64	0.02
Nefazodone	0.618	0.11	400 (depression)	5.62	0.01
Quinidine	0.601	0.11	500 (atrial fibrillation)	5.62	0.01
Sumatriptan	0.521	0.1	6 (migraine)	5.11	0.85

Table 17.1. *Continued*

Compound	UK use (t yr^{-1})	PEC (µg l^{-1})	Dose (mg d^{-1})	I_{70} (mg)	I_{70} (daily dose)
Aminosidin/Neomycin E	0.487	0.09	1 500 (intestinal amoebiasis)	4.60	<0.01
Warfarin	0.476	0.09	3 (thrombo-embolic disorders)	4.60	1.53
Lansoprazole	0.434	0.08	30 (peptic ulcer)	4.09	0.14
Cisapride	0.413	0.08	30 (gastro-oesophageal reflux disease)	4.09	0.14
Chloramphenicol	0.377	0.07	3 000 (bacterial infection)	3.58	<0.01
Famciclovir	0.286	0.05	750 (genital herpes and herpes zostera)	2.56	<0.01
Azithromycin	0.276	0.05	1 000 (Chlamydia infection)	2.56	<0.01
Cetirizine	0.273	0.05	10 (hypersensitivity)	2.56	0.26
Famotidine	0.246	0.05	40 (duodenal ulceration)	2.56	0.06
Ceftibuten	0.095	0.017	400 (urinary/respiratory tract infection)	0.87	<0.01
Lorsatan	0.087	0.016	50 (hypertension)	0.82	0.02
Budesonide	0.081	0.015	0.4 (asthma)	0.77	1.92
Finasteride	0.067	0.012	5 (benign prostatic hyperplasia)	0.61	0.12
Perindopril	0.047	0.009	2 (hypertension)	0.46	0.23
Didanosine	0.039	0.007	400 (HIV infection)	0.36	<0.01
Midazolam	0.037	0.007	15 (hypnotic)	0.36	0.02
Fluticasone	0.034	0.006	0.5 (asthma prophylaxis)	0.31	0.61
Digoxin	0.031	0.006	0.125 (congestive heart failure)	0.31	2.48
Ethinyloestradiol	0.029	0.005	0.010 (menopausal symptoms)	0.26	26
Risperidone	0.021	0.004	4 (schizophrenia/psychoses)	0.20	0.05
Atropine	0.016	0.003	0.2 (gastrointestinal disorders)	0.15	0.03
Carvedilol	0.008	0.001	25 (hypertension)	0.05	<0.01
Alendronic acid	0.007	0.001	10 (post menopausal osteoporosis)	0.05	<0.01
Bicalutamide	0.007	0.001	50 (prostatic cancer)	0.05	<0.01
Salmeterol	0.007	0.001	0.1 (chronic asthma)	0.05	0.5
Dorzolamide	0.004	0.001	20 (glaucoma and ocular hypertension)	0.05	<0.01
Diethystilbestrol	0.002	0.001	1 (prostrate carcinoma)	0.05	0.05
Paclitaxel	0.001	0.001	350 (malignant neoplasms)	0.05	<0.01
Flumazenil	<0.001	0.001	0.5 (reversal of benzodiazepine-induced sedation)	0.05	0.10
Milrinone	<0.001	0.001	~80 (severe heart failure)	0.05	<0.01
Thiotepa	<0.001	0.001	60 (bladder cancer)	0.05	<0.01
Zalcitabine	<0.001	0.001	2.25 (HIV infection)	0.05	0.02

ethinyloestradiol (Rurainski et al. 1977; Aherne et al. 1985; Aherne and Briggs 1989; Kalbfus 1995; James et al. 1998), fenofibrate (Heberer et al. 1997), ibuprofen (Heberer et al. 1997), methotrexate (Aherne et al. 1985), norethisterone (Aherne et al. 1985; Aherne

Table 17.2. Summary of "worst-case" lifetime drinking water exposure

I_{70} (Daily dose equivalent)	I_{70} (Fraction daily dose)	Number	Cumulative frequency (%)
>10	<1:2 500	1	1.5
>5	<1:5 000	2	4.5
>1	<1:25 000	10	19.4
>0.5	<1:50 000	10	34.3
>0.1	<1:250 000	13	53.7
>0.05	<1:500 000	4	59.7
>0.01	<1:2 500 000	9	73.1
≤0.01	>1:2 500 000	18	100
Total	–	67	100

Table 17.3. Observations of human pharmaceuticals in potable water supplies

Compound	Concentration (ng l^{-1})	Reference
Bleomycin	(i) range <5–13 (ii) mean 8.7	Aherne et al. (1990)
Clofibric acid	10–165	Stan et al. (1994)
Clofibric acid	70–7 300[a]	Heberer et al. (1997)
Diazepam	~10	Waggott (1981)
Diclofenac	<LOD–380[a]	Heberer et al. (1997)
Diethylstilbestrol	(i) range 0–0.8 (ii) mean 0.11–0.24	Rurainski et al. (1977)
Ethinyloestradiol	(i) range 0–22.5 (ii) mean 0.69–3.18	Rurainski et al. (1977)
Ethinyloestradiol	<5	Aherne et al. (1985)
Ethinyloestradiol	<1–4	Aherne and Briggs (1989)
Ethinyloestradiol	<0.2	Kalbfus (1995)
Ethinyloestradiol	<0.4	James et al. (1998)
Fenofibrate	<LOD–45[a]	Heberer et al. (1997)
Ibuprofen	<LOD–200[a]	Heberer et al. (1997)
Methotrexate	<6.25	Aherne et al. (1985)
Norethisterone	<10	Aherne et al. (1985)
Norethisterone	<2–<10	Aherne and Briggs (1989)
"Penicilloyl groups"	<10	Richardson and Bowron (1985)
Phenazone	<10–1 250[a]	Heberer et al. (1997)
Propyphenazone	<LOD–1 465[a]	Heberer et al. (1997)

[a] Groundwater supply to drinking water treatment plant.

and Briggs 1989), penicillins (Richardson and Bowron 1985), phenazone (Heberer et al. 1997) and propyphenazone (Heberer et al. 1997).

One of the studies relating to occurrence of pharmaceuticals in water supplies concerns observations of clofibric acid in German potable water. Concentrations ranged from 10–165 ng l^{-1} (Stan et al. 1994). The corresponding refined I_{70} value based on measured observations would be 0.5–8.4 mg. This can be compared to a daily maintenance dose for clofibrate of up to 2 000 mg to give an I_{70} value expressed as 0.004 days. A similar calculation can be made for ethinyloestradiol on the basis of the most recent observed concentrations of <0.4 ng l^{-1} and <0.2 ng l^{-1} in UK and German potable water supplies (James et al. 1998; Kalbfus 1995). This compares to the "worst-case" PEC of 5 ng l^{-1} employed here. The refined I_{70} value of 0.02 mg can be compared with a minimum daily therapeutic dose of 0.01 mg used in the treatment of menopausal symptoms. This equates to an I_{70} value of 2 days when expressed as daily dose. Although concerns have been expressed over the possibility of adverse effects on human reproductive biology arising from the presence of oestrogenic substances in drinking water (Ginsburg et al. 1994), a review of international water use patterns highlighted a lack of homogeneity and suggested that drinking water is consequently unlikely to be a significant factor (Fawell and Wilkinson 1994). The lack of a vitellogenin response on the part of caged fish in UK raw water storage reservoirs, in contrast to sewage effluent discharges, may similarly be interpreted as supporting this conclusion (FWR 1995). After ethinyloestradiol, the compound with the highest initial "worst-case" I_{70} value when expressed as daily dose was paracetamol (9 days). This ignores a high degree (98%) of elimination during wastewater treatment (Ternes 1998) and surface water dilution (default 1:10) of treated wastewater effluent. Incorporation of these factors would yield a refined PEC of 0.7 µg l^{-1} compared to the "worst-case" 367 µg l^{-1} employed here. Refinement of the I_{70} on this basis would result in a value of 35.8 mg or 0.02 days. The conservatism of the initial "worst-case" PEC for paracetamol is confirmed by the lack of observation of paracetamol at detectable concentrations in surface waters in the UK (Richardson and Bowron 1985), Germany (Ternes 1998) and the Netherlands (Van Hoof et al. 2000).

Also contributing to the discrepancy between observed concentrations of pharmaceuticals in potable water and the "worst-case" concentrations employed here are drinking water treatment processes. For example, Hutchinson et al. (1996) details the efficacy of a number of drinking water treatment processes (chlorination, ozonation, coagulation and powdered activated carbon) on a range of steroids on a laboratory scale. Chlorination, ozonation and powdered activated carbon were effective at removing steroids, but coagulation with aluminium sulfate had little effect. A subsequent study (James et al. 1998) employing similar methodologies confirmed the efficacy of chlorination, ozonation and powdered activated carbon (>95% steroidal removal) and the ineffectiveness of coagulation. It additionally demonstrated that filtration was ineffective but aeration was quite effective. Ternes (2000) similarly confirmed the general efficacy of drinking water treatment for a large number of pharmaceuticals.

In considering the fate of pharmaceuticals, several studies have highlighted cytotoxic drugs such as antineoplastics (e.g. Aherne et al. 1985; Richardson and Bowron 1985; Lee 1988; Aherne et al. 1990). Many of these are carcinogenic, mutagenic, embryotoxic or teratogenic, and concerns have been expressed over potential risks to potable water supplies. However, where observations from environmental samples are available, concentrations of cytotoxic drugs are limited. For example, concentrations of methotrexate in river water and potable water samples were all found to be <6.25 ng l^{-1}. This can be compared to a concentration of 1 µg l^{-1} found in a sewer immediately downstream of an oncology clinic (Aherne et al. 1985). Sewage and water treatment, dilution and degradation effectively reduced this level in the river and potable samples. Methotrexate itself is known to be readily metabolised and to undergo hydrolytic decomposition. Bleomycin was chosen for study by Aherne et al. (1990) on the basis of its relative stability. Concentrations of this cytotoxic drug varied from 11–19 ng l^{-1} in effluents to <5–17 ng l^{-1} in river and potable water samples. Aherne et al. (1990) concluded that any risk to public health from such levels of bleomycin in drinking water was unlikely. This followed the calculation that consumption of 2 l d^{-1} of such water would result in the ingestion of one-millionth of the daily adult dose of 20–30 mg d^{-1}. Other antineoplastics detected in the aquatic environment (but not drinking water) include ifosfamide and cyclophosphamide (Steger-Hartmann et al. 1996; Kümmerer et al. 1997). One major concern with antineoplastics is the possibility that a cancer risk may exist at any level of exposure (i.e. there is no threshold dose). In the case of other carcinogenic compounds, mathematical models have been developed to try and predict the hypothetical incremental cancer rate at low doses. These models require the selection of an acceptable cancer risk – typically 1×10^{-5} to 1×10^{-6} (i.e. 1:100 000 to 1:1 000 000). Such an approach maybe appropriate in determining limits on antineoplastics (and other potentially carcinogenic pharmaceuticals) in drinking water supplies. Sources of data relating to the carcinogenicity (or otherwise) of pharmaceuticals in general include IARC (1974, 1977, 1979, 1980, 1981, 1990, 1996, 1999) and Fung et al. (1995).

Implicit in the calculation of I_{70} values is a lifetime exposure over 70 years, i.e. 25 550 days. For the large majority (80%) of compounds with I_{70} values equivalent to <1 day's daily therapeutic dose, this implies a margin of ≥25 000 (2.5×10^4) between indirect exposure and efficacious therapeutic dosage. Refinement of the exposure for the remaining compounds with "worst-case" I_{70} values equivalent >1 day's daily therapeutic dose would undoubtedly lead to smaller values if based on more realistic fate scenarios or measured concentrations. Witness the reduction in the refined I_{70} value for ethinyloestradiol, clofibrate or paracetamol. The relevance of the use of therapeutic dosage as a benchmark can undoubtedly be questioned, but the absence of a readily available comprehensive chronic mammalian NOAEL (no observed adverse effect level) database for pharmaceuticals obliged its use in this study and by Richardson and Bowron (1995). Similarly, caveats need to be voiced concerning the potential issues associated with potential lifelong exposure at low sub-therapeutic levels and what risk assessment paradigm should apply under such circumstances. A subset of the population that is potentially exposed to low sub-therapeutic levels of a pharmaceutical over extended periods includes workers from the pharmaceutical industry. One approach used to derive occupational exposure limits (OELs) for pharmaceuticals is based on the application of a safety factor to the lowest recommended therapeutic dose in order to determine a therapeutically non-effective dose (Ku 2000). This safety factor is typically 100. Whilst there are some issues associated with this approach (i.e. cases of compounds where toxicity is unrelated to pharmacological effects or compounds used in life threatening situations where significant toxicities are acceptable), it does offer some useful perspective and perhaps a basis from which to derive an acceptable exposure limit for the population as a whole. If an additional safety factor of 10 were applied to OELs in order to derive general population exposure limits, a margin of safety would still apply to all compounds with I_{70} values <25 days. In the case of an additional safety factor of 100, a margin of safety would apply to all those compounds with I_{70} values <2.5 days.

17.5
Conclusions

Numerous observations of pharmaceuticals (or their metabolites) in wastewater, surface water and groundwater have given rise to concerns over the possibility of adverse human effects arising from indirect exposure to pharmaceuticals via drinking water. In the absence of regulatory guidance as to how the significance of such contamination to human health may be assessed, quantitative estimates of potential lifetime "worse case" indirect exposure to pharmaceuticals via drinking water have been undertaken and benchmarked against daily therapeutic dosage. Calculated "worst-case" lifetime (70 years) ingestion for pharmaceutical compounds via potable water is <1 day therapeutic dose for at least for 80% of the compounds assessed. This implies a margin of at least 25 000 between indirect exposure and efficacious therapeutic dosage. For compounds where "worst-case" lifetime ingestion was >1 day therapeutic dose, refinement of the exposure for several compounds (i.e. paracetamol, clofibrate and ethinyloestradiol) demonstrated the degree of conservatism associated with the exposure estimations. Overall it appears that indirect exposure to pharmaceuticals via the potable water supply is unlikely to represent a general objective safety issue. It is however, an area that requires further attention.

References

Aherne GW, Briggs R (1989) The relevance of the presence of certain synthetic steroids in the aquatic environment. J Pharm Pharmacol 41:735–736

Aherne GW, English J, Marks V (1985) The role of immunoassay in the analysis of micro-contaminants in water samples. Ecotoxicol Environ Safety 9:79–83

Aherne GW, Hardcastle A, Nield AH (1990) Cytotoxic drugs and the aquatic environment: estimation of bleomycin in river and water samples. J Pharm Pharmacol 42:741–742

Christensen FM (1998) Pharmaceuticals in the environment – A human risk? Reg Toxicol Pharmacol 28:212–221

Dollery CT (ed) (1991) Therapeutic drugs, vol I and II. Churchill Livingstone, Edinburgh

Fawell JK, Wilkinson MJ (1994) Oestrogenic substances in water: a review. J Wat SRT – Aqua 43(5):219–221

FDA-CDER (1998) Guidance for industry – environmental assessment of human drugs and biologics applications. FDA Center for Drug Evaluation and Research, Rockville MD, USA (CMC6 Revision 1, http://www.fda.gov/cder/guidance/index.htm)

Fung VA, Barrett JC, Huff J (1995) The carcinogenesis bioassay in perspective: application in identifying human cancer hazards. Environ Health Perspect 103(7–8):680–683

FWR (1995) Effects of trace organics on fish – Phase 2. Foundation for Water Research, Marlow (Bucks.), UK (FR/D 0022)

Ginsburg J, Okolo S, Prelevic G, Hardiman P (1994) Residence in the London area and sperm density. Lancet 343:230

Heberer T, Dünnbier U, Reilich C, Stan HJ (1997) Detection of drugs and drug metabolites in groundwater samples of a drinking water treatment plant. Fresenius Environ Bull 6:438–443

Hirsch R, Ternes T, Haberer K, Kratz KL (1999) Occurrence of antibiotics in the aquatic environment. Sci Total Environ 225:109–118

Hoof F Van, Genderen J Van, Mons M, Claeys C (2000) Perspective of the drinking water industry. In: KVIV (ed) Proceedings of International Seminiar on Pharmaceuticals in the Environment March 9th 2000 (Brussels). Technological Institute (KVIV), Brussels

Hutchinson J, Harding L, Carlile P, Hart J, Fielding M, Kanda R (1996) Effect of water treatment processes on oestrogenic chemicals. DW-05 Drinking Water Quality and Health. UK Water Industry Research Limited (UKWIR), London

IARC (1974) IARC Cancer Monographs on the Evaluation of Carcinogenic Risk of Chemicals to Humans – Sex Hormones (volume VI). World Health Organisation, International Agency for Research, Lyon, France

IARC (1977) IARC Cancer Monographs on the Evaluation of Carcinogenic Risk of Chemicals to Humans – Some Miscellaneous Pharmaceutical Substances (volume XIII). World Health Organisation, International Agency for Research, Lyon, France

IARC (1979) IARC Cancer Monographs on the Evaluation of Carcinogenic Risk of Chemicals to Humans – Sex Hormones (II) (vol XXI). World Health Organisation, International Agency for Research, Lyon, France

IARC (1980) IARC Cancer Monographs on the Evaluation of Carcinogenic Risk of Chemicals to Humans – Some Pharmaceutical Drugs (vol XXIV). World Health Organisation, International Agency for Research, Lyon, France

IARC (1981) IARC Cancer Monographs on the Evaluation of Carcinogenic Risk of Chemicals to Humans – Some Antineoplastic and Immunosuppressive Agents (vol XXVI). World Health Organisation, International Agency for Research, Lyon, France

IARC (1990) IARC Cancer Monographs on the Evaluation of Carcinogenic Risks to Humans – Pharmaceutical Drugs (vol L). World Health Organisation, International Agency for Research, Lyon, France

IARC (1996) IARC Cancer Monographs on the Evaluation of Carcinogenic Risks to Humans – Some Pharmaceutical Drugs (volume LXVI). World Health Organisation, International Agency for Research, Lyon, France

IARC (1999) IARC Cancer Monographs on the Evaluation of Carcinogenic Risks to Humans – Hormonal Contraception and Post-Menopausal Hormonal Therapy (vol LXXII). World Health Organisation, International Agency for Research, Lyon, France

James HA, Fielding M, Franklin O, Williams D, Lunt D (1998) Steroid concentrations in treated sewage effluents and water courses – implications for water supplies. UK Water Industry Research Limited (UKWIR), London (Report Ref. No. 98/TX/01/1)

Kalbfus W (1995) Belastung bayerischer Gewässer durch synthetische Östrogene. Vortag bei der 50. Fachtagung des Bayerischen Landesamtes für Wasserwirtschaft "Stoffe mit endokriner Wirkung im Wasser" (Abstract). (Effects in Bavarian watercourses through synthetic oestrogens. Presentation at the 50th Seminar of the Bavarian Association for Waters Supply "Substances with endocrine effects in water")

Ku RH (2000) An overview of setting occupational exposure limits (OELs) for pharmaceuticals. Chem Health Safety 7(1):34–37

Kümmerer K, Steger-Hartmann T, Meyer M (1997) Biodegradability of the anti-tumour agent ifosamide and its occurrence in hospital effluents and sewage. Wat Res 31:2705–2710

Lee MG (1988) The environmental risks associated with the use and disposal of pharmaceuticals in hospitals. In: Richardson ML (ed) Risk assessment of chemicals in the environment. The Royal Society of Chemistry, London, pp 491–504

Olejniczak K (1995) Environmental risk assessment for medicinal products in the EU, Phase I. In: Wolf PU (ed) Environmental risk assessment for pharmaceuticals and veterinary medicines. RCC Group, Itingen, CH (Proceedings of the International RCC Workshop held in Basel, Switzerland, February 1, 1995, pp 58–66)

Reynolds JEF (ed) (1996) Martindale – the extra pharmacopoeia (electronic version). The Royal Pharmaceutical Society of Great Britain. Micromedex Inc., Engelwood, CO, USA

Richardson ML, Bowron JM (1985) The fate of pharmaceutical chemicals in the aquatic environment. J Pharm Pharmacol 37:1–12

Rurainski R, Theiss HJ, Zimmermann W (1977) Über das Vorkommen von natürlichen und synthetischen Östrogenen im Trinkwasser. gwf-Wasser/Abwasser 118(6):288–291 (Concerning the occurrence of natural and synthetic oestrogens in drinking water)

Stan HJ, Heberer T, Linkerhägner M (1994) Vorkommen von Clofibrinsäure im aquatischen System – Führt die therapeutische Anwendung zu einer Belastung von Oberflächen-, Grund- und Trinkwasser? Vom Wasser 83:57–68 (Occurrence of clofibric acid in the aquatic system – is the use in human medical care the source of the contamination of surface, ground and drinking water?)

Steger-Hartmann T, Kümmerer K, Schecker J (1996) Trace analysis of the antineoplastics ifosamide and cyclophosphamide in sewage water by two-step solid phase extraction and gas chromatography-mass spectrometry. J Chromatogr A 726:179–184

Stumpf M, Ternes TA, Haberer K, Seel P, Baumann W (1996) Nachweis von Arzneimittelrückständen in Kläranlagen und Fliessgewässern. Vom Wasser 86:291–303

Ternes TA (1998) Occurrence of drugs in German sewage treatment plants and rivers. Chemosphere 32(11):3245–3260

Ternes TA (2000) Pharmaceuticals: occurrence in rivers, groundwater and drinking water. In: KVIV (ed) Proceedings of International Seminiar on Pharmaceuticals in the Environment March 9th, 2000 (Brussels). Technological Institute (KVIV), Brussels

Waggott, A (1981) Trace organic substances in the River Lee. In: Cooper WJ (ed) Chemistry in water reuse. Ann. Arbor Publishers Inc., Ann Arbor, MI, USA, pp 55–99

Webb SF (1998) A data-based perspective on the environmental risk assessment (ERA) of human pharmaceuticals (Abstract). SETAC 19th Meeting The Natural Connection: Environmental Integrity and Human Health. November 15–19, 1998, Charlotte, NC (USA)

Chapter 18

The ECO-SHADOW Concept – A New Way of Following Environmental Impacts of Antimicrobials

T. Midtvedt

18.1
General Introduction

Microorganisms are the dominating part in all ecological systems (ecosystems) and it is well recognised that antimicrobial agents (for convenience, later called antibiotics) are Mother Nature's own weapons for establishment and maintenance of all microbial ecosystems. Consequently, antibiotic resistance is a natural part of the regulatory factors in any ecosystem, and genes coding for resistance have existed as long as microbes have been around. However, during our increased use of antibiotics over half a century, we have selected more and more bad genes in more and more microbial communities. We got what we have asked for and what we have deserved.

Before going deeper into the concept of how to measure antibiotic-related alterations in microbial ecosystems, the "functional evolution" hypothesis of Stone and Williams (1992) of the origin of antibiotics deserves some comments. These authors have argued that secondary metabolites (that is, antibiotics) have a function in the organisms that produce them, favouring the survival of those organisms in the presence of the competing organisms that have receptors for the antibiotics. These receptors have evolved independently of the antibiotics and have nothing to do with antibiotic binding. Initially, the evolutionary precursors of present-day antibiotics had only a weak affinity for their receptors, and binding produced only a weak inhibition of growth. Then followed selection in organisms that produced antibiotics, with more and more avid binding, and thus greater inhibition of growth of the competitors, until eventually antibiotics as we know them emerged.

This hypothesis is useful in explaining several phenomena, including the evolution of β-lactams, penicillin-binding proteins and β-lactamases, as well as the so-called chlamydial anomaly (Midtvedt 1995). However, whatever the "function evolution" hypothesis may explain of the past, it has implications for the future. The action of antibiotics may extend far beyond their use in treating microbial infections; many of them are active for a long time after they have left the target area (patients, animals, etc.) Many antibiotics, such as broad-spectrum β-lactams, tetracyclines and fluoro-quinolones, are not easily broken down, but will stay in the environment where they will meet new microbes. The efflux of antibiotics from microbes is now known to be a mechanism of resistance in many organisms, and it is a very efficient way of meeting a large number of microbes. The presence of antibiotics in the environment will not only influence the selection of resistance, but also affect the natural producers of antibiotics, i.e. several soil microorganisms. They are not any longer favoured by their own production of antibiotics, and consequently, the ecological balance will be altered. In the long run, this may be more serious than a temporary increase in the number of resistant microorganisms in the environment.

It goes without saying that the "functional hypothesis" stresses the importance of using antibiotics with as few other effects on the environment as possible. Theoretically, the major goal has always been to hit nothing but the target microorganism. The development of antibiotics that are increasingly more resistant to microbial breakdown and with increasingly broader spectra has taken us far away from that goal. The need of a strategy focusing upon usage of antibiotics that will hit nothing but the target organism and that are broken down as soon as possible when they reach the environment, is obvious (Arano et al. 1996).

18.2
The ECO-SHADOW Concept[1]

In brief, an eco-shadow (or ecological shadow) can be defined as any alteration in any ecosystem following exposure of the system to an antibiotic (or any compound influencing the system). The alterations can be of variable length and may involve a variable number of species and functions. When possible, the sum of all alterations caused by an antibiotic might be included in an "eco-shadow index".

Measurement of eco-shadows in macroorganisms: All free-living macroorganisms, including humans, are normally born without any microbes and shortly after birth, microbial colonisation begins. At first, with plenty of space and nutrients, microbes with a high multiplication rate may predominate. However, as space and nutrients diminish, every location becomes occupied by the fittest microbes. Normally, the flora and the host will balance each other, that is, an ecological system is established. However, under normal conditions, the microbial part of the ecosystem is never dormant; it is always in a state of balanced unbalance (or unbalanced balance).

The gastrointestinal flora is without doubt the most complex part of normal mammalian flora. The composition of the gastrointestinal flora differs among animal species, among individuals within the same species, and also throughout life within the same individual. However, whatever the differences might be, the flora itself can principally be investigated in three different ways.

1. Enumeration studies
2. "What can the flora do?"
3. "What have the flora done?"

Att. 1. In the past, most attention has dealt with the composition of the flora, and great efforts have been made to isolate, identify and enumerate the hundreds of species now known to be present. In addition, nearly as much effort has been expended in following alterations in the composition and balance of the flora after various external manipulations, such as changes in dietary habit and exposures to antibiotics. Application of modern molecular methods has greatly increased our possibilities for a better characterisation of the flora. However, to the best of my knowledge, a full-scale evaluation of the intestinal flora in a healthy human individual has not been carried out up to now.

---

[1] The ECO-SHADOW concept represents a challenging way to follow alterations in mammalian and environmental ecosystems carried out by exposure of these ecosystems to antibiotics.

Att. 2. Another approach is to study the metabolic capability of the microbial flora – in other words, what can the microbes do? It goes without saying that most of these studies have been carried out in vitro, and over the years, a long series of biochemical microbial transformations has been studied. Some in vivo metabolic capacity tests have been worked out, and a few of them are well established in clinical medicine, such as the bile acid deconjugation test, the lactulose test and the urea breath test.

Att. 3. A third approach is to study more directly the functional status of the flora; that is, what have the microbes done? To do this, it is necessary to clarify which mechanisms and reactions are related to the host and which are related to the microflora itself, respectively. With a slight modification of terms first used by Claude Bernhard, the mammalian organism itself or the host's side of the ecosystem can be defined as milieu interieur (MI), the non-host side as milieu exterieur (ME), and MI and ME together as milieu total (MT).

Studies in mammals, birds, fish, insects, and reptiles with no microbial flora (germ-free individuals) have established basal values for anatomical structures and physiological, biochemical and immunological (when applicable) variables in the MI, that is the macroorganism itself. When such basal values or baselines are established, the normal functions of the flora, as well as alterations in these functions, can be worked out. In such studies, two terms – microflora-associated characteristic (MAC) and germ-free animal characteristic (GAC) – have been shown to be of considerable value. A MAC is defined as the recording of any anatomical structure or physiological, biochemical or immunological function in a macroorganism that has been influenced by the microflora. When microorganisms that influence the variable under study are absent, as in germ-free animals or new-borns or in relation to ingestion of antibiotics, the structure or functions are defined as GACs. Consequently, a collection of GACs describes a MI, and a similar collection of MACs describes a MT. A simple equation is MT minus MI equals ME – or what the microbes have done. Over the years, many MAC/GAC parameters have been studied in conventional and germ-free animals, and some examples are given in Table 18.1 (for review, see Falk et al. 1998 and Midtvedt 1999). During the last 2–3 decades, many studies have also been carried out following alterations in MACs after exposure of the macroorganism to antimicrobial agent(s) (for review, see Midtvedt et al. 1985; Midtvedt 1989; Steinbakk et al. 1992; Norin 1997). Taken together, the results clearly indicate that each antibiotic may create its own MAC/GAC profile of disturbances. In general, antibiotics acting upon anaerobic, gram-positive microorganisms cause most MAC disturbances Obviously, the MAC/GAC concept is a very handy tool for classifying the eco-shadow following exposure to antibiotics.

18.3
Influences of Antibiotics on Environmental Ecosystems

It is well recognised that antibiotics also may cause disturbances in environmental ecosystems. Especially in aquacultures (or fish farming), many studies have been carried out to study half-lives of antibiotics in natural sediments and the development of resistant microbes (Lunestad 1992; Midtvedt and Lingaas 1992; Samuelssen et al. 1992). It has been clearly shown that some groups of antibiotics, especially the newer

Table 18.1. Influence of the microflora on some major anatomical, physiological and biochemical parameters in the intestine

Parameter	MAC	GAC	Microbes
Anatomical/Physiological			
Intestinal wall	Thicker	Thinner	Unknown
Cell kinetics	Fast	Slower	Unknown
Migration motor complexes	Normal	Fewer	Unknown
Caecum size (rodents)	Normal	Enlarged	Partly unknown
Oxygen tension	Low	High (as in tissue)	Several species
Osmolality	Normal	Reduced	Unknown
Colloid osmotic pressure	Normal	Increased	Unknown
Eh (mV)	Low (<100)	High (>100)	Unknown
Biochemical			
Bile acid metabolism	Deconjugation	No deconjugation	Many species
	Dehydrogenation	No dehydrogenation	Many species
	Dehydroxylation	No dehydroxylation	Few species
Bilirubin metabolism	Deconjugation	Little deconjugation	Many species
	Urobilin	No urobilin	One species
Cholesterol	Coprostanol	No coprostanol	Few species
Intestinal gases	Carbon dioxide	Some carbon dioxide	Many species
	Hydrogen	Little hydrogen	Some species
	Methane	No methane	Few species
Mucin	Degraded	No degradation	Many species
Tryptic activity	Little or none	High	Few species
Beta-aspartylglycine	None	Present	Few species

quinolones, are present in the environment for months or years after they have been administered for prophylactic or therapeutic purposes. In fact, the environmental breakdown of these compounds rely upon ultraviolet light (which does not go far below the surface of water and soil) high temperature (only present in the vicinity of volcanoes) or enzymes deriving from very few microbial species mostly present in tropical climate only. Increased usage of these newer fluoroquinolones represents a severe threat to all environmental ecosystems.

It is also well established that usage of antibiotics in animal husbandry, either as growth promoters or as prophylactic agents, may cause the development of resistance in selected microbial species. Far less studies have been carried out in order to follow the impact of antibiotics upon the ecosystems in soil and other terrestrial localisations. Such studies are hampered by the enormous diversity in these ecosystems. In a recent investigation it was shown (utilising DNA reassociation analysis) that bacterial communities in pristine soil may contain more than 10 000 different bacterial types (Chatzinotas et al. 1998). The diversity of the total soil community was at least 200 times higher than the diversity of bacteria isolated from the same soil. This indicates that our culture conditions select for a distinct subpopulation of the bacteria present in the environment. A similar discrepancy between species shown to be present by modern molecular methods and species shown to be culturable has been demonstrated occurring in cultured soil as well (Torsvik et al. 1990).

Thus, the great number of species present and the great difficulties in culturing these species are making attempts to follow antibiotic-induced alterations in these ecosystems up to now close to impossible. Additionally, useful guidelines for studies of functiona alterations in environmental ecosystems ("what the microbes have done?") have, to the best of my knowledge, not been satisfactorily evaluated and presented. The concept of "what the microbes have done" may be the easiest concept to be implemented. A set-up of practical MAC/GAC parameters should be a challenging task for young microbiologists, giving enough data for eco-shadow indexing. The need for future investigations of eco-shadows in environmental ecosystems is obvious.

18.4
Future Tasks

Accepting the mere fact that our knowledge about and methods to follow antibiotic-induced alterations in environmental ecosystems still are limited – and applying a safety-first principle for the future use of antibiotics, the following simple rules are put forward:

1. The antibiotic should rapidly be broken down to non-toxic and microbiologically inactive substances, giving rise to small eco-shadows.
2. Neither the compound itself nor any of the metabolic breakdown product should be concentrated in any particular part of the environment.
3. None of the antibiotics that are of great human interest should be used in non-medical situations.

References

Arano BA, Cebra JJ, Beuth J, Fuller R, Heidt PJ, Midvedt T, Nord CE, Nieuwenhius, P, Manson WL, Pulverer G, Rusch VC, Tanaka, R, Van der Maaij D, Walker RI, Wells CL (1996) Problems and priorities for controlling opportunistic pathogens with new microbial strategies: an overview of current literature. Zentralblatt Bakt 283:431–465

Chatzinotas A, Sandaa RA, Shonhuber W, Amann R, Daae FL, Torsvik V, Zeyer J, Hahn D (1998) Analysis of brad-scale differences in microbial community composition of two pristine forest soils. System Appl Microbiol 21:579–87

Falk PG, Hooper LV, Midtvedt T, Gortdon JI (1998) Creating and maintaining the gastrointestinal ecosystem: wehat we know and need to know from genotobiology. Microbiol Mol Biol Rev 62:1157–1170

Midtvedt T (1989) Influences of antibiotics on biochemical intestinal microflora-associated characteristics in man and animals. In: Gililissen G, Opferkuch W, Peters G, Pulverer G (eds) The influence of antibiotics on the host-parasite relationship III. Springer Verlag, Berlin, Heidelberg, pp 209–215

Midtvedt T (1995) Antibiotic resistance: long ecological shadow. Side Effects of Drugs Annual 19:237–239

Midtvedt T (1999) Microbial functional activities. Nestle Nutrition Workshop Series 42:79–96

Midtvedt T, Lingaas E (1992) Putative public health risks of antibiotic resistance development in aquatic bacteria. In: Symposium Office International des Epizooties (ed) Chemotherapy in aquaculture: from theory to reality. Symposium Office International des Epizooties, Paris, pp 302–314

Midtvedt T, Bjoerneklett A, Carlstedt-Duke B, Gustafsson BE, Hoeverstad T, Lingaas E, Norin KE, Saxerholt H, Steinbakk M (1985) The influence of antibiotics upon microflora-associated characteristics in man and mammals. In: Wostmann BS (ed) Germfree research: micrioflora control and its application to the biomedical sciences. Alan R Liss, New York, pp 241–244

Lunestad BT (1992) Environmental effects of antibacterial agents used in aquaculture. Thesis, University of Bergen, Norway

Norin KE (1997) Influence of antibiotics on some intestinal microflora associated characteristics. Anaerobe 3:145–148

Samuelssen OB, Torsvik V, Ervik A (1992) Long-range changes in oxytetracyline concentration and bacterial resistance toward oxytetracycline in a fish farm sediment after medication. Sci Total Environ 114:25–36

Steinbakk, M, Lingaas E, Carlstedt-Duke B, Hoeverstad T, Midtvedt AC, Norin KE, Midtvedt T (1992) Faecal concentration of ten antibiotics and influence on some microflora-associated characteristics. Microbial Ecology in Health and Disease 5:269–276

Stone MJ, Williams DH (1992) On the evolution of functional secondary metabolites (natural products) Mol Microbiol 6:29–34

Torsvik V, Gogsoyr J, Dae FL (1990) High diversity in DNA of soil bacteria. Appl Environ Microbiol 56:782–87

Part III

Perspectives

Chapter 19

Present Knowledge and Need for Further Research

K. Kümmerer[1]

Drugs and medications are characterised by their strong effect and wide-ranging benefits in certain areas of application. Some of them may affect organisms in the environment and ecosystems. Moreover, antibiotic agents and disinfectants in particular can impair biological wastewater treatment. From the point of view of environmental hygiene, the contamination of groundwater and drinking water is highly undesirable, even if the compounds involved have a low acute human toxicity.

Answers to the following questions are urgently needed:

- What is the state of knowledge concerning the emission of pharmaceuticals into the environment (water and soil)?
- The extent to which the comparison of a short-lived high dose (for diagnosis and treatment) with a long-term low dose (intake via the drinking water) is permissible, is open to question not least because of the polymorphisms in sensitivity and responsiveness of individual persons.
- What are the effects of these substances on organisms and ecosystems? Special emphasis has to be placed on the identification of gaps in our knowledge and on the assessment of risks connected with these emissions and gaps in our knowledge.
- What kind of research is needed?

The discharge of pharmaceutically active substances into the environment does not require any new fundamental approaches. Instead, the experiences made with other chemicals (in particular with pesticides and biocides) need to be utilised and, if necessary, developed further. Besides, drugs, diagnostic agents and active disinfecting substances used in medicine and veterinary medicine must also be included.

Environmental quality objectives need to be determined for drugs and/or their active ingredients. Under the aspect of sustained dealings with the environment, the long-term objective ought to be the zero emission of substances that have no appreciable natural background concentration, while the emission of other substances ought to be kept so low that the natural background concentration is not increased. To ensure that these objectives are operationally viable, the potential long-term effects and precautionary principle dictate a maximum permissible concentration in surface waters and in drinking water of $0.001\ \mu g\ l^{-1}$. This concentration may also be used as a

---

[1] This chapter is a result of the discussions within the ESF-workshop "Pharmaceuticals in the Environment", held on July 14–16, 1999, in Freiburg, Germany. Thank you to all participants.

trigger value: if, as a consequence of the production quantities, a higher concentration may be expected in surface water, further investigations and studies on environmental interaction will be required. If new and lower effective thresholds of drugs become known, the maximum permissible concentration must be lowered accordingly.

The users of drugs, diagnostic agents and disinfectants must be suitably informed on the possible risks to the environment that may be related to the use of these substances or their improper disposal (e.g. safety data sheets, recommendations for use, package inserts, specialist information for pharmacists/dispensing chemists, etc.).

Some initial answers to these questions have been given for some compounds. But the work required is just beginning. Nevertheless, some general conclusions can be drawn.

19.1
Sources of Pharmaceuticals in the Environment

Countries differ in the patterns of use of pharmaceuticals, disinfectants and growth promoters. The reasons for these differences are not clear, but may be due to differences in legislation, doctors' preferences, tradition and social influences. It is well-known that the dissemination of information on the environmental impact of pharmaceuticals among the doctors and the users (patients) should be improved. It is estimated that up to 50% of antibiotics used might be useless due to incorrect diagnosis or lack of diagnosis prior to medication.

Some drugs are forbidden in one country, but may be used in other countries, especially Third World Countries. In Scandinavia, the use of antibiotics is very restricted. There is less restriction in Southern Europe. The patterns of use of antibiotics are well documented in Scandinavian countries. Since the early 1980s, the use of growth promoters in farming and aquaculture has largely been reduced in these countries, but they have not been banned entirely.

No data is available on the use of antibiotics in some industries (e.g. production of beer, cheese, filter tips for cigarettes, cleaning pipelines, etc.). There is a shortage of information on the global usage of antibiotics and other pharmaceuticals. Data on production is not available. The role of manufacturers in supplying the required data has to be clarified with respect to existing substances and new ones. According to EU-legislation, a general absence of these compounds in water is desired.

19.2
Detection of Pharmaceuticals in the Environment: Substances and Concentrations

19.2.1
Analytical Data

While a growing number of analytical results on pharmaceuticals mainly in the aquatic environment have been published, the data available from the literature is neither comparable nor sufficient. The quality of the published data remains somewhat unclear, if the analytical results are compared with the data related to usage and elimination in the environment (so far as data are available). Furthermore, physicochemical data are often lacking. For these reasons, it would be desirable to set up an exchange of experience in the analysis of these mostly polar substances. It would also be desirable to develop new analytical methods and a system of inter-laboratory testing. Methods should be standardised and investigations co-ordinated (e.g. sampling procedures and locations). Furthermore, it should be made possible to compare data on a regional, nation-wide, Europe-wide or even world-wide level.

19.2.2
Selection of Compounds to Be Analysed

A list is required of those chemicals that should be covered. Pharmaceuticals should be divided into pharmaceuticals such as antibiotics, which may produce resistance, or cytotoxics (antineoplastics), which should be covered separately because of their high toxicity, and others.

Criteria for the selection of compounds to be analysed are not yet available. One rationale could be a list of 20–50 priority compounds. Grouping substances according to their medical use/effect and/or chemical structure may be helpful. In a first step, the establishment of at least two subgroups, antibiotics and non-antibiotics, would be useful. The input of antibiotics into the environment favours the selection of resistant bacteria. Resistance could spread without antibiotics present and will be long-lasting. Therefore, antibiotics should be handled as a separate group. Further criteria for substance selection are mutagenic or cancerogenic activity (e.g. antineoplastics, some antibiotics) for another subgroup. Others can be handled as usual for other chemicals.

Effects should be taken into account when selecting the compounds to be analysed. Criteria for the selection of the substances should be the amounts used and the loads emitted into the environment in relation to their effective concentrations on organisms in the environment – in so far as data is available. However, so far it is unclear which organisms should be used for this purpose. The question of which tests are suitable to obtain this data requires clarification. For certain groups of pharmaceuticals such as antibiotics, the development of new test systems might be necessary. Highly mobile molecules or substances, already detected in the environment, are of special interest. As a further criterium, the hydrophobicity, i.e. the potential for bioaccumulation and persistence, i.e. the potential for bio-magnification and enrichment in certain environmental compartments, should be used. The fate and effects of important metabolites, which are still active, have to be investigated. It is also necessary to clarify whether the list has to be specific to regions, countries, or even to Europe and North America.

In order to assess the loads, excretion rates and data on (bio)degradation as well as metabolism by environmental organisms are required. To a great extent this data is lacking. Data from the producer must be provided as well as data concerning the environmental fate and effects of the substances.

19.3
Fate of Pharmaceuticals in the Environment

It is important to study physicochemical data (e.g. acidity, volatility, solubility, distribution coefficients) of the substances and to predict their environmental fate and effects. If they exist at all, these data are only partially available. The quality is mostly unclear. The substances are often highly polar and multifunctional. In this respect, they are comparable to dyes.

An enrichment of some pharmaceuticals in different environmental compartments is possible, e.g. quinolones tend to adsorb onto sewage sludge or soil particles, whereas other substances do not. Different environmental media have to be investigated, including analysis and modelling under spatial and temporal aspects, as well as the exchange and distribution between different environmental media. The same applies to biological data (effects on biodiversity, biodegradability, e.g. in biological test systems). The relevant media (e.g. soil, sewage) for biodegradability studies should be chosen according to use patterns and in some cases after the prediction of environmental behaviour and partitioning by modelling (e.g. fugacity models). There are a lot of models described in the literature, and it is unclear which one should be chosen. Once the behaviour of the substances in the environment has been understood, relevant compartments requiring analysis can be identified, and analytical programmes can be set up on the basis of this knowledge. Mass balances can be used to check the analytical results. Possible food chains can be identified. Also, it may be necessary to study local conditions.

Degradation tests are per se not good models for testing what happens in the real world. OECD tests, such as the Zahn-Wellens test or Closed Bottle test and others are only ranking systems. Standard tests may be performed with realistic drug concentrations. Radioactive markers (^{14}C) can be used to study the biodegradability and partitioning of the substances.

Most pharmaceuticals are manufactured as racemic mixtures, whereas their efficiency and fate in the environment may depend on stereo-chemistry. With the present state of knowledge, stereo-chemistry is not the main problem to be solved first.

19.4
Effects of Pharmaceuticals in the Environment

High (standard) concentrations in (standard) tests may not lead to visible short-term effects. If high concentrations are chosen, unrealistic effects may be produced. Therefore, modifications of the standard tests may be necessary. The role of the biodegradation properties of the substances should be assessed. It is necessary to use new test systems for non-antibiotics as well as antibiotics and for a main degradation route in soils, sediments and sewage treatment.

Resistance is transferred from one country to another by travellers. Growing resistance is a very serious problem in human medicine. Antibiotics and disinfectants present in the environment may produce resistant pathogenic and environmental bacteria. They can diffuse also in the absence of antibiotic substances. Therefore, antimicrobial substances should be grouped in a special list. Perhaps they should have specific criteria defining the problems resulting from their emission into the environment. Cross resistance caused by antibiotics used in medicine and those used in veterinary medicine and growth promoters has to be taken into account. Resistance effects in correlation to concentrations should be investigated.

19.5
Risk

19.5.1
Hazard Assessment

There is a need for quality assurance in analytical chemistry with regard to pharmaceuticals in the environment. Effect studies may only be necessary for antimicrobials or antineoplastics. Disinfectants should be included in the scenario for antibiotics. But others, such as sedative or lipid lowering agents, might also be of interest.

Research on the fate and effects of pharmaceuticals in the environment is urgently needed. The scientific procedures in use will probably need some modification. For antibiotics, the possibility of favouring the development of resistant bacteria needs additional attention, as resistance is growing and may be propagated by the organisms themselves not only in the presence of the substances. Substances with mutagenic effects, such as quinolones and antineoplastics, should also be of special concern. Increasing allergies to antibiotics have to be mentioned. The fate of the substances in drinking water treatment has to be assessed. There is a need for a closer look at various levels (global, regional, and local).

A hazard assessment can be undertaken. It is not clear whether a risk assessment is possible at all due to a lack of data and knowledge.

19.5.2
Impact of Pharmaceuticals in the Environment

The first step for an assessment of the effects is to summarise testing to obtain an overview of the possible effects of the substances. The test organisms used should be divided into two main groups: microbes and other organisms such as animals. In a first assessment, the organisms targeted by the substances should be used. Methods for testing the effects of pharmaceuticals on microorganisms need further discussion. Target *functions* should be basic ones, like effects on carbon and nitrogen cycling, respiration, or enzymatic activity. It is unclear whether there is something like a critical concentration of pharmaceuticals in the environment. The substances exhibit different concentration/response-curves. Some pharmaceuticals have a high response level even in low concentrations.

Effects on biodiversity, i.e. *patterns,* should be included. This should be studied with different methods. Methods for the investigation of microbial biodiversity, for example, are molecular biological methods, such as in situ hybridisation and chemotaxonomy (e.g. lipid and quinone or polyamine analysis).

Local emissions may not only cause short term local but also long term local, regional and global effects. Long-term observations are recommended. Low concentrations should be used to assess effects such as resistance development and long term effects. Possible allergic effects in humans should also be mentioned. As for the fate of pharmaceuticals, more data is needed for an impact assessment. Any drug reaching any part of the environment is a potential hazard. Information on risk management is vital. As long as data is lacking, people either believe there is no risk ("no data, no risk"), or that there is a huge risk ("no data, everything is risky").

19.5.3
Risk Assessment

A differentiation should be made between ecological risk assessment and human risk assessment. The question of whether risk assessment procedures used for pesticides can also serve as a prototype for pharmaceuticals should be examined. In the environment, concentrations occurring over a long period are a concern, whereas in medicine high dosages are used, but only for a short time. There is a lack of knowledge of long-term effects.

19.5.4
Risk Management

For several reasons, the prohibition and phasing out of certain pharmaceutical substances, which may pose a risk to the environment, are not favoured. But doctors/users could, after obtaining proper information, check whether there is an environmentally friendlier substance offering the same medical effectiveness as the one in use. A prerequisite for this is appropriate data and proper information.

For new substances, an examination of their environmental properties should be included in the development of new substances and be part of the registration process. Often, risk management is oriented towards short-term economic aspects rather than towards ecological effects. Costs, which may be incurred following the misuse of substances, should be considered, such as the long term costs for health insurance caused by increasing resistance.

In any case, a solution must be found which will reduce the input of antibiotics and thereby the risks associated with the input. Using the Scandinavian experience with antibiotics, this should be possible by strict management.

Growth promoters could be forbidden as the Swedish and Danish experiences show, but really good arguments are needed, due to their effect on profits and economic interests. For this reason, a political decision is essential. Because of the lack of data on the different questions concerning the effect of pharmaceuticals in the environment, it is important that information is shared.

19.6
Summary

"Pharmaceuticals in the Environment" is a new emerging topic, now receiving more and more attention. In this field, European research is leading the world.

The present knowledge shows that there is an urgent need for further research on the fate and effects of pharmaceuticals in the environment. Special environmental aspects are connected with their use. The huge number of different, often highly polar substances and their mode of action, increases the need for co-ordinated research and networking. In this context, the need for standardisation of methods (e.g. analytical methods and sampling as well as testing and modelling) has to be stressed. Despite the fact that the use of substances varies between countries, the compounds used are quite often the same or at least belong to the same class of substances. These differences are advantageous for further research, because different experiences can lead more rapidly to practical solutions. The experience gathered in Scandinavia with respect to reducing the use of antibiotics is a good example that can be used by other countries and applied to other compounds.

Index

Printing (Computer to Film): Saladruck, Berlin
Binding: Stürtz AG, Würzburg